WORLD HEALTH ORGANIZATION

INTERNATIONAL AGENCY FOR RESEARCH ON CANCER

IARC MONOGRAPHS
ON THE
EVALUATION OF THE
CARCINOGENIC RISK
OF CHEMICALS TO HUMANS

Wood, Leather and Some Associated Industries

VOLUME 25

This publication represents the views and expert opinions
of an IARC Working Group on the
Evaluation of the Carcinogenic Risk of Chemicals to Humans
which met in Lyon,
3-10 June 1980

February 1981

INTERNATIONAL AGENCY FOR RESEARCH ON CANCER

IARC MONOGRAPHS

In 1971, the International Agency for Research on Cancer (IARC) initiated a programme on the evaluation of the carcinogenic risk of chemicals to humans involving the production of critically evaluated monographs on individual chemicals. In 1980, the programme was expanded to include the evaluation of the carcinogenic risk associated with employment in specific occupations.

The objective of the programme is to elaborate and publish in the form of monographs critical reviews of data on carcinogenicity for chemicals and complex mixtures to which humans are known to be exposed, and on specific occupational exposures, to evaluate these data in terms of human risk with the help of international working groups of experts in chemical carcinogenesis and related fields, and to indicate where additional research efforts are needed.

International Agency for Research on Cancer 1981

ISBN 92 8 321225 8

PRINTED IN SWITZERLAND

CONTENTS

4

IARC WORKING GROUP ON THE EVALUATION OF THE CARCINOGENIC

RISK OF CHEMICALS TO HUMANS:

WOOD, LEATHER AND SOME ASSOCIATED INDUSTRIES

Lyon, 3-10 June 1980

Members[1]

E.D. Acheson, MRC Unit of Environmental Epidemiology, Southampton General Hospital, Southampton SO9 4XY, UK *(Chairman)*

R. Althouse, University of Oxford, Clinical Medical School, Radcliffe Hospital, Oxford, UK

F.B. Blackwell, Head, Adhesion, Soling & Chemical Testing Department, Shoe & Allied Trades Research Association, Satra House, Rockingham Road, Kettering NN16 9JH, UK

W.J. Blot, Environmental Epidemiology Branch, Landow Building C307, National Cancer Institute, Bethesda, MD 20205, USA

D. Brink, Forest Products Laboratory, University of California, 47th Street & Hoffmann Blvd, Richmond, CA 94804, USA

E. Buiatti, Centro per lo Malattie Sociali e la Medicina Preventiva, Via Alessandro Volta 171, I-50131 Firenze, Italy *(Rapporteur sections 3.1, 3.2, leather)*

F. Carnevale, Istituto di Medicina del Lavoro, Centro Ospedaliero Clinicizzato di Borgo Roma, I-37100 Verona, Italy

P. Decouflé, Associate Professor of Biostatistics and Epidemiology, School of Health Related Professions, University of Arizona, Tucson, AZ 85724, USA

---

[1] Unable to attend: L. Belin, Allergy Section, Occupational Health Centre, Sahlgren's Hospital, S-413 45 Göteborg, Sweden; P.N. Magee, Director, Fels Research Institute, Temple University, School of Medicine, Philadelphia, PA 19140, USA; G.B. Pliss, Chief, Laboratory of Carcinogenic Agents, N.N. Petrov Research Institute of Oncology, 68 Leningradskaya St., Pesochny 2, Leningrad 188646, USSR

B. Drettner, Department of Otorhinolaryngology, Huddinge University Hospital, S-14186 Huddinge, Sweden *(Rapporteur section 3.3)*

A. Englund, Bygghalsän, Box 26055, S-10041 Stockholm, Sweden *(Vice-Chairman) (Rapporteur section 3.4)*

J. Fajen, National Institute for Occupational Safety and Health, Robert A. Taft Laboratories, 4676 Columbia Parkway, Cincinnati, OH 45226, USA

G. Gavend, Head, Tannery Department, Centre Technique du Cuir, 181 avenue Jean Jaurès, BP 1, 69342 Lyon Cedex 2, France

R. Mäkinen, Director, Lappeenranta Regional Institute of Occupational Health, Pormestarinkatu 1, 53100 Lappeenranta 10, Finland *(Rapporteur sections 3.1, 3.2, wood)*

S. Milham, Population Studies Unit, LB-15, Department of Social & Health Services, Olympia, WA 98504, USA

C. Rappe, University of Umeå, Department of Organic Chemistry, S-90187 Umeå, Sweden

D.P. Rounbehler, New England Institute for Life Science, 125 Second Avenue, Waltham, MA 02154, USA

B. Terracini, Istituto di Anatomia e Istologia Patologica, Via Santena 7, I-10126 Torino, Italy

M. Valsecchi, Ufficio Igiene del Comune di Mantova, Consorzio di Medicina del Lavoro con sede in Montecchio Maggiore (Vincenza), Via Vincenti 9, I-37100 Verona, Italy

L.M. Williams, HM Factory Inspectorate, East Midlands Area, 5th floor, Belgrave House, Greyfriars, Northampton NN1 2LQ, UK

Representative from the US National Cancer Institute

H.F. Kraybill, Scientific Coordinator for Environmental Cancer, National Cancer Institute, Division of Cancer Cause & Prevention, Bethesda, MD 20205, USA

Representative from the American Paper Institute/National Forest Products Association

J. D. Wendlick, Corporate Industrial Hygienist, Weyerhaeuser Company, Tacoma, WA 98477, USA

Observers

U. Engzell, Department of Otolaryngology, Huddinge Hospital, S-14186 Huddinge, Sweden

C. Robinson, National Institute for Occupational Safety and Health, Robert A. Taft Laboratories, 4676 Columbia Parkway, Cincinnati, OH 45226, USA

D. Shortridge, 36 Parkdise Road, Leeds LS6 4QC, UK

Secretariat

C. Agthe, Division of Epidemiology and Biostatistics

H. Bartsch, Division of Environmental Carcinogenesis

J.R.P. Cabral, Division of Environmental Carcinogenesis

B. Dodet, Division of Environmental Carcinogenesis

M. Friesen, Division of Environmental Carcinogenesis

E. Heseltine, Charost, France *(Editor)*

V. Khudoley [1], Division of Environmental Carcinogenesis

A. Likhachev, Division of Environmental Carcinogenesis

D. Mietton, Division of Environmental Carcinogenesis *(Library assistant)*

R. Montesano, Division of Environmental Carcinogenesis

C. Partensky, Division of Environmental Carcinogenesis *(Technical officer)*

I. Peterschmitt, Division of Environmental Carcinogenesis *(Bibliographic researcher)*

R. Saracci, Division of Epidemiology and Biostatistics

L. Simonato, Division of Epidemiology and Biostatistics

L. Tomatis, Director, Division of Environmental Carcinogenesis *(Head of the Programme)*

---

[1] Present address: Laboratory of Chemical Carcinogenic Agents, N.N. Petrov Research Institute of Oncology, 66 Leningradskaya St., Pesochny 2, Leningrad 188646, USSR

E.A. Walker[2], Division of Environmental Carcinogenesis

J. Wahrendorf, Division of Epidemiology and Biostatistics

J.D. Wilbourn, Division of Environmental Carcinogenesis *(Secretary)*

Secretarial assistance

A. Beevers

M.-J. Ghess

S. Reynaud

J. Smith

---

[2] Present address: 62 Rennie Court, Upper Ground, Blackfriars, London SE1, UK

NOTE TO THE READER

The term 'carcinogenic risk' in the *IARC Monograph* series is taken to mean the probability that exposure to a chemical or complex mixture or employment in a particular occupation will lead to cancer in humans.

The fact that a monograph has been prepared on a chemical, complex mixture or occupation does not imply that a carcinogenic hazard is associated with the exposure, only that the published data have been examined. Equally, the fact that a chemical, complex mixture or occupation has not yet been evaluated in a monograph does not mean that it does not represent a carcinogenic hazard.

Anyone who is aware of published data that may alter an evaluation of the carcinogenic risk of a chemical, complex mixture or employment in an occupation is encouraged to make this information available to the Division of Environmental Carcinogenesis, International Agency for Research on Cancer, Lyon, France, in order that the chemical, complex mixture or occupation may be considered for re-evaluation by a future Working Group.

Although every effort is made to prepare the monographs as accurately as possible, mistakes may occur. Readers are requested to communicate any errors to the Division of Environmental Carcinogenesis, so that corrections can be reported in future volumes.

BACKGROUND

In 1971, the International Agency for Research on Cancer (IARC) initiated a programme on the evaluation of the carcinogenic risk of chemicals to humans with the object of producing monographs on individual chemicals. Since 1972, the programme has undergone considerable expansion, primarily with the scientific collaboration and financial support of the US National Cancer Institute. In June 1980, an IARC Working Group met to evaluate for the first time the carcinogenic risk of exposures in certain industries.

The existing criteria used to evaluate the carcinogenic risk of chemicals to humans were established in 1971 and were adopted in essence by the various Working Groups whose deliberations resulted in volumes 1-16 of the *IARC Monographs*. In October 1977, a joint IARC/WHO *ad hoc* Working Group met to re-evaluate these criteria. The cardinal aim of this Working Group was to update and rewrite the Preamble to the *IARC Monographs*, which sets forth the criteria for their preparation. The Preamble which subsequently reflected the results of their deliberations(1), together with those of a further *ad hoc* Working Group which met in April 1978(2), was first adopted by the Working Group which met to evaluate some *N*-nitroso compounds and whose deliberations resulted in volume 17 of the *IARC Monographs*. Since that time, the criteria have been used by individual Working Groups whose deliberations resulted in volumes 18-24 of the *IARC Monographs*.

OBJECTIVE AND SCOPE

The objective of the monographs hitherto published in the programme has been to critically review data on carcinogenicity for individual chemicals to which humans are known to be exposed, to evaluate those data in terms of human risk with the help of international working groups of experts in chemical carcinogenesis and related fields, and to indicate where additional research efforts are needed.

These monographs summarize the evidence for the carcinogenicity of the chemicals and other relevant information. The critical analyses of the data are intended to assist national and international authorities in formulating decisions concerning preventive measures. No recommendations are given concerning legislation, since this depends on risk-benefit evaluations, which seem best made by individual governments and/or other international agencies. In this connection, WHO recommendations on food additives(3), drugs(4), pesticides and contaminants(5) and occupational carcinogens(6) are particularly informative.

Up to February 1981, 25 volumes of the *IARC Monographs on the Evaluation of the Carcinogenic Risk of Chemicals to Humans* had been published or were in press(7). In these volumes, a total of 532 chemicals and 7 occupational exposures were evaluated or re-evaluated. For 39 chemicals, groups of chemicals, industrial processes or industrial exposures, a positive association or a strong suspicion of an association with human cancer has been found. For 26 of the individual chemicals, exposures are predominantly in occupational settings, although the general population may be exposed through environmental contamination. For 10 chemicals, human exposure was related to therapeutic uses; for one compound, exposure occurs *via* the diet. The preponderance of experimental data over epidemiological data on the 532 chemicals is striking: data on humans were available for only 60 of the chemicals, and 130 of them had to be evaluated solely on the basis of experimental data which provided *sufficient evidence* of carcinogenicity in animals.

NEW UNDERTAKING

An *ad hoc* Working Group which met in Lyon in April 1979 to prepare criteria to select chemicals for *IARC Monographs*(8) recommended that the Monograph programme be expanded to include consideration of human exposures in selected occupations. The objective of the programme has therefore now been broadened to include the consideration of mixtures of chemicals which result in complex exposures, as they often occur in human populations. Occupational exposures are a typical example, and wood, leather and some associated industries were selected as the starting point for this expansion in scope of the programme.

These monographs attempt to describe the industries in such a way as to indicate exposures to all known exogenous and endogenous chemicals involved in the processing or use of a material, and review all available epidemiological data in specific occupations within the selected industries. One additional aim of the deliberations of such Working Groups is to identify chemicals that should be evaluated individually for their carcinogenic risk to humans at future IARC Working Group meetings.

SELECTION OF COMPLEX MIXTURES AND OF OCCUPATIONAL EXPOSURES FOR MONOGRAPHS

The complex exposures (mixtures of chemicals) are selected for evaluation on the basis of two main criteria: (a) there is evidence of human exposure, and (b) there are some data relating the exposure to cancer in humans. The occupations to be considered by IARC Working Groups are chosen on the basis that some epidemiological data have suggested that they result in increased cancer risks at various sites. As new data on complex exposures for which monographs have been prepared and new principles for evaluating carcinogenic risk receive acceptance, re-evaluations will be made at subsequent meetings, and revised monographs will be published as necessary.

WORKING PROCEDURES

Approximately one year in advance of a meeting of a working group on individual chemicals, complex mixtures, or occupational exposures, a list is prepared by IARC staff in consultation with other experts. Subsequently, as many chemical, biological and epidemiological data as possible are collected by IARC; in addition to searching the published literature, other recognized information sources on chemical carcinogenesis and related fields such as CANCERLINE, MEDLINE and TOXLINE have been used.

Six to nine months before the meeting, reprints of articles containing relevant data are sent to experts, or are used by the IARC staff, for the preparation of first drafts of the monographs. These drafts are edited by IARC staff and are sent prior to the meeting to all participants of the Working Group for their comments. The Working Group then meets in Lyon for seven to eight days to discuss and finalize the texts of the monographs and to formulate the evaluations. After the meeting, the master copy of each monograph is verified by consulting the original literature, then edited by a professional editor and prepared for reproduction. The monographs are usually published within six to nine months after the Working Group meeting.

Each volume of monographs is printed in 4000 copies, 2500 in soft covers and 1500 in hard covers, and distributed by the WHO distribution and sales service.

DATA FOR EVALUATIONS

With regard to experimental and epidemiological data, only reports that have been published or accepted for publication are reviewed by the working groups, although a few exceptions have been made. The monographs do not cite all of the literature on a particular chemical, complex mixture or occupational exposure; only those data considered by the Working Group to be relevant to the evaluation of carcinogenic risk to humans are included.

Anyone who is aware of additional data that have been published or are in press which are relevant to the evaluation of the carcinogenic risk to humans of chemicals, complex mixtures or occupational exposures for which monographs have appeared is urged to make them available to the Division of Environmental Carcinogenesis, International Agency for Research on Cancer, Lyon, France.

THE WORKING GROUP

The tasks of the Working Group are five-fold: (a) to ascertain that all data have been collected; (b) to select the data relevant for the evaluation; (c) to ensure that the summaries of the data enable the reader to follow the reasoning of the committee; (d) to judge the significance of the results of experimental and epidemiological studies; and (e) to make an evaluation of the carcinogenic risk of the chemical, complex mixture or occupational exposure.

Working Group participants who contributed to a particular volume are listed, with their addresses, at the beginning of each publication. Each member serves as an individual scientist and not as a representative of any organization or government. In addition, observers are often invited from national and international agencies, organizations and industries.

GENERAL PRINCIPLES FOR EVALUATING THE CARCINOGENIC RISK OF EXPOSURES IN OCCUPATIONS

Evidence of carcinogenicity in humans

Evidence of carcinogenicity in humans, whether it relates to an individual chemical, to a complex exposure or to an occupational exposure, can be derived from three types of study, the first two of which usually provide only suggestive evidence: (1) reports on individual cancer patients (case reports), including a history of exposure to the supposed carcinogenic agent or agents; (2) descriptive epidemiological studies in which the incidence of cancer in human populations is found to vary (spatially or temporally) with exposure to the agent(s); and (3) analytical epidemiological studies (e.g., case-control or cohort studies) in which individual exposure to the agent(s) is found to be associated with an increased risk of cancer. Since occupation is typically recorded on death certificates, routine or specially tabulated reviews of mortality by occupational category often provide a means of generating or testing hypotheses about cancer in occupational or industrial groups. Death certificate statements, however, provide no information on duration, change or details of employment, and may not include data on other factors (e.g., cigarette smoking) that may be related to cancer risk.

An analytical study that shows a positive association between exposure and a cancer may be interpreted as implying causality to a greater or lesser extent if the following criteria are met: (a) There is no identifiable positive bias. (By 'positive bias' is meant the operation of factors in study design or execution which lead erroneously to a more strongly positive association between an agent(s) and disease than in fact exists. Examples of positive bias include, in case-control studies, better documentation of exposure to the agent(s) for cases than for controls, and, in cohort studies, the use of better means of detecting cancer in individuals exposed to the agent(s) than in individuals not exposed.)   (b) The possibility of positive confounding has been considered. (By 'positive confounding' is meant a situation in which the relationship between an agent and a disease is rendered more strongly positive than it truly is as a result of an association between the agent and another agent which either causes or prevents the disease. An example of positive confounding is the association between coffee consumption and lung cancer, which results from their joint association with cigarette smoking.)   (c) The association is unlikely to be due to chance alone. (d) The association is strong. (e) There is a dose-response relationship.

In some instances, a single epidemiological study may be strongly indicative of a cause-effect relationship; however, the most convincing evidence of causality comes when several independent studies done under different circumstances result in 'positive' findings.

Analytical epidemiological studies that show no association between exposure and cancer ('negative' studies) should be interpreted according to criteria analogous to those listed above: (a) There is no identifiable negative bias. (b) The possibility of negative confounding has been considered.   (c) The possible effects of misclassification of exposure or outcome have been weighed.

In addition, it must be recognized that in any study there are confidence limits around the estimate of association or relative risk. In a study regarded as 'negative', the upper confidence limit may indicate a relative risk substantially greater than unity; in that case, the study excludes only relative risks that are above its upper limit. This usually means that a 'negative' study must be large to be convincing. Confidence in a 'negative' result is increased when several independent studies of sufficient size carried out under different circumstances are in agreement.

Finally, a 'negative' study may be considered to be relevant only to dose levels within or below the range of those observed in the study and is pertinent only if sufficient time has elapsed since first human exposure to the agent(s). Experience with human cancers of known etiology suggests that the period from first exposure to a chemical carcinogen to development of clinically observed cancer is usually measured in decades and may be in excess of 30 years. This also implies that the analysis of data from epidemiological studies must explicitly take into account time from first exposure according to life-table principles.

Experimental data

There are few experimental data from long-term and/or short-term tests on complex mixtures (e.g., soot and tar, smoke condensate) or on exposures to a variety of chemicals that mimic those of humans in occupational environments. Such data are limited in general to the effect of a single chemical and refer in only a few instances to more than one identified chemical.

The evaluations made in the present monographs therefore rely almost entirely on epidemiological data which take into account the effects of the entire spectrum of human exposures in a given situation. One of the aims of the present monographs is to identify the possible contributing roles of individual chemicals in the carcinogenic effect of a known or suspected exposure to a complex mixture.

If experimental data on chemicals so identified exist, they will either already have been considered in an *IARC Monograph*, in which case suitable reference is made, or they will be included for consideration in future monographs. If, however, no experimental data exist, recommendation will be made that the chemical suspected of playing a role in the causation of human cancer be submitted to carcinogenicity testing.

The criteria used in analysing experimental data and in assessing their relevance to the evaluation of carcinogenic risk to humans(8) are described in detail in the preambles to volumes 17-24 of the *Monographs*(7).

REFERENCES

1.   IARC (1977) IARC Monograph Programme on the Evaluation of the Carcinogenic Risk of Chemicals to Humans. Preamble. *IARC intern. tech. Rep. No. 77/002*

2.   IARC (1978) Chemicals with *sufficient evidence* of carcinogenicity in experimental animals - *IARC Monographs* volumes 1-17. *IARC intern. tech. Rep. No. 78/003*

3.   WHO (1961) Fifth Report of the Joint FAO/WHO Expert Committee on Food Additives. Evaluation of carcinogenic hazard of food additives. *WHO tech. Rep. Ser., No. 220*, pp. 5, 18, 19

4.   WHO (1969) Report of a WHO Scientific Group. Principles for the testing and evaluation of drugs for carcinogenicity. *WHO tech. Rep. Ser., No. 426*, pp. 19, 21, 22

5.   WHO (1974) Report of a WHO Scientific Group. Assessment of the carcinogenicity and mutagenicity of chemicals. *WHO tech. Rep. Ser., No. 546*

6.   WHO (1964) Report of a WHO Expert Committee. Prevention of cancer. *WHO tech. Rep. Ser., No. 276*, pp. 29, 30

7.   IARC (1972-1981) *IARC Monographs on the Evaluation of the Carcinogenic Risk of Chemicals to Humans*, Volumes 1-25, Lyon, France

Volume 1 (1972) Some Inorganic Substances, Chlorinated Hydrocarbons, Aromatic Amines, *N*-Nitroso Compounds and Natural Products (19 monographs), 184 pages

Volume 2 (1973) Some Inorganic and Organometallic Compounds (7 monographs), 181 pages

Volume 3 (1973) Certain Polycyclic Aromatic Hydrocarbons and Heterocyclic Compounds (17 monographs), 271 pages

Volume 4 (1974) Some Aromatic Amines, Hydrazine and Related Substances, *N*-Nitroso Compounds and Miscellaneous Alkylating Agents (28 monographs), 286 pages

Volume 5 (1974) Some Organochlorine Pesticides (12 monographs), 241 pages

Volume 6 (1974) Sex Hormones (15 monographs), 243 pages

Volume 7 (1974) Some Anti-thyroid and Related Substances, Nitrofurans and Industrial Chemicals (23 monographs), 326 pages

Volume 8 (1975) Some Aromatic Azo Compounds (32 monographs), 357 pages

Volume 9 (1975) Some Aziridines, *N-, S-* and *O*-Mustards and Selenium (24 monographs), 268 pages

Volume 10 (1976) Some Naturally Occurring Substances (32 monographs), 353 pages

Volume 11 (1976)   Cadmium, Nickel, Some Epoxides, Miscellaneous Industrial Chemicals and General Considerations on Volatile Anaesthetics (24 monographs), 306 pages

Volume 12 (1976)   Some Carbamates, Thiocarbamates and Carbazides (24 monographs), 282 pages

Volume 13 (1977)   Some Miscellaneous Pharmaceutical Substances (17 monographs), 255 pages

Volume 14 (1977)   Asbestos (1 monograph), 106 pages

Volume 15 (1977)   Some Fumigants, the Herbicides 2,4-D and 2,4,5-T, Chlorinated Dibenzodioxins and Miscellaneous Industrial Chemicals (18 monographs), 354 pages

Volume 16 (1978)   Some Aromatic Amines and Related Nitro Compounds - Hair Dyes, Colouring Agents, and Miscellaneous Industrial Chemicals (32 monographs), 400 pages

Volume 17 (1978) Some N-Nitroso Compounds (17 monographs), 365 pages

Volume 18 (1978)   Polychlorinated Biphenyls and Polybrominated Biphenyls (2 monographs), 140 pages

Volume 19 (1979)   Some Monomers, Plastics and Synthetic Elastomers, and Acrolein (17 monographs), 513 pages

Volume 20 (1979) Some Halogenated Hydrocarbons (25 monographs), 609 pages

Volume 21 (1979) Sex Hormones (II) (22 monographs), 583 pages

Volume 22 (1980) Some Non-Nutritive Sweetening Agents (2 monographs), 208 pages

Volume 23 (1980) Some Metals and Metallic Compounds (4 monographs), 438 pages

Volume 24 (1980) Some Pharmaceutical Drugs (16 monographs), 337 pages

Volume 25 (1981) Wood, Leather and Some Associated Industries (7 monographs), 412 pages

8.   IARC (1979) Criteria to select chemicals for *IARC Monographs*. *IARC intern. tech. Rep. No. 79/003*

1. Reasons for choice of industries

The wood, leather and some associated industries were selected for review mainly because of a series of reports dating back to 1965 which indicated unusually high relative risks of nasal cancer (in the nasal cavities and sinuses) in workers in certain segments of both industries, in particular the furniture and cabinet-making industry and boot and shoe manufacture and repair. The results of these studies were so striking and so consistent that they strongly suggested the presence of carcinogenic materials in those work environments. These monographs thus proceed from the existence of epidemiological evidence associating a specific tumour site with employment in a particular trade, without necessarily pinpointing specific causative agent(s). Observations of an increased incidence of the same respiratory tumour in workers in two industries in which airborne dusts of natural materials are found also suggest a similarity in etiology. In addition, many chemicals are common to the two industries. Other tumour sites have also been found to occur in excess in workers in these industries, and data on those are reviewed. Sections of the wood and leather industries, other than those in which nasal tumours were originally found, are also considered.

2. Estimations of employment in wood and leather industries

The wood and leather industries can be subdivided into several (or many) specific trades, depending upon the source of data. For instance, the *United Nations Yearbook of Industrial Statistics* (United Nations, 1977) provides figures for the following sectors: leather and products (not further specified), footwear, wood products, furniture and fixtures, paper and paper products, pulp and paper, etc. The employment figures given can provide crude estimates of the populations at risk but are probably best interpreted as upper bounds of the numbers of workers in each industry, since not every worker may experience the relevant exposure(s). Caution should be exerted in relating any of the descriptions in the tables to the occupations described in the monographs.

The data in these tables do not always indicate secular trends in employment, which have been noteworthy, at least in the leather industry: for example, there has been a steady decrease over time in the number of leather workers in the United States and in England and Wales, whereas that industry has begun to proliferate in certain developing countries.

3. Possible differences in technology among and within countries, and evolution of the industries over time

Industries are not always unique, well-defined entities, i.e., there may be more than one way to manufacture and use a particular product, and industries usually change over time. These factors produce a heterogeneity of processes within the same industry.

Differences in processes may be associated with different exposures: thus, two epidemiological studies of the 'same' industry could in fact relate to two entirely different sets of exposures. This fact may account for some of the divergence in the results from different epidemiological studies of the same industry.

The following are specific factors that account for qualitative and quantitative differences within an industry:

(a)   introduction of a new technology (e.g., the movement of plant indoors from outdoors, or the introduction of more powerful machines),

(b)   continual modernization of processes,

(c)   the size of factories,

(d)   differences in work practices.

4.   Difficulties in determining exposures

The contribution of each of the specific agents found in the wood, leather and associated industries to the unusual cancer experience associated with certain occupations is not fully understood. The first reason for this situation is the great *multiplicity of exposures* of workers in these industries. Various factors account for this:

(a)   A large number of different chemicals are used; often these are referred to only by trade names so that it is impossible to know when changes in the composition of compounds have come about.

(b)   Changes occur over time in the raw materials and additives used (e.g., benzene has been replaced by other chemicals in the shoe industry).

(c)   Within certain segments of the wood industry, individual workers routinely handle different types of wood.

(d)   In some countries, a number of processes within an industry are carried out in the same plant (e.g., in a tannery that makes its own dyes there may be associated exposure to the dye intermediates).

(e)   An industrial process may result in the formation of new materials, as by-products, or in interactions of known chemicals to produce other entities (e.g., *N*-nitrosamines in leather tanneries).

The second reason behind the poor understanding of exposure-effect relationships in these industries is the *missing link between occupational titles and exposures.* The epidemiologist usually relies on occupational descriptions (job title or title of industry), of varying degrees of specificity, for an indirect, qualitative assessment of possible exposures. In contrast, the industrial hygienist focuses on the actual exposures that occur in the workplace. What is missing is a historical and up-to-date data source that cross-references job titles within specific industries and specific exposures. For example, 'carpenter' might appear to be a simple, well-defined job title on the surface; but two individuals whose occupation can be described in that way may work in two entirely different exposure milieux.

Finally, industrial hygienists find practical difficulties in *'keeping up' with continually changing work environments.* Data gathered at one point in time may not be representative of the industry over the twenty- or thirty-year time span covered by an epidemiological study.

The Working Group considered that, while recognizing the importance of the problem of effluents, it was outside the scope of the evaluations made in the present volume to discuss in detail the chemicals which may be present in those from the industries considered. It was noted, however, that the wide use of chlorination processes for treatment of effluents from the pulp and paper industry gives rise to transformation of molecular species into chemicals that may be carcinogenic or mutagenic.

5.   Deposition of inspired particles

Deposition in the nose depends on the size, shape and density of the particles and the turbulence and velocity of the airflow. Variations in the physiological and anatomical patency of the nasal airways are also of importance.

The latter factors are relatively constant in an individual, thus the size of the particles dictates their deposition in the nose. Particles of 5 μm or more in diameter are, according to most reports (Hilding, 1977), deposited in the nose almost completely; particles 2 μm in diameter are retained to about 60%; and almost all those smaller than 1 μm pass through the nose to the the lower airways. Very small particles, of 0.5 μm in diameter, may, to a great extent, leave the respiratory tract on expiration; and they are therefore retained neither in the upper nor in the lower airways. The term 'respirable', usually applied to dust of < 5 μm, refers to the fraction that reaches the tracheobronchial and pulmonary airways to a greater extent; this term has no application to the nasal passages.

Wood-dust particles are irregular in shape; however, most of the particles found in the furniture industry are 5 μm or more in diameter. Deposition therefore occurs largely in the nose, although particles larger than 5 μm may also reach the airways below the nose to some extent. The particle size of wood dust found in furniture industries in the High Wycombe, UK, area varied from 5.6-11.5 μm (Hounam & Williams, 1974). According to Andersen et al. (1977), particle size distribution has a maximum at between 6 and 10 μm, and the mean specific gravity is about 0.8.

Leather dusts can contain both fibres and grains; the fibres can vary from 30-1200 μm in length and from 10-30 μm in diameter. Grains are usually <10 μm in diameter. In several surveys in Italy, more than 50% of the total dust in tanneries had a particle diameter of < 5 μm.

The relative distribution of particles between the alveolar and the tracheobronchial regions of the lung was investigated experimentally by Pavia & Thomson (1976) in healthy human beings by inhalation of polystyrene particles of different sizes and using a radio-active technique. In the first six hours after aerosol inhalation, the mean rate of lung clearance increased considerably with particle size. Deposition in the tracheobronchial region in relation to that in the whole lung was dependent on particle size: thus, 31% of particles of 2 μm and 54% of those 5 μm in diameter were deposited in the tracheobronchial tree; and the alveolar/tracheobronchial ratio decreased with increasing particle size.

Mucociliary clearance

The deposition of wood dust in the nose strongly influences its mucociliary transport. So far nothing is known about which substances in wood are thus transported.

Black et al. (1974) examined the nasal mucociliary transport of radioactive particles in nine woodworkers in the furniture industry and in 12 controls. They found that only one of the woodworkers had a clearance rate within the normal range, and he had been exposed for only six years; the other woodworkers had very slow clearance or almost complete stasis. Andersen et al. (1977) examined nasal mucociliary transport time with a saccharin/sky-blue technique and found that the transport time in furniture workers had two maxima, one exceeding 40 minutes, which was equivalent to mucostasis, and one of about 14 minutes. When these values were analysed in relation to the wood dust concentration, a direct correlation between the incidence of mucostasis and the concentration of wood dust was found: in the group with the highest concentration of wood dust (25.5 mg/m^3), 63% had mucostasis; while in the group with the lowest dust concentration (2.2 mg/m^3), only 11% had mucostasis. If the values are expressed in relation to wood-dust concentrations below or above 5 mg/m^3, 20 and 49%, respectively, had mucostasis. Mucostasis may be transient, because examinations carried out after 48 hours without exposure to wood dust revealed normal mucociliary transport in six of nine persons.

Andersen *et al*. (1979) recently showed that inhalation for 5 hours of inert dust consisting of polymerized plastic dust containing carbon black, with dust concentrations of 2, 10 and 25 mg/m^3 and with particle sizes between 1.8 μm and >12.5 μm, had no effect upon the nasal mucociliary clearance rate. The effect of wood dust on mucociliary transport thus appears to be due to some soluble component of the wood and not to a direct mechanical effect. In that report it was also found that nasal penetration of particles was about 55% for the smallest particles and 20% for the largest. No reports of short-term, experimental exposures of healthy volunteers to wood dust have been found in the literature. Hadfield (1970) found that in an overwhelming number of subjects dust was deposited in two areas of the nasal mucosa. The first was an oval area measuring 1 x 0.5 cm on the anterior-lower part of the nasal septum and the second was on the anterior end of the middle turbinates and measured about 1 cm in diameter. There was a greater deposition of dust on that side of the nose in which the airways were more open.

Metaplastic changes but no tumours were found in 10% of samples of epithelial cells obtained by direct sampling from the middle meatus of furniture workers (Drettner & Stenkvist, 1978). A good correlation was reported between rhinoscopy and cytological examination of nasal secretions of 135 furniture workers; metaplasia was found in 33 and dysplasia in 2 (Mozzo *et al*., 1978).

No reports have been found in the literature concerning mucociliary transport in the lower respiratory airways in woodworkers or about mucociliary clearance in the nose and bronchial tree in workers in leather and associated industries. Equally, no publications have been found concerning defence mechanisms against the entry of wood particles other than mucociliary transport. The fate of particles which remain for a long time on the mucosa is thus obscure.

6.   Recommended and legislated exposure levels applicable to wood, leather and associated industries

Threshold limit values (TLVs) and other, comparable regulations apply to pure wood and leather dusts only. The most commonly used TLV values are those of the American Conference of Governmental Industrial Hygienists; these are re-published, for example, in the UK by the Health & Safety Executive. If the dust contains other substances which are more toxic than the dust itself, the TLVs of those substances are applied. TLVs for some of the chemicals used in wood, leather and associated industries are given by the International Labour Office (1977). No TLVs or recommended values have been established for spores or other biological factors.

Wood industry

In 1964, Hanslian & Kadlec in Czechoslovakia recommended certain provisional limits for wood dust exposure on the basis of clinical studies of exposed workers. Woods could be differentiated into three categories, they suggested, dependent upon their biological activity: (1) woods with low toxicity, e.g., oak, beech, maple, ash, birch and lime; (2) woods with high toxicity, e.g., pine, larch, ebony and mahogany; and (3) strongly allergenic woods, e.g., yew, box and mansonia. Corresponding to these classifications, exposure limits of 10 mg/m^3, 5 mg/m^3 and 1 mg/m^3, respectively, were recommended.

Following the establishment of the Occupational Safety and Health Act of 1970 in the United States, worker wood dust exposures were unofficially regulated in the same category as so-called 'inert or nuisance dusts', at levels of 15 mg/m^3 total dust and 5 mg/m^3 for the respirable fraction. A field directive to all regions of the Occupational Safety and Health Administration in February 1978 officially designated the nuisance dust category to include dusts such as wood dust as well as inorganic dusts. The nuisance dust classification is applied to those substances which, when inhaled as particulates at levels no greater than listed regulations, will: (a) not change the architecture of the lungs; (b) not result in the production of collagen; and (c) produce no irreversible tissue reactions. In addition, the nuisance dust classification stipulates that free silica content be no greater than 1%. USSR health authorities have taken similar cognizance of free silica contamination and adopted maximum allowable concentrations of 2 mg/m^3 for wood dust containing 10% or more of free silica, and 4 mg/m^3 for wood dust containing below 10% (International Labour Office, 1974).

A TLV of 5 mg/m^3 non-allergenic wood dust (total) was recommended by the American Conference of Governmental Industrial Hygienists (ACGIH) in the autumn of 1970 (after the Occupational Safety and Health Act became law in the United States). The information supporting this recommended change in wood dust exposure limits was published in the ACGIH documentation of Threshold Limit Values in 1971. In the United States and Canada, such values, when adopted, have significance, since state or provincial health and safety regulation enforcement agencies are free to include them in their programmes if the values are at least as stringent as the federal regulations. The ACGIH recommended wood dust limit of 5 mg/m^3 was adopted in 1973 in the states of Oregon, Washington and California and in 1974 in the province of British Columbia in Canada. In recognition of the difference between certain biologically active species and species which are properly designated nuisance particulates, the Workers' Compensation Board of British Columbia established in 1976 a separate regulation for 'wood-dust, allergenic' at 2.5 mg/m^3 total (which applies to western red cedar, certain true mahoganies and teak).

The ACGIH added a new category for TLV exposure limits in 1976 which considered the health effects of short-term exposures as well as of the conventional full work shift (8 or 10 hours) time-weighted averages. For wood dust, the short-term exposure limit was set at 10 mg/m^3 for any 15-minute period during the shift, provided that such excursions did not cause the time-weighted average of 5 mg/m^3 to be exceeded. Later, in 1979, the ACGIH included an intended change for wood dust, hardwood (as in furniture-making) of 1 mg/m^3 (American Conference of Governmental Industrial Hygienists, 1979). As discussed previously, this limit will become part of the adopted values list in April 1981 if no comments are received to suggest that the value should be changed.

Lists of present wood dust regulations, on the basis of toxicological data other than that on carcinogenicity, and proposed limits for work place wood dust exposure, are given in Tables 1 and 2.

Leather industry

There are no TLVs or other regulations specific for the various kinds of leather dust. The current regulations and TLV for 'nuisance dusts' are not appropriate because of epidemiological evidence that leather dust produced during shoe manufacture or repair may be harmful.

7.   Structures of wood and leather

Wood

Many features tend to unify the physical structure of wood, yet wood species may be classified by dichotomous keys on the basis of visual characteristics; thus, woods may vary by subtle differences in anatomy, even within narrowly related groups. Such differences affect substantially the manner in which wood failure will occur when it is reduced to small particulates by various machining processes.

Numerous treatises describe the anatomical structure of plants. Specific reference is made to the excellent treatment of the subject by Esau (1953). Only a cursory treatment of those aspects of wood anatomy that are pertinent to the subject of wood dust and its formation will be undertaken here.

Anatomy provides the basis for a natural phylogenetic system for classification of plants. Arborescent species of the highest phylum of the plant kingdom, Spermatophyta, are present in both classes, Gymnospermae and Angiospermae, and these comprise the materials used in the manufacture of lumber. Significantly, the chemical compositions of cell-wall materials and extractives are consistent with the taxonomic classification. Indeed,

Table 1. Regulations concerning exposure to wood dust

Country	Threshold limit value (mg/m^3)	Comments & reference
Finland	5	
Federal Republic of Germany	10	Fine; inert dust
German Democratic Republic	10	Domestic wood dust only[a]
United Kingdom	5	
United States		
Washington	5	
Oregon	10	Presently at 10 mg/m^3, moving towards 5 mg/m^3
California	5[b]	
Canada		
British Columbia	5[b]	Non-allergenic (Workers' Compensation Board, 1978)
	2.5	Allergenic (Workers' Compensation Board, 1978)
Alberta	5[b]	All wood dust
India	15	Total
USSR	2	>10% free silica (ILO, 1974)
	4	<10% free silica (ILO, 1974)
Sweden	4	
Poland	10	Containing no free silica
Yugoslavia	10	Total; containing no free silica
	3	Respirable; containing no free silica
Switzerland	20	Total
	8	Fine

[a]Pine, oak, fir, beech

[b]Short-term exposure limit, 10 mg/m^3

Table 2. **Proposed regulations or recommendations concerning exposure to wood dust**

Country	Threshold limit value (mg/m^3)	Comments & reference
United States	15	Total (ACGIH, 1971)
	5	Respirable (ACGIH, 1971)
	5^a	Non-allergenic (ACGIH, 1979)
	1	Hardwood; ACGIH (1979) intended change
Italy	5	(Ente Nazionale Prevenzione Infortuni; Societa Italiana di Medicine del Lavoro)

a Short-term exposure limit, 10 mg/m^3

chemotaxonomic studies have resolved questions of classification where anatomical studies were unable to provide the required distinctions.

(i)   The stem of arborescent species: a woody stem comprises a vascular system with two major parts: namely, the xylem and the phloem.

Phloem comprises the bark, and this is removed early in the manufacturing process. In physical structure it resembles that of the xylem. One of its distinctive features, however, is that it has a substantially higher content of extractives. The principal function of the phloem is the translocation of products of photosynthesis from the leaf to the growing tissue of the stem and root of a plant.

Xylem comprises the woody component of the stem and root and is that part which is converted by manufacturing processes into products including lumber, plywood, flakes used in particleboard, and pulp. Wood normally amounts to 85 - 90% of the stem of gymnosperms and has two principal functions. One is the translocation of water and mineral matter essential in plant growth from the soil to the root, the stem and finally to the site of photosynthesis, the leaf. A second function is to support the plant and enable it to compete for the sunlight that is the energy source required in photosynthesis.

The terms commonly applied to xylem and phloem in arborescent species are 'wood' and 'bark', respectively. Similarly, the terms commonly applied to arborescent species of Gymnospermae and Angiospermae are 'softwoods' and 'hardwoods', respectively.

(ii)   Structure of secondary xylem (wood):   secondary xylem is composed of two inner penetrating systems of longitudinal (or axial) and transverse (or radial) cells. These systems are integrated with respect to origin, structure and function.

The longitudinal system is composed of one or more cell types, including tracheidal elements, fibres, and parenchyma. The axes of these cells coincide with the axis of the stem. Tracheidal elements, in general, include tracheids in softwoods and vessel members or vessel elements in hardwoods; both are water-conducting tissues. Tracheids are imperforate cells, communicating in translocation of water through pit pairs (bordered pits) on their common walls (described later). In contrast, a vessel member communicates with a second vessel member with which it is in contact through perforations in the cell wall. These perforations, generally in the end walls, may be simple openings or scalariform (ladder-like) with multiple openings. Fibres comprise thick-walled cells with simple or near-simple pits; these are highly specialized cells which provide support for the plant. Fibres and tracheids interact to form cells which are called fibre-tracheids. Axial parenchyma, derived from the same type of cambial initials as the tracheidal elements and fibres, serves for food storage. Parenchymal cells communicate with other cells by means of pits, the structures of which are consistent with the type of cell with which the parenchyma is in communication.

The radial system is composed of parenchymal cells which normally have their long axes parallel to the radii of the cylindrical stem. Therefore, when wood is sectioned in the longitudinal direction, the lengths of the rays are exposed on the radial faces, whereas the cross-sections of the rays are exposed on the tangential faces. A section cut perpendicular to the axis of a stem is known as a cross-section. Rays extend lengthwise along the radii from the pith to the cambium. The height of a ray is the dimension parallel to the axis of the stem, and its width is the dimension perpendicular to the plane defined by the length and height of the ray. Rays one cell in width are uniseriate; those more than one cell in width are multiseriate.

Translocation of aqueous solutions takes place between two contiguous cells through perforations or through pits. Pits are formed by perforations in the secondary walls of contiguous cells when the primary walls remain intact. Simple pits are formed by abrupt interruption of secondary wall growth. A bordered pit is formed when the secondary wall toward the cell lumen arches over the opening left by the secondary wall at its point of contact with the primary wall. This differential growth produces a pit cavity and an effect of two concentric circles when viewed perpendicular to the pit. The central portion of the membrane of the bordered pit becomes densified and thickened, with the formation of an impenetrable 'torus'. The membrane, known as the 'margo', retains many openings between the fibrils of the primary walls of the contiguous cells, which allow translocation of water between cells.

As the stem grows during a given season, secondary xylem cells are formed by differentiation in the vascular cambium. Cells formed during vigorous growth periods (spring and early summer) have thin walls and large diameters: these cells form the early wood or spring wood. Toward the end of the growing period, cell growth is less vigorous, cell walls become thicker and cell diameters diminish: this wood is known as late wood or summer wood. The total growth for one season, especially in the temperate zone, is recognized as an annual ring.

The life of tracheidal elements and fibres is short; their protoplasts are lost as the cells mature and become lignified. The parenchyma continues to live and serve its function of food storage for a number of years; however, it ceases to function as a living cell when transformation from sapwood to heartwood takes place. At the same time, the tracheidal elements cease their function of water translocation. The transformation from sapwood to heartwood in many species is also accompanied by a distinctive change in colour. The water content of the wood diminishes, food stored in parenchymal cells is consumed, and various organic products are deposited either by impregnation of the cell walls or by deposition within the cell lumina. The nature of these organic products is highly species dependent; in total, they comprise a wide spectrum, including oils, gums, resins, tannins, aromatics and pigments. These materials are not part of the cell wall and are known generically as 'extractives' or 'extraneous materials'. They are responsible for the distinctive colour, odour and taste of various woods.

The secondary xylems of gymnosperms and angiosperms are distinct and are considered separately.

The xylem of gymnosperms (softwoods) is made up of a number of elements, which are listed in Table 3. The axial or longitudinal system in the xylem of gymnosperms is composed entirely or mostly of tracheids (Table 4). These cells vary from 0.5 - 11 mm in length but are normally within a range of 3 - 6 mm in length and from 0.01 - 0.07 mm in diameter. Thus, the ratio of length to diameter is in the order of 100.

The framework of tracheids is composed of cellulose; hemicelluloses and lignins provide a matrix of encrusting substances. Cellulose is a linear macromolecule composed exclusively of several thousand D-glucose units that are β-linked. Cellulose molecules aggregate into microfibrils, the dimensions of which have been the object of considerable study over a period of three decades.

Table 3. Elements of softwood xylem[a]

	Longitudinal system	Transverse system
Prosenchymatous	Tracheids	Ray tracheids
Parenchymatous	Epithelial cells (lining longitudinal resin canals)	Ray parenchyma Epithelial cells (lining transverse resin canals)

[a]From Panshin & de Zeeuw (1970)

Table 4. Typical properties and dimensions of cell types, in xylem[a]

| Cell type | Volume (%) | | Dimension (mm) | | | |
| | | | length | | tangential diameter | |
	min.	max.	min.	max.	min.	max.
Softwoods[b]						
Tracheids	89	94.8	1.3	9.3	0.025	0.065
Rays	5.0	10.0	-	-	-	-
Resin canals	0.1	0.8	-	-	-	-
Douglas fir						
	(average)					
Tracheids	92.5		1.7	7.0	0.035	0.045
Rays	7.3		-	-	-	-
Resin canals	0.2		-	-	-	-
Hardwoods[c]						
Vessels	11.6	55.6	0.22	1.32	0.02[d]	0.30[d]
Fibres	26.8	69.4	0.8	1.9	0.010	0.040
Axial parenchyma	trace	7.0	-	-	-	-
Rays	6.1	20.0	-	-	-	-

Table 4 (contd)

Cell type	Volume (%)	Dimension (mm)		
		length	tangential diameter	
		American beech		
	(average)	(average)		
Vessels	31	0.61	-	-
Fibres	44	1.2	0.016	0.022

[a]Data summarized from Isenberg (1963)

[b]From 12 selected softwoods in the US

[c]From 13 selected hardwoods in the US

[d]Data from Panshin & De Zeeuw (1970)

Mühlethaler (1965) described one school of thought which proposed that the width of cellulose microfibrils is 3.5 nm. Preston (1974) discussed a second theory, that cellulose microfibrils in higher plants have dimensions of 8.5 x 4.5 nm, with a cortex of 70 cellulose chains. The cortex is defined as a paracrystalline sheath of molecular chains lying parallel to the microfibril but not otherwise stacked in the crystalline array. Côté (1977) noted that the diameter of microfibrils could range from an estimated minimum of 1.7 nm to over 50 nm. He suggested that the larger size diameter observed results from aggregations of smaller sized units; or, alternatively, smaller sized units are created by mechanical means from larger strands. The length of the cellulose microfibril is indefinite.

There is general agreement concerning the structure formed by cellulose microfibrils. The tracheid consists of a primary wall (P) and a secondary wall (S). Esau (1953) discussed the nature of xylem development, and Preston (1974) presented a hypothetical model of disposition of the cell wall.

In the growth of any cell, the primary wall is first deposited, and the cell then essentially acquires its full length. This wall is relatively low in cellulose, and its microfibrils are oriented randomly. In those cell types that develop a secondary wall, the cellulose microfibrils are deposited in a highly oriented laminar structure. Cellulose comprises the major percentage of this cell wall. The secondary wall is deposited in distinct layers as it grows. The outer layer that is contiguous with the primary wall is designated the S_1 layer; the intermediate layer, usually comprising the major amount of material, is designated the S_2 layer; and, when formed, the inside layer, immediately adjacent to the cell lumen, is designated the S_3 layer. Each of these layers is formed by sequential deposition of microfibrils as lamellae. The microfibrillar orientations and thicknesses of the respective cell-wall layers of softwood tracheids are given in Table 5. Harada (1965) discussed the occurrence of crossed lamellae and intermediately oriented microfibrils between lamellae, which serve as potential zones of delamination. He demonstrated that the anatomical structure of the ray parenchyma of *Cryptomeria japonica* was similar to that of the tracheids in this species.

The xylem of angiosperms (hardwoods) differs from that of softwoods in several respects. The cell wall is formed in the same way, and all of the longitudinal elements are derived from the same cambial initials. However, there is substantially more differentiation than in the more primitive softwoods. The elements of hardwoods (Table 6) thus reflect the greater complexity of hardwood structure (Isenberg, 1963).

Table 5. Cell wall of softwood tracheids[a]

Cell-wall layer[b]	Microfibrillar orientation angle with fibre axis (°)	Thickness (μm)
Middle lamella	none	0.1 - 0.2
P	random	0.03 - 0.10
S_1	35 - 75	0.10 - 0.20
S_2	10 - 35	0.50 - 8.0
S_3	70 - 90	0.07 - 0.10

[a]From Janes (1969)

[b]See text for descriptions of layers

Average values for the volume percentages, lengths and tangential diameters of cell types present in 13 species of hardwoods were given in Table 4. It may be noted that the vessels and fibres of hardwoods serve the same functions as tracheids in softwoods. The hardwood fibres, and especially the vessel segments, are substantially shorter than tracheids. The transverse system in hardwoods may comprise a substantially greater volume percentage than in softwoods. A further distinction with respect to hardwoods is that the rays in many species are multiseriate (two or more cells in width).

Inclusions, namely tyloses and cellular secretions, in vessel elements are particularly worthy of note. Tyloses are outgrowths of the protoplasm from adjacent parenchymal cells through pit cavities adjoining the two cells and into the cavity of the vessel element; such growths may completely fill the vessel cavity. Tyloses are normally formed upon transformation of sapwood to heartwood or may result from a trauma such as low water content, mechanical injury, fungal growth or virus infection. The second type of inclusion is made up of secretions of gummy substances, apparently in lieu of tylosis formation. These inclusions may form lumps on the inner wall of the vessel or may completely occupy the cavity of the vessel segment. The colour of the secretions varies from light yellow to deep red, brown or even black, and their texture varies from gummy to chalk-like.

Vascular tracheids are very similar to small late wood elements, but their blunt ends are imperforate. Their latest walls may contain numerous border pits and, in certain genera, such as *Ulmus* (elm) and *Celtis* (hackberry), conspicuous spiral thickenings.

Vasicentric tracheids are short, irregularly-shaped cells with closed ends. They are found in such ring-porous woods as oak and chestnut in association with longitudinal parenchyma. Their lateral walls are heavily pitted and their ends are tapered or rounded.

Table 6. Elements of hardwood xylem

Longitudinal system	Transverse system
Prosenchymatous	none
Vessel elements	(in US hardwoods)
Tracheids	
Vascular	
Vasicentric	
Fibre	
Fibre tracheids	
Libriform fibres	
Parenchymatous	
Axial parenchymal strands	Ray parenchyma
Fusiform	Procumbent cells
Epithelial cells (lining gum cells)	Upright cells
	Epithelial cells (lining transverse gum canals)

Fibres may be of three types. Fibre tracheids are similar to late wood tracheids of softwoods, with thick cell walls, pointed ends and bordered pits. Libriform fibres differ from fibre tracheids in that they have simple pits. Fibre tracheids and libriform fibres may comprise over 50% of the wood volume.

Tropical timber and, rarely, temperate-zone wood may have septate fibres. The septum may be a thin transverse wall, or it may be a false septum resulting from the deposition of gummy or resinous material. Gelatinous fibres, modified by changes in chemical constitution, are present in tensile wood. The S_2 and/or S_3 layers may be replaced, or a layer may be deposited in addition to the layers usually present in the secondary wall.

The parenchymatous elements in hardwoods, as shown in Table 6, include cell types in both the longitudinal and transverse systems. The parenchyma is composed largely of isodiametric cells with only simple pitting, and functions in conduction, storage of food and deposition of extractives.

The longitudinal parenchymal system includes three types of cell: strand, fusiform and epithelial. Of these types, strand parenchyma contributes the greatest volume percentage of the wood, varying from 1 - 18% in temperate-zone woods and to over 50% in tropical woods. These cells are derived by transverse division of fusiform cambial daughter cells, such that the entire strand retains the shape of the original fusiform mother cell. Strand parenchyma, in turn, may be classified into three types: apotracheidal (arranged independently of the vessels), paratracheidal (associated with vessels or vascular tracheids) and banded (forming concentric lines or bands). Fusiform parenchyma is derived from fusiform cambial initials without subdivision; if present, it comprises only a very small percentage of the wood. Epithelial parenchyma encircles the longitudinal canals. Such resin canals are not present in temperate-zone woods (of America) but are found in some tropical woods.

Ray parenchyma comprises the transverse parenchymal system and originates from ray initials in the cambium as either a xylem ray or a phloem ray. Rays increase in number as the diameter of the stem increases, so that the proportion of rays in a given species remains fairly constant. Size and spacing of rays is extremely variable in hardwoods. Ray parenchyma is normally procumbent (homocellular rays), i.e., with the long axes of the cells in the transverse direction. In some species the rays are bordered by marginal upright parenchymal cells with their long axes in the longitudinal direction (heterocellular rays). In a few species rays are uniseriate, but in the majority of species they are multiseriate. Woods such as oaks in the temperate zone may have rays over 30 cells and 300 μm in width. Combinations of uniseriate with multiseriate rays are common, for example, in some maples, beeches and oaks. Large rays impart qualities to the wood which make it desirable for use in making furniture.

Parenchymal cells are repositories for various included materials. These inclusions comprise materials that are either crystalline (especially mineral) or amorphous. The amorphous materials include a wide variety of gums, resins, tannins, oils, latexes, colouring matter, and nitrogenous materials such as alkaloids. Silica, although sometimes present as crystalline inclusions in cell cavities, usually occurs in the cell walls. Other crystalline inclusions include calcium oxalate as rhomboidal, acicular or raphide (needle-shaped) crystals. In heterocellular rays crystals are normally found in the upright cells; they are also commonly found in the procumbent cells of homocellular rays. Strand parenchyma sometimes function as crystal repositories.

Gum canals in angiosperms are of two types: normal and traumatic. Normal gum canals, formed by epithelial parenchyma of both longitudinal and transvere types, are equivalent to resin canals in some softwoods. However, these are not found in temperate-zone hardwoods of America except in sweetgum *(Liquidambar styraciflua)*. They are found in dipterocarp woods, including Philippine mahogany, but not in American mahogany *(Swietenia spp)* or in African mahogany *(Khaya spp* and *Entandrophragma spp)*. Traumatic gum canals form only in the horizontal parenchyma by either one or a combination of two mechanisms: (a) cells separate at the middle lamella (schizogenous), as in the formation of resin canals in conifers; (b) cell walls disintegrate (lysigenic); or (c) a combination of the two mechanisms (schizolysigenic). The formation of traumatic gum canals is unusual in temperate-zone woods.

Leather

Leather is the product obtained by tanning skins and hides by any one of several methods. By convention, the term 'hide' generally refers to the skin covering of larger animals (cows, steers, horses, buffaloes, etc.), while those of smaller animals (calves, sheep, goats, pigs, etc.) are called 'skins'. The hides or skins from different animals possess unique physical properties that are inherent to the particular animal or breed of animal, due largely to differences in climate, type of feed, etc. to which the animal is exposed. They are thus used for different specific purposes (Table 7).

Although the physical properties of these different skins vary, their basic histological and chemical characteristics are similar. A review was made by O'Flaherty & Stubbings (1966).

(i)   Animal skin histology and chemistry

Animal skin is made of cells and fibres, with a certain amount of amorphous material in between. Skin is composed of three layers: the epidermis, or outer surface; the corium, or bulk of the skin, which consists chiefly of fibres; and the loose 'flesh' or connective tissue on the under surface, which serves to attach the skin to the underlying tissues of the animal. The space between the epidermis and the beginning of the corium, equal to the full length of the hair follicle, is referred to as the 'grain layer', while the outer surface from which the hair or wool protruded during life is referred to as the 'grain surface'. With thick hides, the leather is frequently split into two or more layers; it is desirable to retain some of the corium with the grain layer to provide sufficient strength. The loose tissue on the under-surface of the skin is removed in preparatory processes.

Table 7. Leather uses in relation to type of hide or skin[a]

Skin origin	Use
Cow and steer	Shoe and boot uppers, soles, insoles, linings; patent leather; clothing; work gloves; waist belts; luggage and cases; upholstery; transmission belting; sports goods; packings
Calf	Shoe uppers; slippers; handbags; wallets; hat sweatbands; bookbindings
Sheep and lamb	Grain and suede clothing; shoe linings; slippers; dress and work gloves; hat sweatbands; bookbindings; novelties
Goat and kid	Shoe uppers and linings; dress gloves; clothing; handbags
Pig	Shoe suede uppers; dress and work gloves; wallets; fancy leather goods
Deer	Dress gloves; moccasins; clothing
Horse	Shoe uppers; straps; sports goods
Reptile	Shoe uppers; handbags; fancy leather goods

[a]From New England Tanners' Club (1977)

At the bottom of the corium are the main blood vessels which nourish the skin. At the junction of the corium and the flesh are fat cells containing triglycerides.

The skin is made up chiefly of proteins, although it also contains lipids, carbohydrates, inorganic salts and water. The proteins of the skin are the most important components from the point of view of leather manufacture. These include collagen, which constitutes the bulk of the fibrous portion, and reticulin, which is similar to collagen but differs from it in its ability to combine readily with silver salts. Elastin, also a fibrous protein, is present in very small quantities, chiefly in the grain area and to a small extent in the blood vessels. Non-fibrous plasma proteins - albumins, globulins - are also present in fresh animal skin, along with small quantities of glycoproteins and carbohydrates. Keratin is present in the hair or wool and epidermis.

Most of the non-collagenous proteins are removed during pretanning operations, which are effectively a means of preparing a matrix of relatively pure collagen fibres which will subsequently be stabilized by tanning. The precise technology used determines the extent to which individual non-collagenous components are removed; these mechanisms include chemical and enzymatic processes coupled with extraction by aqueous solvents, e.g., brine, lime-water.

The lipids consist of triglycerides located in fat cells, and small amounts of fatty acids, phospholipids and traces of waxes in the grain area. Extensive studies of the original lipids in animal skin and the changes they undergo during processing were reported by Koppenhoefer & Highberger (1934) and Koppenhoefer (1938, 1939). The carbohydrates are of little importance in leather manufacture and occur only in very small fractions associated with the collagen and the mucoids. The usual physiological salts are present, constituting less than 1% of the skin. The water content of fresh hides may be as high as 80%; in cured hides it is reduced to about 40%; and in finished leather only 10-15% remains.

The matrix of fibres present in the skin varies both topographically and stratigraphically in dimensions and orientation but is essentially a three-dimensional non-woven sheet material. A consequence of this structure is a high degree of flex resistance and resistance to tearing and puncturing (New England Tanners' Club, 1977). These properties were essential to protect the animal during its life and should be retained after tanning.

(ii)   Leather chemistry

In simple terms, tanning is any process which renders animal hides or skins imputrescible without impairing their flexibility after drying. The most widely used technical criterion of tannage is the increased hydrothermal stability of leather in comparison with skin collagen. When a strip of skin is heated in a neutral aqueous environment there is a marked contraction in length at a temperature of 60-65°C; this is associated with the development of rubber-like elasticity in the contracted material. Depending on the materials used for tanning, leather may have a hydrothermal shrinkage temperature of 70-120°C.

The concept of classifying tannins according to their chemical reactivity dates back to the nineteenth century: catechol tannins were those which give a green colour with ferrous ions, and pyrogallol tannins those which give a blue colour with ferrous ions. Later research showed that the tannins fall into two broad chemicals groups. *Hydrolysable tannins* are mainly glucosides, i.e., glucose esterified with polyhydroxyl phenyl carboxylic acids such as gallic and ellagic. These readily ferment to release the free acid used in primitive tanning processes to control acidity. Many of these hydrolysable tannins give a blue colour with ferrous ions. *Condensed tannins* are more complex chemical structures and are more likely to be found in the bark or wood of a tree, whereas the hydrolysable tannins predominate in the leaves and fruits; it has been suggested that hydrolysable tannins may be the precursors of the condensed tannins. The chemistry of condensed tannins is extremely complex, but the current view is that they are oligomers containing 4-10 flavonoid units, each containing 4-6 hydroxy groups. Molecular weights in non-aqueous solvents range from 1000 - 3000, although measurements in aqueous solution suggest aggregation or association to give an effective molecular weight of approximately 10,000. Most give a green colour with ferrous ions, due to the presence of two adjacent hydroxyl groups on the B ring. The commercially important mimosa extract is anomalous in that it gives a blue colour with ferrous ions due to a pyrogallol structure on the B ring of the flavonoid unit.

The reaction mechanism between vegetable tannins and collagen is not completely understood. The literature abounds with plausible explanations, most of which can be faulted on some point or other. No significant new work has appeared for almost thirty years; the general consensus now appears to be that multipoint hydrogen bonding takes place (Tu & Lollar, 1950), concurrently with loss of the water previously associated with both the collagen and the vegetable tannin. (For a review on vegetable tannage, see Shuttleworth & Cunningham, 1948.) The shrinkage temperature of vegetable-tanned leather ranges from 70-80°C, according to the extract used and the process conditions.

The mechanism of chrome tannage is better understood. In solution, the chromium [III] ions form polynuclear complexes involving, typically, four chromium atoms. Ring structures containing coordinated sulphate and hydroxyl ligands are formed, giving an effective ionic weight of approximately 800. When skins are immersed in a solution of basic chromium sulphate, carboxyl side chains on the collagen enter the coordination sphere of the chromium to form an insoluble complex. This reaction, which invariably involves cross-linking, is the basis of chrome tanning. The hydrothermal stability of chrome-tanned leather, as measured by its shrinkage temperature, is 90-120°C.

When leather is analysed, it is finely divided (originally by dicing into small cubes with a knife, but currently using cutting mills which cause no significant generation of heat), and then the proportion of the total leather mass which is soluble in an organic solvent and water is determined. The analytical techniques are empirical but reproducible; extraction conditions are specified by the International Union of Leather Technologists' and Chemists' Societies and subsequently incorporated into national standards. The organic solvent used is dichloromethane; and although it is primarily a solvent for fats present in the leather, it may remove other components, e.g., some dyes. The water extraction step removes both inorganic salts and water-soluble organic matter. For most purposes, such as quality control and to establish specifications, only total extractives are recorded. Occasionally, more detailed analyses of the extracts have been undertaken; in vegetable-tanned leather, some unbound plant phenolics are extracted, generally with low molecular weights.

8.   **Experimental data on endogenous substances in wood, wood shaving and wood dust**

The Working Group noted the paucity of data on the long-term effects of wood and leather dusts and of endogenous substances in wood.

Podophyllin, a crude extract from the roots of the mandrake *(Podophyllum peltatum L.)* and from dried needles of the red cedar *(Juniperus virginiana L.)* and other juniper species, has been shown, in preliminary and incompletely reported studies in male BALB/c mice, to increase the incidence of hepatomas and lymphomas (O'Gara, 1968).

Several studies have been undertaken in which experimental animals were exposed throughout life to bedding consisting of certain wood shavings and the incidence of tumours compared with that among control groups. These experiments do not allow an assessment of the potential carcinogenicity of the different types of wood shavings (Sabine *et al.*, 1973; Heston, 1975; Sabine, 1975; Vlahakis, 1977; Jacobs & Dieter, 1978).

In a study designed to assess the toxicity of wood dust *in vivo*, 16 male, random-bred guinea-pigs (average weight, 300 g) received a single intratracheal injection of 75 mg mango or sheesham wood dust in 1.5 ml saline. Serial killings took place 60 and 90 days after inoculation; in those lungs that were examined, disintegration of giant cells, centrilobular emphysema and fibrosis were observed (Bhattacharjee *et al.*, 1979).

9.   **Comments on the epidemiological studies**

It is important to point out that there are certain limitations to the epidemiological data presented in these monographs. However, because each limitation may apply to several reports, they are described here in a general way, rather than mentioning specific limitations for each study cited.

(a)   Types of epidemiological studies

Most of the epidemiological reports available for review consist of case-control studies, descriptive surveys and case reports. Some of these are fairly straightforward in their interpretation, but many others are equivocal. For example, in most of the studies presented here, information on occupations of cancer patients was obtained from death certificates rather than by interviewing patients or their relatives. Many of the data on occupational mortality were derived from tabulations based on extensive national and state vital statistics; these are summarized in Appendix 1.

(b)   Occupational title designations

Some of the epidemiological reports that relate to one of the two broad industries (wood, leather) do not pinpoint specific occupational titles. Their results could not therefore be allocated to a monograph on a specific occupation. In such cases, special sections have been constructed in which these reports are considered (Appendices 2 and 3). Examples of such designations include 'woodworkers', 'leather industry', and reports in which specific occupations are combined in such a way that it is impossible to separate the individual results.

Another problem arises when different meanings exist for the same occupational title in different countries (e.g., 'joiner'), or when it is not clear exactly what type of work is implied by a particular term. Thus, the term 'shoemaker' could refer to a job on a production line in a large factory or to an owner-run shop in which shoe repairing is also done.

(c)   Non-occupational factors

Cigarette smoking is a major risk factor for cancer of the lung and certain other sites. However, many of the epidemiological reports cited in the individual monographs do not give data on cigarette smoking habits. Thus, results on oral and pharyngeal, laryngeal, lung and bladder cancer in which no data on smoking are given should be interpreted with caution.

10.   Areas in which no data were available

A number of occupations that are found within the wood, leather and associated industries were not considered by the Working Group due to lack of data. Examples are wood-panel makers, floor layers, coffin-makers, wheelwrights, musical instrument makers and glove makers.

The Working Group considered that several areas require attention in the further elucidation of cancer risks within the wood and leather industries. The largest gap in our knowledge is characterization of exposure-response relationships, beginning with identification of specific job titles and of specific carcinogenic agents. It is apparent, for instance, that further research is necessary on the chemical composition of leather dust and on its potential health hazards.

It became evident from the meeting of this Working Group that in carrying out future research in this area, the collaboration of occupational hygienists, toxicologists and epidemiologists is essential.

References

American Conference of Governmental Industrial Hygienists (1971) *Threshold Limit Values for Chemical Substances Adopted by ACGIH for 1971,* Cincinnati, OH

American Conference of Governmental Industrial Hygienists (1979) *Threshold Limit Values for Chemical Substances and Physical Agents in the Workroom Environment with Intended Changes for 1979,* Cincinnati, OH

Andersen, H.C., Andersen, I. & Solgaard, J. (1977) Nasal cancers, symptoms and upper airway function in woodworkers. *Br. J. ind. Med., 34,* 201-207

Andersen, I., Lundqvist, G.R., Proctor, D.F. & Swift, D.L. (1979) Human response to controlled levels of inert dust. *Am. Rev. resp. Dis., 119,* 619-627

Bhattacharjee, J.W., Dogra, R.K.S., Lal, M.M. & Zaidi, S.H. (1979) Wood dust toxicity: *in vivo* and *in vitro* studies. *Environ. Res., 20,* 455-464

Black, A., Evans, J.C., Hadfield, E.H., Macbeth, R.G., Morgan, A. & Walsh, M. (1974) Impairment of nasal mucociliary clearance in woodworkers in the furniture industry. *Br. J. ind. Med., 31,* 10-17

Côté, W.A. (1977) *Wood ultrastructure in relation to chemical composition.* In: Loewus, F.A. & Runeckles, V.C., eds, *Recent Advances in Phytochemistry,* Vol. 11, *The Structure, Biosynthesis and Degradation of Wood,* New York, Plenum Press, pp. 1-44

Drettner, B. & Stenkvist, B. (1978) *Nasal cytology in woodworkers for early diagnosis of ethmoidal adenocarcinoma.* In: *International Symposium on the Control of Air Pollution in the Working Environment,* Part I: *Opening, Research Methods, Measurement Techniques, Stockholm, 1977,* Geneva, International Labour Office, pp. 266-276

Esau, K. (1953) *Plant Anatomy,* New York, Wiley

Hadfield, E.H. (1970) A study of adenocarcinoma of the paranasal sinuses in woodworkers in the furniture industry. *Ann. R. Coll. Surg. (UK), 46,* 301-319

Hanslian, L. & Kadlec, K. (1964) Timber and timber dust (Czech.). *Prac. Lék., 16,* 276-282

Harada, H. (1965) *Ultrastructure and organization of gymnosperm cell walls.* In: Côté, W.A., Jr, ed., *Cellular Ultrastructure of Woody Plants,* Syracuse, NY, Syracuse University Press, pp. 215-233

Heston, W.E. (1975) Testing for possible effects of cedar wood shavings and diet on occurrence of mammary gland tumors and hepatomas in C3H-A^{vy} and C3H-A^{vy} fB mice. *J. natl Cancer Inst., 54,* 1011-1014

Hilding, A.C. (1977) *Nasal filtration.* In: Perkins, E. & Hill, D.W., eds, *Scientific Foundations of Otolaryngology,* Chicago, Year Book Medical Publishers, pp. 502-512

Hounam, R.F. & Williams, J. (1974) Levels of airborne dust in furniture making factories in the High Wycombe area. *Br. J. ind. Med., 31,* 1-9

International Labour Office (1974) *Occupational Health and Safety,* Vol. 2, Geneva, p. 1507

International Labour Office (1977) *Occupational Exposure Limits for Airborne Toxic Substances (Occupational Safety and Health Series No. 37),* Geneva

Isenberg, I.H. (1963) *The structure of wood.* In: Browning, B.L., ed., *The Chemistry of Wood,* New York, Interscience, pp. 7-55

Jacobs, B.B. & Dieter, D.K. (1978) Spontaneous hepatomas in mice inbred from Ha:ICR Swiss stock: effects of sex, cedar shavings in bedding, and immunization with fetal liver or hepatoma cells. *J. natl Cancer Inst., 61,* 1531-1534

Janes, R.L. (1969) *The chemistry of wood and fibres.* In: MacDonald, R.G., ed., *Pulp and Paper Manufacture,* Vol. 1, *The Pulping of Wood,* 2nd ed., New York, McGraw-Hill, p. 41

Koppenhoefer, R.M. (1938) Lipids of sheepskin. I. Lipids of fresh sheepskin. *J. Am. Leather Chem. Assoc., 33,* 203-215 [*Chem. Abstr.,32,* 4376 (2)]

Koppenhoefer, R.M. (1939) The lipids of steer hide. V. The effect of sulfide liming on the lipids of steer hide. *J. Am. Leather Chem. Assoc., 34,* 380-396 [Chem. Abstr., *33,* 7609 (9)]

Koppenhoefer, R.M. & Highberger, J.H. (1934) Grease stains on leather. III. Lipids of fresh steer hide. *J. Am. Leather Chem. Assoc., 29,* 598-623 [*Chem. Abstr., 29,* 1676 (5)]

Mozzo, W., Cavazzani, M., Zampieri, P. & Viola, A. (1978) Nasal exfoliative cytology for early diagnosis of preneoplastic and neoplastic lesions in wood workers (Ital.). *Nuovo Arch. Ital. Otol. Rinol. Laringol., 6,* 299-305

Mühlethaler, K. (1965) *The fine structure of cellulose microfibril.* In: Côté, W.A., Jr, ed., *Cellular Ultra-structure of Woody Plants,* Syracuse, NY, Syracuse University Press, pp. 191-198

New England Tanners' Club (1977) *Leather Facts,* Peabody, MA, pp. 28-32

O'Flaherty, F. & Stubbings, R.L. (1966) *Leather.* In: Kirk, R.E. & Othmer, D.F., eds, *Encyclopedia of Chemical Technology,* 2nd ed., Vol. 12, New York, Wiley, pp. 303-343

O'Gara, R.W. (1968) Biologic screening of selected plant material for carcinogens. *Cancer Res., 28,* 2272-2275

Panshin, A.J. & de Zeeuw, C. (1970) *Textbook of Wood Technology,* Vol. 1, *Structure, Identification, Uses and Properties of the Commercial Woods of the United States and Canada,* 3rd ed., New York, McGraw-Hill, pp. 111, 526-537

Pavia, D. & Thomson, M.L. (1976) The fractional deposition of inhaled 2 and 5 μm particles in the alveolar and tracheobronchial regions of the healthy human lung. *Ann. occup. Hyg., 19,* 109-114

Preston, R.D. (1974) *The Physical Biology of Plant Cell Walls,* London, Chapman & Hall, pp. 163-191

Sabine, J.R. (1975) Exposure to an environment containing the aromatic red cedar, *Juniperus virginiana*: procarcinogenic, enzyme-inducing and insecticidal effects. *Toxicology, 5,* 221-235

Sabine, J.R., Horton, B.J. & Wicks, M.B. (1973) Spontaneous tumours in C3H-A^{vy} and C3H-A^{vy} fB mice: high incidence in the United States and low incidence in Australia. *J. natl Cancer Inst., 50,* 1237-1242

Shuttleworth, S.G. & Cunningham, G.E. (1948) The theory of vegetable tannage. *J. Soc. Leather Trades Chem., 32,* 183-209 [*Chem. Abstr.,42,* 6147d]

Tu, S.-T. & Lollar, R.M. (1950) A concept of the mechanism of tannage by phenolic substances. *J. Am. Leather Chem. Assoc., 45,* 324-349 [*Chem. Abstr., 44,* 1147(*g*)]

United Nations (1977) *Yearbook of Industrial Statistics, 1975 Edition,* Vol. 1, *General Industrial Statistics,* New York, Department of Economic and Social Affairs, Statistical Office of the United Nations

Vlahakis, G. (1977) Possible carcinogenic effects of cedar shavings in bedding of C3H-A^{vy} fB mice. *J. natl Cancer Inst., 58,* 149-150

Workers' Compensation Board (1978) *Industrial Health & Safety Regulations,* Vancouver, British Columbia, p. A-17

THE MONOGRAPHS

WOOD

1. HISTORICAL OVERVIEW OF THE INDUSTRY

Use of the saw as a hand tool dates back many thousands of years. The Dutch are considered to be the inventors of machine saws, since they built wind-operated saws in around 1000 AD. By the end of the Middle Ages, water power was frequently used, and this soon became the most common driving force for saws. Water-driven saws are known to have been used in Germany, in Augsburg in 1337 and in Breslau in 1427; in Norway, Sweden and Finland the first water-driven saws were built in the sixteenth century.

The move from water-driven saws to saws driven by steam engines at the end of the eighteenth and beginning of the nineteenth century heralded a period of vigorous construction and development. During this period many large steam-sawmills were constructed, mainly at the mouths of rivers. The Scandinavian sawmill machine industry dates to the 1850s when the first frame saws were manufactured.

The beginning of the present century brought more changes to the industry, when electric saws were introduced. Nevertheless, steam-driven saws were used side by side with the new electric saws for a long time. The basis of the operation of modern sawmills was created in the 1930s with the application of, for example, hydraulics and pneumatics. The processes and machines of that period are still in use in many sawmills.

The advent of new techniques and technology ushered in an age of greater capacity: that of a steam-driven frame saw was usually less than 2 m^3/hr; today, as a rule, the capacity is more than 15 m^3/hr. Large, modern sawmills that produce over 200,000 m^3/year may have hundreds of workers. However, there still exist many small sawmills using circular saws which produce wood mainly for local needs; the number of workers in such sawmills may be ten or less.

The total world production of sawn wood in 1977 was about 440 million m^3. Coniferous wood (spruce, pine, fir, parana pine, deodar or Himalayan cedar, ginkgo, larch, chir, kail, etc.) accounted for 336 million m^3. The major producers of coniferous wood were the USSR, $\sim$ 97 million m^3; the US, 73 million m^3; Canada, 41 million m^3; Japan, $\sim$ 29 million m^3; the People's Republic of China, $\sim$ 11 million m^3; and Sweden, 11 million m^3. World production of non-coniferous sawn wood (maple, birch, aspen, oak, alder, ebony, beech, lignum vitae, poplar, sal, teak, etc.) was 99 million m^3. The most important producers were the US, 15 million m^3; the USSR, $\sim$ 14 million m^3; Japan, $\sim$ 9 million m^3; the People's Republic of China, $\sim$ 6 million m^3; Brazil, 6 million m^3; Peninsular Malaysia, 5 million m^3; and France, 4 million m^3 (Food & Agricultural Organization, 1979).

2. DESCRIPTION OF THE INDUSTRY

2.1 Processes used previously and changes over time

(a) Handling of logs

The manner of transporting and storing logs remained unchanged for a long time. In the eighteenth and nineteenth centuries, techniques of floating were primitive, and the logs were brought to the mill over only short distances. Later the logs were transported as boom rafts, hauled by horses; horses were also used to lift the logs from the water and to shift them to the sawmill. No other methods were developed until the twentieth century, and the greatest improvements have been made over the last 30 years. Now, transport by rail and road has become general.

Debarking machines such as we know them were developed in the 1950s.

(b) Sawing

The first water-driven saws were frame saws. A connecting rod fastened to the axle of a water wheel moved a thick, ferrous saw blade back and forth; the log was fastened to a log carriage which pushed it through the frame of the saw. By this method, the sawing of one log could last for over an hour. The Dutch began to use more than one saw blade in their frame saws, and they also invented the thin saw blades which became used generally in the northern countries at the beginning of the eighteenth century. The change to steam engine-driven saws increased capacity, so that the sawing of one log lasted 'only' 15 - 20 minutes. In the period of steam saws, double-cut sawing, edging and cut-off sawing were brought into use; however, there were no conveyers, and sawing waste had to be carried out. Conveyors and chain-driven log-transferring devices were introduced at the beginning of the twentieth century, since the increasing capacity of the saws now required a continuous input of logs. The application of electricity, hydraulics, pneumatics and other improvements has greatly increased the efficiency of sawing during the last decades.

The bandsaw was patented in 1795, but it did not come into general use until the 1850s; however, by the end of the nineteenth century, many kinds of bandsaws were in use. Double-cutting log bandsaws were introduced. American log and rip-bandsaws were more efficient than European bandsaws; they were used mostly for sawing coniferous and broad-leaved trees, whereas in European sawmills, bandsaws were used mostly in the sawing of broad-leaved and imported tropical trees. Technical improvements during the twentieth century have made bandsaws as efficient and as ubiquitous as frame saws were in their own time. Bandsaws are especially popular in Africa, Australia, Asia and South America. In Scandinavia, bandsaws have become used more generally, but the frame saw is still the most common type of saw.

The use of circular saws for sawing logs was developed in the 1930s. In general, circular sawing is used for the edging and cross-cutting of boards. Circular sawing of logs has become popular, particularly in smaller Swedish sawmills; small gangsaw mills use circular saws almost exclusively.

(c) Stain control

Before the Second World War, little attention was paid to protecting wood from blue-stain fungi and moulds. The boards were air-seasoned in timber yards and bluing was general. About 40 years ago, the organic mercury compounds were found to be effective in the surface treatment of newly-sawn timber, and a little later, chlorophenol preparations were introduced. Since then those compounds have been the most commonly used antistaining agents. However, the toxicity of mercury compounds for humans and for animals is high and they tend to accumulate in the environment. Substitution of ethylmercury with phenylmercury and of the acetate with the oleate did not improve the situation sufficiently, and nowadays mercurial preparations are, in most countries, prohibited or not recommended. Chlorophenol compounds are used in many countries, but since the 1970s many alternative inorganic and organic preparations have also been available.

Chemical treatment is carried out before dimensional sorting in the loading bridge. In newer systems, bundles of boards are dipped into a basin filled with a solution of antistaining agent or are sprayed.

(d) Seasoning

Until the 1920s, when artificial seasoning was developed, sawn timber was seasoned outdoors in timber yards. The first kilns were operated with a natural draught and the results were unsatisfactory. The next improvement was the compartment kiln, which contained a long shaft equipped with blowers. In the 1940s, when kiln drying became more general, the shaft with blowers was replaced by separate electric blowers. Continuous tunnel kilns were developed for larger sawmills. Today, most sawn wood is dried artificially.

(e) Other phases of production

Other phases of sawmill work underwent no marked development until the past few decades, when physical work was replaced more and more by machines and automatic control devices. Sawing, edging and pre-trimming are followed by dimensional sorting, which can be done by hand or with a sorting machine. Stacking after sorting used also to be done by hand at the loading bridge or at a separate stacking place; today, it is generally carried out by machine at a separate plant. After stacking and seasoning, the boards go to another plant, where they are trimmed, graded for quality and packaged by machines.

2.2 Processes used currently

(a) The production line of a modern sawmill

An example of a production line and various phases of work at a typical Scandinavian sawmill are shown in Figure 1.

Fig. 1. Example of the production line at a typical Scandinavian sawmill, with occupations at each point

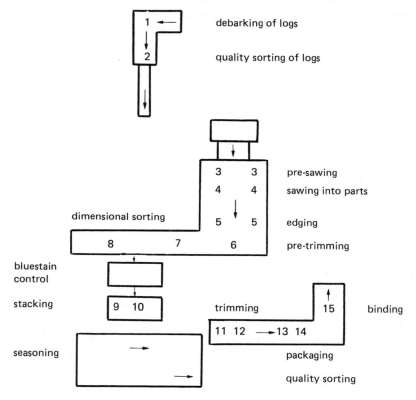

Occupations:

1. Controller at debarking plant	9. Machine stacker
2. Quality sorter of logs	10. Assistant machine stacker
3. Sawyer with pre-frame saw	11. Butt-end trimmer
4. Sawyer with parting-frame saw	12. Quality sorter at trimming-grading plant
5. Edger	13. Packager
6. Pre-trimmer	14. Assistant packager
7. Quality sorter at sawhouse	15. Binder
8. Dimensional sorter (loader)	

(b)   Handling of logs

Logs may be stored at the sawmill in water or on land. In water storage, logs are grouped in boom rafts as loose logs or in bundles. In land storage, logs are piled into heaps with log lifts. When logs are to be stored for a long time, pesticides are used for insect control.

Almost all timber is debarked before sawing. The debarking of logs is most often done with a hole-rotor debarking machine in which rotating blades rub the bark off. The logs are then sorted according to diameter and species of tree. Sorting is done in log ponds or in a log sorting plant. The older of these two methods is pond sorting, in which logs are sorted according to their thickness into lockers in front of the sawmill before sawing. In a mechanical sorting plant, the diameter of the log is measured, the class of thickness is registered by pressing a button, the log is transported to the right locker along a conveyor and is dropped into it. The diameter can also be measured automatically.

(c)   Sawing, edging and pre-trimming

In frame sawing, logs are brought into the sawhouse on a chain conveyor. The use of such built-in saws results in heavier exposure to dust and vapours than was experienced previously when saws were used out of doors. Logs are fed into the frame saw on a log carriage or automatically, with monitoring. Frame sawing involves a single or double cut. In a single cut, the log is sawed into parts with many blades in one phase. A double cut takes place in two phases: first, the log is sawed from two sides, and then the cant is turned 90° and it is sawed into parts with another frame saw. In a double cut, the heartwood of the log need not be edged. Side boards are edged with an edger, usually consisting of two parallel circular saws. After edging, the conveyor carries the boards to the pre-trimming table, where the tops and ends of wane-edged boards are trimmed with circular saws.

With bandsawing, many saw combinations are available. The canter-chipper-double-bandsaw, for example, is a machine consisting first of two rotating cutters and then of two parallel bandsaws. The cutters convert the log to a cant, and then the bandsaws cut one board from each side of the cant. Side boards are edged and pre-trimmed as in frame sawing.

In circular sawing methods, the basic machine is a circular saw with one or several blades. Logs are fed to the saws on a table that moves back and forth at a controllable speed. Circular sawing with one blade can be done in various ways according to the thickness of the log. When several blades are used, the log is first converted to a cant with a canter-chipper and then sawn into parts with two-bladed or several-bladed circular saws. Edging and pre-trimming are done as in frame and band sawing.

(d)   Dimensional sorting

Dimensional sorting is still carried out by hand in many sawmills. The boards move along a loading bridge, from which loaders select them according to their dimensions and transfer them to carriages. One type of mechanical loading consists of an automatic sorting table: the boards first come to a measuring device, with which their width and thickness are measured; these values are transmitted to a regulator which drops the boards into the appropriate lockers.

(e)   Stain control

In North America, antistain agents are generally used only on lumber that is seasoned outdoors. In Scandinavia, antistain agents may be used before either outdoor or kiln seasoning, except during the winter months. The two methods of antistain application generally in use today are dipping and spraying.

Dimensionally sorted bundles of boards may be dipped into a basin for a short period of time using an overhead crane or a specially designed dipping device. Dipping is usually done before stacking but may also be done afterwards. The bundles drip while suspended over the basin or over an earth concrete foundation; in some cases, dripped solution is collected and pumped back into the basin. In general, treated wood need not be handled while wet; however, boards that enter the stacking plant may still be damp if they have not been allowed to drip off completely.

In older systems, boards are dipped one at a time before loading. A conveyor carries the boards through a trough, and then loaders take them out wet and place them in the sorting lockers (the trough-dipping method). This work is so wet that loaders have to use protective gloves, aprons and rubber boots.

In spraying, boards are sprayed one at a time on a conveyor which goes through a spraying chamber. Another method is the spraying of stacked bundles with a special device before kiln drying.

(f)   Stacking

Stacking can be done by hand or by machine. Machine stacking is more common in larger sawmills: the bundle is brought by an overhead crane or truck to a table, spread and moved along a conveyor to a stacking machine. The machine stacks the boards and slats in layers. After each layer has been placed, the lift automatically lowers the stacked bundle so that the following layer can be stacked. When the whole bundle has been stacked, the lift lowers it to the ground, from where it can be transported to a kiln.

(g)   Seasoning

Sawn wood can be seasoned in timber yards; but in bigger sawmills it is usually done artificially in a kiln. There are many kinds of kilns: compartment kilns and high-temperature kilns are serial kilns; in continuous kilns, stacked bundles can move through the kiln in a perpendicular or parallel position, and the direction of air movement can be perpendicular or parallel to the boards. In Scandinavia, the temperature in kilns is generally 40-60°C, and the lumber may have been previously treated with antistain agents. In North America, kiln temperatures are generally higher, 90-100°C, and kiln-seasoned lumber has not generally been pretreated with antistain agents. Artificial drying is currently carried out automatically, according to a programme which takes into account the moisture content and dimensions of the wood. The main task of a kiln worker is to follow the progress of the drying by watching meters and regulating the process when necessary. He enters the kiln when loading and unloading it, but at these times the temperature in the kiln is usually low.

(h)   Trimming, surfacing and grading

The dried wood is further processed in the trimming-grading plant. The phases of work are as follows:

- spreading stacked bundles
- removing slats (stickers)
- trimming tops and ends
- surfacing, grading
- stamping and packaging
- binding.

Bundles are spread and are shifted to the conveyor by a lift. End-trimming is carried out with circular saws. Grading can be done either by hand or automatically at the same time as the trimming and/or surfacing. Graded boards are moved along the conveyor to the paper lockers. When one locker is full, the boards either drop automatically or a lockerguard drops them down. The bundle is re-spread, and the boards are transferred by conveyor to a packaging machine. The package is bound with metal bands and transported by motor truck or conveyor to storage.

(i)   Further processing

In some sawmills, boards may also be sorted according to length or planed. Debarked logs, sleepers and sawn wood may also be impregnated with chemicals, used as preservatives against rotting (moulds and other fungi) and wood-destroying insects, in specialized sawmills or treatment plants. In some countries in the last ten years, such impregnation has been done in closed cylinders, using CCA-salts (copper, chrome and arsenic oxides), creosote oil, chlorophenols or other chemicals. (See section 2.3 (*d*), p. 77 .)

(j)   Production of cork

Cork is obtained from the bark of the cork-oak tree *(Quercus suber)*, a medium-sized tree with a very bulky bark, which is found principally in the western Mediterranean basin, since it requires a certain level of humidity and mild winters. About 70% of the world's cork (24 million kg/yr) is produced in the Iberian Peninsula, with two-thirds from Portugal and one-third from the south-western part of Spain. It is also produced in Algeria, France, Italy, Greece, Turkey and the USSR.

In 1963, Portugal had 980 cork factories employing 20,500 workers (De Carbalho Cancella, 1963); Spain had 249 cork factories in 1976, employing about 4000 workers. In both countries, production has decreased in recent years due to the replacement of cork in traditional uses by other materials.

The occupational categories found in the cork production industry are strippers, agricultural workers who strip the bark from the trees, using jack-knives, once every nine years; those who prepare cork sheet, by scraping with knives, boiling and quality-grading; those involved in processing cork to the final product (see below); and workers who extract tannin from the bark.

Bark stripped from the trees is stacked outside for about a year, then cut to size, baled, boiled in water and restacked until required, often in damp, poorly ventilated warehouses.

There are two principal types of cork processing plant. The 'natural' plant uses cork that has been stripped of its hard outer layer for the production of bottle corks, crown closure inserts, cork paper for cigarette tips, balls, rings, buoys, etc. A work flow diagram for such a plant is shown in Figure 2. The 'reconstituted' cork plant uses whole cork, including the hard outer layer, which is ground into particles then bonded together with an adhesive to produce floor coverings, panels and special sections for thermal and acoustic insulation. A work flow diagram for such a plant is shown in Figure 3.

The exact composition of cork is not yet well known, although tannins can be extracted from it. It seems, however, to be comprised of a mixture of fatty acids of high molecular weight, some of which are either not saponifiable or insoluble, and others of which are of as yet unknown composition. The outer part of the cork contains a certain amount of silica, probably deposited by the wind, since the cork oak grows mainly on poor soils with a high silica content (International Labour Office, 1976).

Fig. 2. Work flow diagram for a 'natural' cork processing plant;
= end products[a]

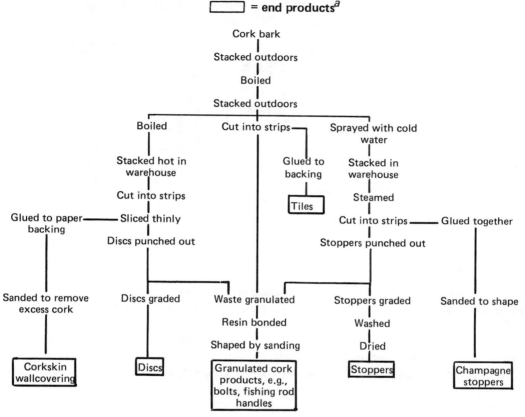

[a]From Lacey (1973)

De Carbalho Cancella (1963) reported finding 0.18-9.8% particles total silica and 0.9-3.1% particles free silica in a sample of 'not pure' cork dust collected in cork factories. The dust concentration was 165-1260 particles/m^3, showing a range in diameter from 0.45-1.4 μm.

2.3 Qualitative and quantitative data on exposures

The most important hazardous substances in sawmills are wood dust, antistain agents and other preservatives, sawing vapours and fungal spores. Other possible sources of hazardous substances include exhaust gases and oil mists associated with sawblade lubrication, but no quantitative data were available. A list of the chemicals used in the sawmill and lumber industries is given in Appendix 4.

Fig. 3. Work flow diagram for a 'reconstituted' cork plant: A, natural cork;
B, grinding; C, classifying; D, silo storage; E, coal, tar, pitch; F, grinding; G, melting;
H, drying; I, mixing; J, pressing (block production); K, slicing, sawing, moulding;
L, blocks, slabs; M, finished parts[a]

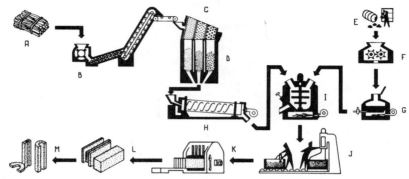

[a]From International Labour Office (1976)

(a) Dust

McKenzie (1967) outlined some of the basic aspects of machining wood. Wood is highly anisotropic, being about 50 times stronger along the fibre axis than normal to it. It is preferable to cut wood longitudinally, using a high concentration of energy, and to remove debris and heat efficiently. The number of variables is formidable, even when reduced to simplest terms: groups of variables include the geometry of cutting, the properties of the wood and the physics of cutting. Because of the anisotropic properties of wood, cutting direction relative to fibre orientation is of major importance. The two cardinal orientations of the cutting edge and motion vector, i.e., 0° and 90°, give rise to three sets of orientation resulting in maximum difference in cutting: 0/90, 90/0 and 90/90 (Table 1). Each of these sets is subdivided into three or four subcategories. At the expense of great oversimplification, it can be said that the effects of cutting are to strip elongated sections parallel to the fibre axis or to cut cubical fragments perpendicular to the fibre axis. As wood density increases, more energy is required; as moisture content increases, less energy is required, but deformation of the wood is greater. High density, low moisture content, high speeds of cutting, and shallow depth per cut tend to minimize the dimensions of the chips formed but also increase the conversion of mechanical energy to thermal energy.

Vorreiter (1953) investigated sawdust produced by rip-sawing pine using a frame saw and a circular saw. The frame saw, with side edges cutting according to the 0/90 and main edges according to the 90/90 orientation sets given in Table 1, produced splintery particles with their longitudinal axis in the direction of the wood grain. The circular saw, with side edges cutting according to the 90/0 and main edges cutting according to the 90/90 orientation sets, produced granular-shaped particles which were approximately cubicular. It

Table 1. Maximum orientation in cutting patterns

Symbol	Tool relative to grain direction		Related cutting operations
	Edge	Motion	
0/90	parallel	perpendicular	veneer peeling, slicing; side edges of band and frame saws
90/0	perpendicular	parallel	planing; side edges of circular saws
90/90	perpendicular	perpendicular	shear cross-cutting; main edge of saws

was shown that the cubicular particles, even though more coarse, gave a higher density than the elongated particles, due to their better packing.   Density increased as particle size diminished; as the size of the particle decreased to a grain size less than that of the smallest cell cavity of the wood, i.e., to about 0.1 μm, the specific weight became approximately that of the density of cell wall substance, or about 1.51 g/cm^3.   The specific areas calculated for particles of standard screen sizes are shown in Table 2 for grain sizes 1000-fold or more greater than that of the 0.1 μm particle size. The densities of some of the grain sizes are also shown.

In subsequent articles, Vorreiter (1960) discussed the properties, manufacture and applications of wood flour.   Particle shapes are described as comprising:

(i)   powders of uniform particle shapes

(ii)   fine splinters or bundles of fibres

(iii) granular or grille-like particles

(iv)   very fine lamellar particles manufactured in ball mills.

Shape and size depend on the type of saw used, the nature of the original wood, and its moisture content.   Softwoods produce fibrous particles, whereas hardwoods or kiln-dried and embrittled softwoods produce powdered or granular wood flour. Wood flour with grain sizes as small as 1 μm can be produced. Wood flour (Table 3) is graded according to the mesh size through which particles will pass (-) or be retained (+).

Since cell cavities vary in size from about 1 to 650 μm, the density of wood flour within any given mean range is affected. Formulae are given for calculating the bulk weight of wood flour and the falling or sedimentation velocity of wood flour suspended in a gas.   The chemical reactivity of wood flour was attributed to its total surface and surface irregularities.

**Table 2. Internal surface and density of cubical wood particles
as a function of particle size[a]**

Mesh/cm^2	Grain size (mm)	No. of particles x 10^{-3} per cm^3	Internal surface (cm^2/cm^3)	Density (g/cm^3)
1	8.0	0.001	36	
9	2.5			0.100
16	1.5			0.110
36	1.0	0.905	54.3	0.125
100	0.6	4.3	86	0
144	0.5	7.6	114	
256	0.4			0.173
400	0.3	34.8	188	
900	0.2	120	288	
3600	0.1	980	588	
	0.004-0.025			0.94[b]
	0.001			1.35[b]
	0.0001			1.51

[a]From Vorreiter (1953)

[b]From Vorreiter (1960)

Table 3. Grades of wood flour

Grade	Clearance between meshes[a] (μm)
Very coarse	-800 +400
Coarse	-400 +200
Fine	-200 +100
Very fine	-100 +50
Extra fine	-50 +20
Colloidal	-10 +10.1

[a]Particles smaller than screen openings (-); particles larger than screen openings (+)

Reineke (1966), in a paper on wood flour, gave a classification based on the principle of air elutriation and some data on particle size distribution. He indicated that bag filters remove essentially all fine particles.

The exposure of sawmill workers to wood dust has also been studied in Sweden and Finland. Söderqvist & Ager (1975) measured and estimated exposures to wood dust during different phases of work in Swedish sawmills and divided the exposures into four classes on the basis of the measured or estimated dust concentrations. If the concentration at a working place seemed to be very low, no measurements were taken. If the dust concentration was suspected to be higher, it was measured using personal sampling, in which a filter connected to a battery-driven pump was placed in the breathing zone for at least half a day. Thirty-six samples were taken in all. According to their results (Table 4), 2% of workers were exposed to wood-dust concentrations over 5 mg/m^3, 18% to concentrations of 2.1-5.0 mg/m^3 and 80% to concentrations below 2 mg/m^3. Concentrations over 5 mg/m^3 were measured, for example, in sawing, packaging and trimming operations. The workers themselves considered that dust exposure was greatest in cleaning and chipper-controlling posts; many packagers, assistant sawyers, and edgers also considered their work to be dusty. Measurements showed that the occupations with the highest dust levels were chipper controllers, cleaning personnel and slat controllers.

Kauppinen et al. (1979) measured wood dust concentrations in five relatively large sawmills in eastern Finland. Sampling was conducted at static points and in the breathing zone, using the usual filter method, during phases of work which were estimated to be dustier than normal. A total of 61 samples were taken. The results are presented in Table 5. Concentrations over 5 mg/m^3 were measured in 11% of the phases, concentrations of 2-5 mg/m^3 in 19%, and less than 2 mg/m^3 in 70% of the phases. Concentrations of over 5 mg/m^3 were found in cleaning, slat-positioning, butt-end trimming, quality sorting by hand and bandsawing operations and near sorting lockers. The measurements showed that cleaning was the dustiest phase of work; the concentration was particularly high in the trimming-grading plant during the cleaning of dry sawing waste.

The use of carbide-tipped circular saws has gained favour in recent years, since it reduces maintenance and improves timber production. One result of this evolutionary change has been that dusts different from those produced previously are now encountered, although the wood-saw interface is heated less. Since non-carbide-tipped saws tend to dull more quickly, the dust they produce has a particle size distribution that shifts towards finer particles over time until the next sharpening.

Table 4. Distribution of sawmill workers on the basis of exposure to total dust concentration in different phases of production[a]

Phase of work	Number of workers	% of workers exposed to:			
		'Small'[b]	<2 mg/m^3	2.1-5.0 mg/m^3	>5.0 mg/m^3
Grinding	23	0	57	43	0
Sawing	134	4	57	34	5
Packaging	46	24	41	31	4
Trimming	61	18	58	21	3
Several production phases	9	33	45	22	0
Handling of timber and barking	83	48	30	22	0
Storage and timber yard tasks, loading	57	16	70	14	0
All other production phases	53	21	68	9	2
Pre-trimming and dimensional sorting	69	54	39	6	1
Drying	15	33	60	7	0
Maintenance	61	20	78	2	0
Stacking	36	44	56	0	0
Handling of logs	42	81	19	0	0
Total	689	28	52	18	2

[a]From Söderqvist & Ager (1975)

[b]If the concentration at a working place appeared to be very low, no measurements were taken.

**Table 5. Concentrations of total dust in different phases of work
in five Finnish sawmills[a]**

Phase of work	Concentration of dust (mg/m^3)		
	Range	Mean	Median
Frame sawing	0.4-3.8	1.2	0.8
Edging	0.1-3.4	1.6	1.9
Stacking (by machine)	0.4-2.7	1.3	0.8
Trimming	1.3-9.6	3.2	1.9
Grading (by hand)	1.9-5.6	3.3	2.9
Grading lockers	0.5-2.9	1.5	1.2
Packaging	0.1-1.8	1.1	0.9
Binding	0.4-1.3	0.7	0.4
Sorting lockers in longitudinal packaging plant	1.0-6.3	2.9	1.4
Cleaning	3.1-15	7.4	4.0

[a]From Kauppinen et al. (1979)

A series of compounds has been identified from various wood products. Different species yield different products, and consequently wood dust from various sources is chemically different. Such extractives include tannins and other polyphenolics, colouring matters, essential oils, fats, resins, waxes, gums, starch and simple metabolic intermediates. The quantities in which they are found range from roughly 5-30%.

(b) Antistain agents

Salts of chlorophenols are the antistain agents most commonly used in sawmills. The surface of the wood is treated with a 1-2.5% water solution of chlorophenates, generally during the warm seasons in North America, the Scandinavian countries, the USSR and central Europe. The use of chlorophenates in Sweden has been forbidden since the beginning of 1978.

Chlorophenols

A monograph on the chemistry, pharmacology and environmental toxicology of pentachlorophenol (PCP) has been published (Rao, 1978). The carcinogenic risks of PCP and of 2,4,5- and 2,4,6-trichlorophenols were evaluated recently (IARC, 1979).

Chlorinated phenols constitute a series of 19 compounds consisting of mono-, di-, tri- and tetrachloroisomers and one pentachlorophenol. The compounds of major interest for this review are 2,4,6-tri-, 2,3,4,6-tetra- and, especially, PCP.

Most chlorophenol preparations are contaminated to a greater or lesser extent with a variety of other products. In addition to other chlorophenols, they contain 1-5% of poly-halogenated phenoxyphenols, also called predioxins (Rappe & Nilsson, 1972; Nilsson *et al.*, 1978). Polychlorinated diphenyl ethers, dioxins and dibenzofurans are often present in the range of 200-2000 μg/g; the levels and identity of these toxic contaminants depend on the route of synthesis and purification (Nilsson *et al.*, 1978). (See also below, 'Levels of PCDDs and PCDFs in chlorophenols'.)

The use of chlorophenols as wood preservatives began in the 1930s, although they came into general use in the US in the 1940s and in Europe in the 1950s. PCP and its sodium salt (Na-PCP) are probably the most versatile pesticides now available. In the US, they are the second most heavily used pesticides; annual consumption is about 25,000 tonnes.

Technical chlorophenols are used predominantly in the wood industry: in the US and Canada, more than 80% of PCP is used for wood preservation and wood protection (Cirelli, 1978; Hoos, 1978). PCP, dissolved at a level of about 5% in various solvents (mineral spirits, fuel oil, kerosene, liquid petroleum gas and dichloromethane), is applied using pressure and vacuum cycles to obtain deep and optimum retention, in order to preserve products that will have a long period of service, such as railway ties, pilings and telephone poles.

A substantial proportion of processed wood does not require long-term preservation. Fresh-cut lumber may be protected against attack by fungi and moulds by treatment, in spray tunnels or by dipping, with Na-PCP (US, Canada) or with 2,3,4,6-tetra- and 2,4,6-trichlorophenol (Scandinavia). Chlorophenols are also found in paints used in the wood industry, at levels of 5-10%.

*Polychlorinated dibenzo-*para-*dioxins and polychlorinated dibenzofurans*

(i) Chemical and biological properties: Polychlorinated dibenzo-*para*-dioxins (PCDDs) and dibenzofurans (PCDFs) are series of tricyclic aromatic compounds, which

exhibit similar physical and chemical properties (for a review, see IARC, 1978). Some of these compounds are highly toxic and have been the subject of much concern. They have been involved in accidents like that at Yusho in Japan in 1968, intoxication at horse arenas in Missouri, USA, in 1971, and the accident near Seveso, Italy, in 1976.

The chemical structures and numbering of these hazardous compounds are as follows:

PCDFs   PCDDs

The number of chlorine atoms in these compounds can vary from one to eight. In all, there are 75 PCDD and 135 PCDF isomers, ranging from mono- to octachloro compounds.

PCDDs and PCDFs were discovered largely because of the extremely toxic properties of some of their members; the toxicity of these compounds has been the subject of several recent reviews (IARC, 1978; Ramel, 1978; Nicholson & Moore, 1979). The toxicity of individual congeners is strikingly dependent on the position and number of the chlorine substituents, and seems to peak with the tetra- and pentachloro compounds. The 2,3,7,8-tetrachloro isomers appear to be the most toxic.

Individual isomers of PCDDs and PCDFs have been found to vary greatly in acute toxicity and biological activity (McConnell et al., 1978; Poland et al., 1979): and that of closely related isomers like 2,3,7,8- and 1,2,3,8-tetra-CDD may vary by factors of 1000-10,000. Consequently, the separation, identification and quantitation of individual isomers is highly relevant. Some PCDFs are as toxic or biologically active as the most toxic PCDDs (Moore et al., 1979). The most toxic isomers appear to be the 2,3,7,8-tetra-, 1,2,3,7,8-penta-,1,2,3,6,7,8- and 1,2,3,7,8,9-hexa-CDDs, and the 2,3,7,8-tetra, 1,2,3,7,8- and 2,3,4,7,8-penta-CDFs.

PCDDs and PCDFs are potent inducers of enzyme systems, particularily in the liver. Poland & Glover (1973) reported that some PCDDs are powerful inducers of δ-amino-laevulinic acid synthetase (ALAS) and of aryl hydrocarbon hydroxylase (AHH) in chick embryos. The potency of AHH induction was shown to be strongly correlated with the general toxic responses to the PCDD being studied.

(ii) *Levels of PCDDs and PCDFs in chlorophenols:* Firestone et al. (1972) analysed the levels of PCDDs and PCDFs in commercial US chlorophenols received during the period

1967-1970 (Tables 6 and 7). The highest value reported was 100 μg/g. A technical-grade PCP sample examined in 1973 (Villanueva et al., 1973) contained hexa-, hepta- and octa-CDDs at levels of 42, 24 and 11 μg/g, respectively.

Table 6. Polychlorinated dioxins (PCDDs) in mono-, di-, tri- and tetrachlorophenols[a]

Sample of chlorophenol	Year	PCDD	Level (μg/g)
2-mono-	1967	ND[b]	-
2,4-di-	1970	ND	-
2,6-di-	-	ND	-
2,4,5-tri- (Na-)	1967	ND	-
2,4,5-tri- (Na-)	1969	2,7-di-	0.72
		2,3,7,8-tetra-	1.4
2,4,5-tri- (Na-)	1969	1,3,6,8-tetra-	0.30
		2,3,7,8-tetra-	6.2
2,4,5-tri-	1970	penta-	1.5
2,4,5-tri-	1970	ND	-
2,4,5-tri	1970	2,3,7,8-tetra-	0.07
2,4,6-tri-	-	2,3,7-tri-	93
		1,3,6,8-tetra-	49
2,3,4,6-tetra-	-	hexa-	15
		hexa-	14
		hepta-	5.1
		octa-	0.17
2,3,4,6-tetra-	1967	hexa-	4.1
2,3,4,6-tetra-	-	ND	-

[a]From Firestone et al. (1972)
[b]None detected

Table 7. Polychlorinated (PCDDs) in pentachlorophenols (PCPs)[a]

Sample of PCP	Year	PCDD	Level (μg/g)
Na-PCP	1967	hexa-	14
		hepta-	5.4
		hepta-	9.1
		octa-	3.8
Na-PCP	1969	hexa-	20
		hexa-	1.3
		hepta-	10
		octa-	3.3
PCP	1970	hexa-	0.96
		hexa-	38
		hepta-	10
		hepta-	39
		octa-	15
PCP	1970	hexa-	35
		hepta-	23
PCP	1967	hexa-	0.03
		hexa-	0.14
PCP	1969	hexa-	13
		hepta-	12
		hepta-	35
PCP	1970	hexa-	0.91
		hepta-	0.50
		hepta-	1.6
		octa-	5.3
PCP	1970	hexa-	15
		hepta-	23
		octa-	15

[a]From Firestone et al. (1972)

Manufacturers of PCP have attempted to decrease the concentration of dioxins in their commercial products. However, one purification step (recrystallization) results in an increase in dioxin levels in the discharged fraction. Two reports from Dow Chemical (Michigan) indicate that their product, Dowicide EC-7, contained less than 0.5 μg/g hexa-CDDs, 0.3-11 μg/g hepta-CDDs, and levels of octa-CDD between 0.5 and 33 μg/g (Blaser et al., 1976; Pfeiffer et al., 1978). That company has now stopped production of this chlorophenol.

Buser & Bosshardt (1976) made a survey of the PCDD and PCDF contents of PCP and Na-PCP from commercial sources in Switzerland. The samples could be grouped into two series: those containing < 1 ppm hexa-CDD, and those containing >> 1 ppm. Samples with high levels of PCDDs also had high levels of PCDFs. For most samples, these contaminants occurred in the order tetra- <penta- < hexa- < hepta- < octa-CDD and tetra- $\simeq$ penta- <hexa- <hepta- $\simeq$ octa-CDF. The combined levels of PCDDs and PCDFs were in the ranges 2-16 and 1-26 μg/g, respectively, for the first series of samples, and 120-500 and 85-570 μg/g, respectively, for the second series of samples. The maximum levels of octa-CDD and octa-CDF were 370 and 300 μg/g, respectively (Buser, 1978).

In none of these investigations did the analytical technique used allow the identification and quantitation of individual PCDD and PCDF isomers; this would be of importance for total risk evaluation.

Analysis of some of the Na-PCP samples showed the unexpected presence of 0.06-0.25 μg/g of a tetra-CDD (Buser & Bosshardt, 1976); this impurity was later identified by Buser & Rappe (1978) as the unusual 1,2,3,4-tetrachloro-substituted isomer PCP. Na-PCP samples with a high PCDD content (hexa-CDD >> 1 ppm) were reanalysed on a high-resolution gas-chromatographic column for the presence of individual PCDD isomers (Buser, 1978). As reported earlier, all samples showed an almost identical pattern of hexa- and hepta-CDD isomers. The major hexa-CDD isomers were identified as the toxic 1,2,3,6,7,8-hexa-CDD, and, in addition, 1,2,4,6,8,9- and 1,2,3,6,7,9-hexa-CDD. These three isomers were always present in an almost constant isomeric ratio of 50:40:10. Both of the hepta-CDD isomers were present in these samples in a ratio of 15:85, with 1,2,3,4,6,7,8-hepta-CDD as the major constituent. All hexa-CDD isomers found in these samples were dimerization products of 2,3,4,6-tetrachlorophenol, the assumed precursor of PCP in the chlorination process starting from phenol. Although the actual methods by which these samples were produced were not known, this result indicates that phenol-chlorination processes were probably used.

Rappe et al. (1978a) reported the analysis of two commercial chlorophenate formulations from Scandinavian sources: 2,4,6-trichlorophenate and another product containing mainly 2,3,4,6-tetrachlorophenate and 5-10% 2,4,5-tri- and pentachlorophenates. The combined levels of PCDDs and PCDFs (tetra- to octa-) were 12 and 160 μg/g in the 2,3,4,6-

tetrachlorophenate, <3 and 60 μg/g in the 2,4,6-trichlorophenate and 1000 and 280 μg in the pentachlorophenate, respectively. Differences were also seen in the distribution of the individual PCDD isomers in these two sample types. The main hexa-CDD isomers in the Scandinavian samples were 1,2,4,6,7,9- and 1,2,3,6,8,9-hexa-CDD (or their Smiles-rearranged products), and 1,2,3,4,6,8-hexa-CDD. The latter compound was completely absent from the PCP samples analysed earlier. The toxic 1,2,3,6,7,8-hexa-CDD, which was the major hexa-CDD isomer in the PCP samples, occurred to only a minor extent in the Scandinavian samples. A similar difference was seen in the case of the hepta-CDDs: the major isomer in the Scandinavian samples was the 1,2,3,4,6,7,9-hepta-CDD, whereas in all of the PCP samples it was the 1,2,3,4,6,7,8-substituted isomer (Rappe *et al.*, 1978b).

Using the same analytical technique, Rappe *et al.* (1978a) quantified and identified the major PCDFs in the Scandinavian 2,4,6-tri- and 2,3,4,6-tetrachlorophenate samples. A Na-PCP formulation from the US was also analysed. Quantitative results are shown in Table 8.

Table 8. Levels of polychlorinated dibenzofurans (PCDFs) in commercial chlorinated phenol samples (μg/g) taken in 1975[a]

| | PCDFs | | | | |
	tetra-	penta-	hexa-	hepta-	octa-
2,4,6-Trichlorophenate (Scandinavia)	1.5	17.5	36	4.8	-
2,3,4,6-Tetrachlorophenate (Scandinavia)	<0.5	10	70	70	10
Pentachlorophenate (USA)	0.9	4	32	120	130

[a]From Rappe *et al.* (1978a)

The chlorophenols in the formulations analysed differed in their degree of chlorination and were probably synthesized in different ways. Nevertheless, the same penta-, hexa- and hepta-CDF isomers were found to be the main PCDF components in all three samples, although they occurrred in somewhat different proportions.

(iii) Formation of PCDDs and PCDFs from chlorophenols: The photochemical dimerization of chlorophenols to PCDDs was studied by Crosby & Wong (1976). The only PCDD formed in this study was the octa-CDD. Other PCDDs can be formed by a photochemical cyclization of chlorinated *ortho*-phenoxyphenols, also called predioxins

(Nilsson *et al.*, 1974). These predioxins are very common impurities (1-5%) in commercial chlorophenols (Nilsson *et al.*, 1978), but cyclization is only a minor reaction pathway, the main reaction being the photodechlorination of the predioxin (Nilsson *et al.*, 1974).

Another photochemical process of potential importance is dechlorination of the higher chlorinated PCDDs and PCDFs, octa-CDD and octa-CDF. The products formed in solution photolysis of octa-CDD have now been identified by Buser & Rappe (1978). By comparison with standards, it was found that the main tetrachloro isomer was the 1,4,6,9-tetra-CDD; the major pentachloro compound is assumed to be the 1,2,4,6,9-isomer. The main hexa- and heptachloro compounds were the 1,2,4,6,7,9 (or 1,2,4,6,8,9) and the 1,2,3,4,6,7,9 isomer, respectively (Buser, 1976). The reaction scheme deduced from these data shows that chlorine atoms are removed preferentially from the lateral positions on the carbon rings. Consequently, the most toxic PCDD isomers, such as 2,3,7,8-tetra-CDD, are not likely to be formed from solution photolysis of the higher PCDDs. In the case of the octa-CDF, photo-chemical loss of chlorine seems to be a non-specific reaction, as all four possible hepta-CDFs were formed in approximately similar amounts.

PCDDs and PCDFs have been identified as trace contaminants in fly ash and flue gases (Olie *et al.*, 1977; Buser *et al.*, 1978a,b). This observation strongly indicates that these hazardous compounds can be formed in pyrolytic processes or by burning. A recent report indicated that 2,3,7,8-tetra-CDD and other dioxins are ubiquitous products of combustion processes (Smith, 1978), although this hypothesis has been criticized (Hay, 1979). The amounts of PCDDs and PCDFs formed during combusion depend on temperature, retention time in the hot zone and the flow rate of air. PCDDs have been detected in scrubber water from even the most effective industrial incinerators (Dow Chemicals, 1978).

Rappe *et al.* (1978b) have studied the burning of materials impregnated with various salts of chlorophenols. Both very carefully purifed 2,4,6-tri- and pentachlorophenates and a commercial formulation of 2,3,4,6-tetrachlorophenate were studied. The results are summarized in Table 9. The authors observed that in addition to the expected dimerization products, present at levels of mg/g chlorophenate burned, the highly toxic 2,3,7,8-tetra-CDD and 1,2,3,7,8-penta-CDD were also present in the burning extracts from penta- and 2,3,4,6-tetrachlorophenate. Although they were only minor constituents, in individual experiments both were found at levels exceeding 10 μg/g chlorophenate. The burning of a piece of lumber (plank, board, post) that has taken up 100 ml of a 20% chlorophenol solution might therefore generate more than 20 μg each of 2,3,7,8-tetra- and 1,2,3,7,8-penta-CDD, in addition to much larger amounts of other, less toxic dioxins.

Rappe *et al.* (1978a) also studied the levels of PCDFs found in the burning extracts: levels of most PCDFs were generally much decreased (in contrast to PCDDs), although the levels of a few individual PCDFs increased; e.g., that of the major tetra-CDF (an unknown isomer) increased during burning by more than 100-fold, and two isomers were found that

Table 9. Polychlorinated dioxins (PCDDs) in extracts from the burning of chlorophenate[a]

	Purified 2,4,6-trichloro-phenate	Commercial 2,3,4,6-tetra-chlorophenate	Purified pentachlorophenate
Tetra-CDDs	2100 μg/g	96 μg/g	5.2 μg/g
Number of isomers	2	14	14
Major isomers	1,3,6,8- and 1,3,7,9-	1,3,6,8- and 1,3,7,9-	2,3,7,8- and two others
2,3,7,8-Tetra-CDD	no	yes	yes
Penta-CDDs	5 μg/g	120 μg/g	14 μg/g
Number of isomers	-	9	10
Major isomers	-	unknown	unknown
1,2,3,7,8-Penta-CDD	-	yes	yes
Hexa-CDDs	1 μg/g	110 μg/g	56 μg/g
Number of isomers	-	8	8
Major isomers	-	1,2,3,6,8,9-	1,2,3,6,7,8- and two others
1,2,3,6,7,8- and 1,2,3,7,8,9- Hexa-CDDs	-	yes	yes
Hepta-CDDs	3 μg/g	65 μg/g	172 μg/g
Number of isomers	-	2	2
Octa-CDDs	6 μg/g	1.2 μg/g	710 μg/g

[a]From Rappe et al. (1978b)

had not been identified in the starting materials. 2,3,7,8-Tetra-CDF, which is considered to be the most toxic of all PCDFs, was only a minor component in all the samples.

Kauppinen et al. (unpublished results) have measured the concentrations of chlorophenates present in ten Finnish saw mills. Samples were collected in an absorptive solution and were analysed by gas chromatography. Because chlorophenates can be absorbed through the skin, urine samples were also taken and analysed. The preparation being used for wood treatment in these sawmills was the Finnish KY-5, which is a sodium salt of tri-, tetra- and pentachlorophenols (mainly sodium tetrachlorophenate). The concentration of the treatment solution was usually 1-1.5%. Exposure to chlorophenates or dust containing chlorophenates can occur during preparation of the treatment solution, while working near the dipping basin, when shifting wet bundles on motor trucks, in stacking and kiln drying and in the trimming-grading plant or during further processing (see Table 10). The highest concentrations, up to 17 mg/m^3, were measured inside the kiln during drying. Nowadays, kiln workers very rarely go inside the kiln during drying; the chlorophenol concentrations in their urine were therefore low. Concentrations in the air at work places near the dipping basin were below 0.2 mg/m^3; however, higher concentrations may occur, particularly in the immediate vicinity of the basin when the air is moving towards the workers. The concentrations at the loading bridge and stacking plant were 0.005-0.2 mg/m^3. In the trimming-grading plants and in one longitudinal packaging plant, the chlorophenol concentrations in the dust were 0.2-9.3 mg/m^3; the concentrations of chlorophenate attached to the wood dust were 0.0005-0.01 mg/m^3.

The concentrations of chlorophenols in the urine (Table 11) were found to be highest in samples from two loaders (0.11-3.7 µg/ml). These exceed the recommended threshold limit value established by the Finnish Institute of Occupational Health: i.e., 12 µmol/l, corresponding to 2.8 µg/ml of tetrachlorophenol or 3.2 µg/ml of pentachlorophenol. The chlorophenol concentrations in urine samples from other workers in these mills were much lower.

Levin (unpublished data) has studied the levels of PCP in the urine of Swedish workers exposed in a variety of occupational settings (Table 12). The low values observed for saw-mill workers reflect the fact that chlorophenols are no longer allowed to be used as fungicides in sawmills in Sweden. The workers are exposed only by contact with imported lumber that has been treated with chlorophenols before export to Sweden.

Arsenault (1976) reported the results of analyses of workers occupationally exposed to PCP: concentrations ranged from 0.05-0.34 µg/ml. The author considered that these values fall well within the range found for non-occupationally exposed people, 0.003-1.84 µg/ml. Another series of investigations showed that contamination of the general population with PCP at levels of 0.01-0.02 µg/ml (in urine, blood and adipose tissue) is quite general in industrialized societies (see also Dougherty, 1978).

Wyllie et al. (1975) studied the levels of PCP in blood and urine from workers employed in a small wood-treatment plant (Table 13) and found good agreement between serum and urine values. Contrary to the results of Arsenault, they found high levels in a pressure treater and in a welder-labourer. In rare phases of work (handling and destruction

Table 10. Concentrations of chlorophenates in the air at 10 Finnish sawmills[a]

Phase of work or place (no. of measurements)	Range (mg/m^3)	Median value (mg/m^3)	Mean value (mg/m^3)	Remarks
Preparation of treatment solution (N=6)	0.005-0.21	0.033	0.066	Duration, 2-12 min; sporadic exposure
Work places near dipping basin (N=5)	0.012-0.17	0.019	0.064	Depending on location of basin, air movement, etc.
On loading-bridge above dipping trough (N=14)	0.003-0.15	0.030	0.055	Depending on air movements, board jams, etc.
Inside kiln during drying (N=10)	0.10-17.4	3.35	5.83	Depending on phase of drying, dimensions of boards, etc.; sporadic exposure
During stacking (N=7)	0.033-0.12	0.076	0.075	Depending on dripping time of boards
Work places in the trimming-grading plant (N=18)	0.001-0.010	0.005	0.004	Attached to wood dust

Other phases of work or places:

Spray chamber method

- inside the spraying room (N = 3)   0.19 - 0.36 mg/m^3

- nearest work places   0.057 and 0.095 mg/m^3

Spraying in bundles

- near the spraying place (N=3)   0.007-0.045 mg/m^3

- nearest work places   0.007 and 0.019 mg/m^3

- spraying-machine operator   0.045 mg/m^3

Kiln

- inside the kiln when not in operation (N=4)   0.018-0.75 mg/m^3

- at cooling place of dried bundles (N=3)   0.019-0.049 mg/m^3

Longitudinal packaging plant

- handling of boards   0.004 mg/m^3 (attached to wood dust)

[a]From Kauppinen et al. (unpublished data)

Table 11. Concentrations of chlorophenols in urine samples taken from
workers at 10 Finnish sawmills[a]

Type of work (no. of measurements)	Range (µg/ml)	Median value (µg/ml)	Mean value (µg/ml)	Remarks
Preparing treament solution (N=7)	0.01-0.18	0.11	0.11	Sporadic exposure
Work near dipping basin (motor truck drivers, loaders) (N=8)	0.01-0.07	0.03	0.04	Depending on air movement, dripping system, road-dust in air
Loading (directly after trough dipping) (N=26)	0.11-3.7	0.46	0.73	Depending on protective clothing and condition of skin of hands
Kiln operators (N=7)	0.01-0.13	0.03	0.05	Sporadic exposure to high concentrations possible
Stackers and assistant stackers (N=10)	0.01-0.15	0.07	0.07	Depending on dripping time of boards
Workers at trimming-grading plant (N=13)	0.005-0.15	0.03	0.04	Chlorophenates attached to wood dust

[a]From Kauppinen et al. (unpublished data)

Table 12. Levels of pentachlorophenol in the urine of workers
exposed in various occupational settings[a]

Occupation	Range (µg/ml)	Mean (µg/ml)	Number of workers
Sawmill workers	0.03-0.50	0.20	22
Cable factory workers	0.02-0.04	0.03	5
Leather workers	0.10-10.5	2.7	20
Textile workers (impregnation of fabrics)	0.01-0.80	0.30	15
Seamstresses	0.01-0.35	0.20	20
Seamstresses (unexposed)	0.01-0.05	0.02	38

[a]From Levin (unpublished data)

Table 13. Pentachlorophenol (PCP) residues in serum, whole blood and
urine (5 samples of each) from workers in a PCP treatment plant[a]

Occupation	Exposure (years)	Serum		Urine	
		Range (µg/ml)	Mean (µg/ml)	Range (µg/ml)	Mean (µg/ml)
Officer manager	10	0.42-0.75	0.64	0.04-0.11	0.06
Outside loader	2	0.35-1.63	0.83	0.11-0.16	0.13
Welder-labourer	2[b]	1.24-3.96	1.96	0.08-0.26	0.17
Pressure treater	5	1.51-3.55	2.30	0.09-0.76	0.30
Owner	11	0.69-3.00	1.50	0.11-0.47	0.24
Outside labourer	2	0.41-2.01	1.00	0.04-0.15	0.07
Chemist (control)	-	0.04-0.07	0.05	0.003-0.004	0.003

[a] From Wyllie *et al.* (1975)

[b] Plus 6 summers

of sludge from the dipping basin, welding of chlorophenate-contaminated surfaces), workers may have some exposure to chlorinated phenoxyphenol compounds and to PCDDs and PCDFs. These compounds may occur as impurities in the technical chlorophenates or they may be formed by the heating of chlorophenates. However, exposure to these impurities was not measured.

Lamberton *et al.* (1979) found a 34% increase in octa-CDDs when analysing a recirculating PCP solution from a pressure process. The octa-CDD level in the sludge was 90% higher than in the fresh solution and 42% higher than in the recirculating PCP solution.

Levin *et al.* (1976) also analysed the concentrations of chlorophenates, chlorophenoxyphenols and PCDFs during different phases of work in two trimming-grading plants. One of the plants used a dipping and the other a spraying method. The results are presented in Table 14. In the plant using the spraying method, PCDFs were concentrated to some extent in the wood dust; no increase in PCDFs was found in dust in the plant where the dipping method was used, but the sludge of the dipping basin contained 0.0007%. The sawdust concentrations in the plant were, on the average, 1.5-2.0 mg/m^3 and the chlorophenate concentrations, 0.00003 - 0.0016 mg/m^3.

Table 14. Chlorinated contaminants (ppm) in sawdust from 2 trimming-grading plants[a]

Position	Tetrachlorophenol (μg/g)	Chlorophenoxyphenols (μg/g)	Chlorodibenzofurans (μg/g)
Sawmill A, spraying method			
Trimming	300	30	6
Grading	100	10	3
Packaging	70	10	1
Sawmill B, dipping method			
Trimming	450	13	<0.5
Grading	50	8	<0.5
Packaging	125	15	<0.5

[a]From Levin *et al.* 1976)

The degradation of chlorophenols in wood dust depends on environmental factors like temperature and ultra-violet irradiation. The major elimination pathways are vaporization and photochemical degradation. When the chlorophenols have effectively penetrated wood, however, they may persist for years.

Another risk is associated with the burning of wood, wood shavings or wood dust containing chlorophenols, since this can release chlorinated dioxins into the air (Rappe *et al.*, 1978a) (see p. 70   ).

Other antistain agents have also been used, but up until recent years, to only a limited extent. In Sweden, where chlorophenates have been banned, other compounds, including Benomyl[®] (a benzimidazole derivative), sodium and potassium difluorides and guazatine [*N,N*-(iminodi-8,1-octanediyl)bis-guanidine], are used (Rappe & Levin, 1976). In Finland, ziram (zinc dimethyldithiocarbamate), thiophenates, difluorides and Benomyl[®] are used, besides chlorophenates. Exposure to these substances can occur, in principle, in the same phases of work as when chlorophenates are used, since the methods of surface treatment are almost the same. No reports on measurements of exposure to these substances were available to the Working Group.

(c)   Sawing vapours

The composition of such vapours varies according to the type of wood being sawn and depends on what volatile extractives are present.

Levin (1978) measured the exposure of sawmill workers in seven sawmills to substances that are vaporized from pine during sawing or chipping. A total of 77 samples were taken from the breathing zone with activated carbon tubes, and analysis was carried out with gas chromatography and gas chromatography-mass spectrometry. Sawing vapours from pine were found to consist of the following terpene compounds: α-pinene, β-pinene and △-carene, in an average ratio of about 10:1:5. Small amounts of other monoterpenes and some aromatic alkyl compounds were also found. Exposure to such vapours occurs mainly during sawing (presawing and sawing into parts), edging, trimming and handling wood chips. The concentrations of α-pinene and △-carene are presented in Tables 15 and 16. The concentrations were about the same for water-stored and land-stored pine. Total concentrations were usually 100-400 mg/m^3; sawyers and edgers were exposed to concentrations of 200-300 mg/m^3. In many of the sawmills, the highest concentrations were measured during chipping, because considerable amounts of terpenes may be released from fresh chips.

(d)   Wood preservatives (See also pp. 63-76).

Wood preservatives fall into two general classes: oils, such as creosote and petroleum solutions of PCP, and water-borne salts that are applied as aqueous solutions.

Preservative oils

Such compounds are used to protect wood from weathering outdoors. One drawback to their use is that they may travel from, e.g., treated studs or subflooring, along nails and discolour adjacent plaster or floorboards.

Coal-tar creosote, made by distilling tar, is one of the oldest wood preservatives. It is relatively insoluble in water and has low volatility, so that it persists for a long time after application. The composition of creosotes varies according to the method of distillation and the temperature range in which the creosote fraction is collected. Special creosotes are available for non-pressure treatments. They differ from ordinary commercial coal-tar creosote in (1) being crystal-free to flow freely at ordinary temperatures and (2) having low-boiling distillation fractions removed to reduce evaporation in thermal (hot-and-cold) treatments in open tanks (US Forest Products Laboratory, 1974). Freshly creosoted timber can be ignited easily and will burn readily, producing a dense smoke, until, after a few months, the more volatile parts of the oil disappear from near the surface.

Other creosotes, distilled from tars other than coal, are used to some extent in wood preservation. These include wood-tar creosote, oil-tar creosote and water-gas-tar creosote.

Coal-tars are seldom used alone for preserving wood because good penetration is usually difficult to obtain.

Table 15. Concentrations of α-pinene in different phases of work after sawing[a]

| | Concentration of α-pinene (mg/m^3) | | | |
	Sawing	Edging	Pre-trimming	Chipper
Water-stored pine	178	control room	116	217
	141	41	-	175
	97	control room	45	131
	145	168	46	71
	91	84	73	90
Land-stored pine	109	199	79	91
	-	92	-	-
	183	137	102	85
	52[b]	36[b]	81	119

[a]From Levin (1978)
[b]Partially ventilated control room

Table 16. Concentrations of $\triangle$-carene in different phases of work after sawing[a]

| | Concentration of $\triangle$-carene (mg/m^3) | | | |
	Sawing	Edging	Pre-trimming	Chipper
Water-stored pine	161	control room	104	198
	126	38	-	162
	69	control room	32	91
	64	78	26	33
	38	33	29	44
Land-stored pine	56	101	42	49
	-	33	-	-
	79	59	45	37
	32[b]	21[b]	51	72

[a]From Levin (1978)
[b]Partially ventilated control room

Creosote solutions consist of a mixture of either coal-tar or petroleum oil with coal-tar creosote, in various proportions. They have been used particularly for cross-ties. Most creosote solutions contain from 50-80% coal-tar distillate. Compared with creosote itself, the solutions may have a greater tendency to accumulate on the surface of the treated wood (bleed).

Pentachlorophenol solutions are discussed in detail under 'Antistain agents', above. The performance of PCP and the properties of the treated wood are influenced by the properties of the solvent used. A heavy petroleum solvent is used for maximum protection, particularly when the treated wood is to be in contact with the ground. Heavy oils enable the PCP to remain in the wood for a long time. Volatile solvents, such as liquified petroleum gas and dichloromethane, are used when the natural appearance of the wood must be retained or the treated wood is to be painted or otherwise finished. A 'bloom' preventive, such as ester gum or oil-soluble glycol, is generally required with volatile solvents to prevent crystals of PCP from forming on the surface of the wood. Although PCP has similar preservative properties to creosote, it is ineffective against marine borers and cannot be used for the treatment of marine piling or timbers used in coastal waters.

Water-repellent preservatives containing copper 8-hydroxyquinoline have been used in non-pressure treatment of wood containers, pallets and other products for use in contact with foods. Copper 8-hydroxyquinoline is also used in volatile solvents to pressure-treat lumber for decking of trucks and cars or for related uses involving harvesting, storage and transportation of foods.

Waterborne preservatives

These compounds are often used in combinations for special uses; dual treatment, with waterborne, copper-containing salt preservatives followed by coal-tar creosote, is highly effective in protecting wood against all types of marine borers.

Acid copper chromate [VI] (Celcure) contains (US Federal Supply Service, 1974a) 31.8% copper oxide and 68.2% chromium [VI] trioxide. Equivalent amounts of copper sulphate, potassium dichromate or sodium dichromate may be used in place of copper oxide.

Ammoniacal copper arsenite (Chemonite) contains (US Federal Supply Service, 1974b) approximately 49.8% copper oxide, or an equivalent amount of copper hydroxide, 50.2% arsenic pentoxide, or an equivalent amount of arsenic trioxide, and 1.7% acetic acid.

Chromated copper arsenate (CCA) is available in three types (US Federal Supply Service, 1974c), with the following compositions (parts by weight):

	Type I	Type II	Type III
Chromium trioxide	61	35.3	47
Copper oxide	17	19.6	19
Arsenic pentoxide	22	45.1	34

These types permit substitution of potassium or sodium dichromate for chromium trioxide; of copper sulphate, basic copper carbonate or copper hydroxide for copper oxide; and of arsenic acid or sodium arsenate for arsenic pentoxide. Type I (Erdalith, Greensalt, Tanalith, CCA) is used widely in the US on poles, posts and stakes. Type II (Boliden K-33) has been used commercially in Sweden since 1950 and is now used throughout the world; commercial use in the US started in 1964. Type III (Wolman CCA) is a composition arrived at by technical committees of the American Wood-Preservers' Association in encouraging a single standard for chromated copper arsenate preservatives. Commercial preparations of similar composition have been tested and used in the UK since 1954 and more recently in Australia, New Zealand, Malaysia, and in various countries of Africa and central Europe (US Forest Products Laboratory, 1974).

Chromated zinc chloride was developed in about 1934. US Federal Specification TT-W-551 requires that it contain 80% zinc oxide and 20% chromium trioxide; zinc chloride may be substituted for the zinc oxide and sodium dichromate for the chromium trioxide. Its principal advantages are its low cost and ease of handling at treating plants.

Fluor chrome arsenate phenol (FCAP) is covered by US Federal Specification TT-W-535, whereby it contains 22% fluoride, 37% chromium trioxide, 25% arsenic pentoxide and 16% dinitrophenol. Sodium pentachlorophenate is substituted in equal amounts for dinitrophenol when the compound is to be used on building materials, to avoid staining. Sodium or potassium fluoride may be used as the source of fluoride; sodium chromate or dichromate may be used in place of chromium trioxide; and sodium arsenate may be used in place of arsenic pentoxide.

Application methods

Wood-preserving methods are of two general types: (1) pressure processes, in which the wood is impregnated in closed vessels under pressures considerably above atmospheric, and (2) non-pressure processes, which vary widely as to procedures and equipment used.

In commercial practice, wood is most often treated by pressure processes. The wood, on cars, is run into a long steel cylinder, which is then closed and filled with preservative. Pressure forces preservative into the wood until the desired amount has been absorbed.

Non-pressure methods are used when more thorough methods are either impractical or unavailable or when exposure conditions are such that little preservative protection is required. The simplest treatment is to apply the preservative - creosote or other oils - with a brush or a spray nozzle. Cold-soaking well-seasoned wood for several hours or days in low-viscosity preservative oils, or steeping green or seasoned wood for several days in waterborne preservatives is sometimes used on fenceposts, lumber and timbers. The latter method has been used for many years in Europe.

In the hot-and-cold bath (referred to commercially as thermal treatment), with coal-tar creosote or pentachlorophenol in heavy petroleum oil, the wood is heated in the preservative in an open tank for several hours, then quickly submerged in cold preservative and allowed to remain for several hours. With coal-tar creosote, hot-bath temperatures up to 113°C may be employed, but usually a temperature of 99-104°C is sufficient. The immersion time in the baths depends on the ease with which the timber takes treatment: with well-seasoned timber, a hot bath of 2-3 hours is adequate, but much longer periods are required for resistant woods.

Another process is to subject timber to a low initial vacuum, immerse it briefly in preservative, then subject it to a high final or recovery vacuum. A number of other non-pressure methods have been used to a limited extent. Several of these involve the application of waterborne preservatives to living trees. The Boucherie process for the treatment of green, unpeeled poles has been used for many years in Europe. The process involves attaching impermeable caps to the butt ends of the poles and then forcing in a water-borne preservative through a pipeline or hose under hydrostatic pressure. A simple adaptation of this process is to fasten tightly around the butt end of the post a section of used inner tube to make a bag that holds a solution of preservative.

Mixtures of CCA salts are being used to an increasing extent as long-term wood preservatives, in a pressure treatment process generally carried out in a facility separate from sawmills. Worker exposure to Cr[VI] and As[V] could conceivably occur in such a facility. However, no exposure data on this or other processes were available to the Working Group. (A partial list of active fungicidal and insecticidal products used, with their method of application, is given on pp. 104-105.)

2.4 Biological factors

Logs and sawn timber may contain moulds, rotting fungi, bluestaining fungi and bacteria. Damp wood can support a wide variety of fungal growths; in fresh wood, sapstain is the first defect that may occur, as Ascomycetes and Fungi Imperfecti develop in the residual moisture of the tree. Most bluestaining appears to be caused by Ascomycetes of the genus *Ceratocystis (Ceratostomella)*; however, a number of Fungi Imperfecti also cause

staining of coniferous wood, the most important being *Aureobasidium (Pullularia) pullulans,*
Hormiscium gelatinosum, Cladosporium herbarum, Cadophora fastigiata, Diplodia spp. and
Graphium spp. Sapstain in Scots pine, European redwood or spruce appears to be due to
Ceratocystis pilifera, C. coerulescens, C. piceae and *Aureobasidium pullulans.* Sapstain is
almost invariably associated with superficial discolouration caused by moulds which form
greenish or black, occasionally yellow, powdery growths. A very wide range of species
can develop in this way on damp surfaces of wood, including common genera such as
Penicillium, Aspergillus and *Trichoderma.*

Belin (1978) has analysed moulds in Swedish sawmills and found that the respirable
dust in trimming-grading plants contained moulds of the genera *Rhizopus, Paecilomyces*
and *Mucor.* Some unidentified yeasts were also present.

In Sweden, allergic alveolitis among sawmill workers has occurred mostly in trimming-
grading plants. The increased presence of fungal spores in such areas is suspected to be due
to:

-   the use of more kiln drying (the high temperature and moisture found in kilns are
    favourable conditions for many moulds);
-   the fact that timber is now stored in sawmills for longer periods than before;
-   trimming-grading plants are heated and often have poor ventilation; and
-   there are now better methods for detecting moulds (Belin, 1978).

In one sawmill in Finland, *Paecilomyces, Penicillium, Rhizopus, Aureobasidium* and
Aspergillus moulds and some Actinomycetes and yeasts were found, using a simple Petri dish
method (Haahtela *et al.,* 1979).

The ambient air in the working environment of one allergic alveolitis patient was
analysed using an Andersen-sampler and found to contain a considerable number of spores,
both of fungi and Actinomycetes (Table 17). The most common fungal genus was
Aspergillus; Thermoactinomyces vulgaris predominated among the actinomycetal flora
(Terho *et al.,* 1979).

Lacey (1973) reported finding both cork particles and fungal spores in the air of a
'natural' cork factory in Portugal. In areas where cork was being handled and shaped, fungal
spores were usually more common than cork particles. The most abundant species were
Penicillium frequentans Westling, *P. granulatum* Bain., *Aphanocladium album* (Preuss) W.
Gams, *Monilia sitophila* (Mont.) Sacc. and *Mucor plumbeus* Bon. In a warehouse in which
cork had become mouldy, up to 54×10^6 spores/m^3 were detected, but workers handling
the mouldy cork were exposed to as many as 128×10^6 spores/m^3. Cork particles were
most abundant close to cutting and sanding machines, but their concentration seldom
exceeded 2×10^6 particles/m^3 air.

Table 17. Concentrations of spores in workroom air in one
Finnish trimming-grading plant[a]

Genus or group	Grading lockers		Trimming-grading plane	
	no./m^3	%	no./m^3	%
Moulds and yeasts				
Aspergillus	1800	60	1150	50
Aureobasidium	150	5	230	10
Mucor	150	5	115	5
Paecilomyces	600	20	460	20
Penicillium	-	-	115	5
Other fungi	150	5	115	5
Yeasts	150	5	115	5
Total	**3000**	**100**	**2300**	**100**
Actinomycetes				
Thermoactinomyces vulgaris	1200	80	560	70
Other Actinomycetes	300	20	240	30
Total	**1500**	**100**	**800**	**100**

[a]From Terho *et al*. (1979)

2.5 Current regulations and recommendations on exposures

(a) Wood dust and chemicals

See 'General Remarks on Wood, Leather and Some Associated Industries', p. 23.

(b) Sawing vapours

The major terpenes found in sawing vapours are nearly the same as those in turpentine, and the TLV of 'turpentine' or 'turpentine oil' is often applied to sawing vapours. In 1979, the TLV of turpentine was 560 mg/m^3 (100 ppm) in the US (American Conference of Governmental Industrial Hygienists, 1979), Finland (Sosiaali- Ja Terveysministeriö, 1975) and in many other countries (International Labour Office, 1977). In 1978, the TLV in Sweden was 450 mg/m^3 (80 ppm) (Arbetarskyddsstyrelsen, 1978); and that in the USSR

(Kettner, 1979) and in some other eastern European countries (International Labour Office, 1977) was 300 mg/m^3. In some countries the remark 'sensitizing' is added to the TLV.

2.6 Number of workers involved

See 'General Remarks on Wood, Leather and Some Associated Industries', p. 19.

3. TOXIC, INFLAMMATORY AND ALLERGIC EFFECTS IN HUMANS

Toxic effects attributed to a particular wood are described below in relation to the occupation with which they have been associated most frequently or most conspicuously. However, it may be expected that whenever the same type of wood is used in other occupations, similar adverse effects could occur.

3.1 Respiratory diseases (other than cancer)

In Europe, pulmonary diseases due to dusts are usually referred to as 'allergic alveolitis'; in the US, they are generally designated 'hypersensitivity pneumonitis'. A large number of descriptive terms has been developed; however, these only indicate different occupational situations in which more or less the same type of reaction has occurred. Such occupations are those in agriculture and in the wood and forest industries.

Respiratory disorders that have been attributed to wood dust are suberosis, sequoiosis and maple-bark disease. Combined type I, III and IV allergic reactions are thought to be the immunomechanism, and the inflammatory reaction is to a certain extent a result of complement activation (Gell & Coombs, 1963).

Suberosis is a form of pneumoconiosis that affects cork workers. It starts as a mild acute affliction; however, after 10-15 years' exposure to concentrations of cork dust (ranging in a Portuguese cork factory from 165-1260 particles/cm^3) it progresses to a chronic form characterized by bronchitis and emphysema, accompanied by changes in pulmonary function. Some degree of pulmonary impairment appears to be universal if exposure is sufficiently long (De Carbalho Cancella, 1963; Avila, 1972).

Sequoiosis is a chronic interstitital pneumonitis resulting from inhalation of redwood sawdust containing fungal particles. It appears to be related to 'farmer's lung' disease, an acute or chronic inflammatory reaction in the lungs caused by hypersensitivity to the thermophilic Actinomycetes in mouldy hay or grain or other organic dusts. Anti-redwood precipitins have been demonstrated in cases of sequoiosis (Cohen et al., 1967).

In Sweden, allergic alveolitis among sawmill workers has occurred mostly in trimming-grading plants and has been related to an increase in fungal spores. A survey of 17 sawmills revealed a 10-20% prevalence of repeated acute allergic alveolitis in more than half of the wood trimmers. Evidence of immunostimulating mould exposure was found in more than 50% of the workers, as evaluated by the occurrence of precipitating and complement activating antibodies in the serum (Belin, 1978, 1980; Wimander & Belin, 1980).

Allergic alveolitis has also been reported in relation to exposure to wood chips; the diagnosis was established by the demonstration of precipitation antibodies to various moulds, mainly *Aspergillus fumigatus* (Terho *et al.*, 1979). These authors sampled and analysed the ambient air of the working environment of one allergic alveolitis patient. On the basis of microbiological and serological data, it was concluded that the causative agent(s) of the disease in this case were either *Thermoactinomyces vulgaris* or species of the genus *Aspergillus* (see Table 17 and p. 82).

Marple-bark disease is a granulomatous lesion of the lung induced by inhalation of spores of the fungus *Cryptostroma (Coniosporum) corticale* found in diseased maple trees. The lesion has been observed in workers in paper mills where logs are sawed or where there is manual peeling of the bark. Exposures are greatest in the winter months when work is enclosed and are related to very high spore counts, which may comprise 85% of the dust counts. Pulmonary effects are believed to be due to a combination of a foreign body reaction and a delayed effect resembling protein sensitization (Emanuel *et al.*, 1962, 1966).

3.2 Irritating effects

Irritant chemicals that cause dermatitis and conjunctivitis are found in the sap or latex of trees of certain families, such as Moraceae, Urticaceae, Euphorbiaceae and Apocynaceae (see also Table 18). Some trees (brigalow, tagayasan, araroba) contain irritating powders in the bark or in cracks in the wood (Woods & Calnan, 1976).

Biologically active substances have been detected in the bark of many trees (barberry, missahda, ironwood, sophora, laburnum, wenge, Knysna boxwood, opepe), exposure to which has been reported to be associated with the following symptoms: giddiness, drowsiness, visual disturbances, colic, muscle cramps and cardiac arrhythmias (Woods & Calnan, 1976).

3.3 Skin effects

The bark of many woods appears to contain skin sensitizers, which have been traced to liverworts and lichens. Sesquiterpene lactone has been identified as a strong allergen from liverworts (Mitchell & Chan-Yeung, 1974), which were found to be responsible for 2-4% of all contact dermatitis in the south-west of France (Le Coulant *et al.*, 1966).

Table 18. Principal toxic timbers[a]

Common name	Botanical name	Symptoms[b]	Active substances
Arbor vitae	*Thuja standishii*	M	Tropolones
Ayan	*Distemonanthus benthamianus*	D	Oxyayanins
Blackwood, African	*Dalbergia melanoxylon*	D	Dalbergiones
Boxwood, Knysna	*Gonioma kamassi*	M G	Yohimbine (quebra-chamine)
Cedar, Western red	*Thuja plicata*	(D) M	Tropolones
Cocobolo	*Dalbergia retusa* et spp.	D	Dalbergiones
Cocus	*Brya ebenus*	D	Quinones?
Dahoma	*Piptadeniastrum africanum*	M	?
Ebony	*Diospyros* spp.	D M	Quinones
Guarea	*Guarea thompsonii* et spp.	M	?
Ipé (lapacho)	*Tabebuia ipe* et spp.	D M G	Desoxylapachol
Iroko	*Chlorophora excelsa*	D (M)	Stilbene
Katon	*Sandoricum indicum*	M G	?
Mahogany, African	*Khaya ivorensis* et spp.	D (M)	Anthothecol
Mahogany, American	*Swietenia macrophylla* et spp.	D	?
Makorė	*Tieghemella heckelii*	D M	Saponin
Mansonia	*Mansonia altissima*	(D) M G	Mansonones (quinones), glycosides
Obeche	*Triplochiton scleroxylon*	(D) M	?
Opepe	*Nauclea trillesii*	D M	?
Peroba rosa	*Aspidosperma peroba*	D M G	Alkaloids
Peroba, white	*Paratecoma peroba*	D M	Desoxylapachol?
Ramin	*Gonystylus bancanus*	D	?
Rosewoods	*Dalbergia* spp., *Machaerum* spp.	D	Dalbergiones
Satinwood, Ceylon	*Chloroxylon swietenia*	D	Alkaloid, furocoumarins
Satinwood, West Indian and African	*Fagara flava* et spp.	D	Alkaloid (?), furocoumarins

Table 18 (contd)

Common name	Botanical name	Symptoms[b]	Active substances
Sequoia	*Sequoia sempervirens*	M G	?
Stavewood	*Dysoxylum muelleri*	M G	?
Teak	*Tectona grandis*	D	Desoxylapachol
Liverworts and lichens on bark	*Frullania*, etc.	D	Sesquiterpene lactones

[a]From Woods & Calnan (1976)

[b]D - dermatitis; M - mucosal irritation; G - general symptoms; parentheses indicate suspicion only

'Cedar'-poisoning, an ill-defined term given to certain skin reactions in British Columbia, Canada, was found in 21 out of 43 forest workers to be a manifestation of epidermal sensitization to lichen components. Eight out of the 21 showed positive patch tests to usnic acid and other chemicals derived from lichen (Mitchell, 1965).

4. CARCINOGENICITY DATA[1]

(a)   Nasal cancer

Ball (1967, 1968) found no increase in nasal cancer incidence among lumber workers, loggers or sawyers, i.e., 11 out of 28 among cases and 9 out of 24 among controls. (See also monograph on the furniture and cabinet-making industry, p. 128 .)

Mosbech & Acheson (1971) reported a series of 7 cases of nasal cancer, one of which was in a sawyer. (See also monograph on the furniture and cabinet-making industry, p. 131 .)

Ironside & Matthews (1975) studied 99 cases of malignant tumours of the nose or paranasal sinuses indexed at the Cancer Institute of Victoria, Australia. Nineteen were adenocarcinomas, of which one occurred in a lumber worker and one in a sawmill proprietor. (See also monograph on carpentry and joinery, p. 151 .)

Brinton *et al*. (1977) studied 37 cases of nasal cancer in North Carolina, USA, ascertained through death certificates. They were compared with 73 controls matched for

---

[1] This section should be read in conjunction with Appendices 1 and 2, pp.295 and 301.

age at death, sex, race and county and year of death. Three of the cases (8%) and 3 of the controls (4%) had been lumber or sawmill workers (RR = 2). (See also monograph on the furniture and cabinet-making industry, p. 130 .)

Haguenauer *et al.* (1977) reported one case in a forestry worker and one in a sawmill worker among 30 cases of adenocarcinomas (and 2 cases of adenocarcinoma-reticulo-sarcoma) of the ethmoid sinus in woodworkers in a French clinical series.

Roush *et al.* (1980) identified 301 nasal cancer cases in the Connecticut, USA, Tumor Registry among males who died at the age of 35 or more years between 1935 and 1975 and compared their occupations with those of 857 randomly selected males who died at 35 or over during the same period. Eight cases (3%), including 2 lumber workers and 1 sawmill worker, and 7 controls (0.8%), including 4 lumber workers, were woodworkers. The odds ratio is 3.8 for woodworkers and 2.5 for sawmill and lumber workers.

(b)   Lung cancer

Blot & Fraumeni (1976) found that in US counties in which lumber industries were situated, there were lower lung cancer rates than expected. No data were given on smoking habits. (See also monograph on the pulp and paper industry, p. 191 .)

Occupational statements on the death certificates of 858 white male lung cancer cases from coastal Georgia (USA) counties were compared with those of 858 control records matched for sex, race, age at death (within 1 year), year of death (within 6 years) and county of residence. No increased risk of lung cancer was found in 'wood and paper' workers in the urban areas, but a relative risk of 3.3 was found for rural counties. The increased risk was greatest among sawmill, lumber and forestry workers. No data were given on smoking habits (Harrington *et al.*, 1978).

Milham (1974) studied 16,443 deaths that occurred in 1969-1970 among members of a large North American labour union (American Federation of Labor-Congress of Industrial Organizations, United Brotherhood of Carpenters and Joiners of America). The union has a death benefit plan which requires submission of a death certificate. Counts of membership by age, occupation, duration of membership, cause of death, residence and union local number were available. When age-specific mortality rates were computed, lumber workers, sawmill workers and millmen showed an age-adjusted lung cancer SMR of <80. No data were given on smoking habits.

(c)   Stomach cancer (see Appendix 1).

(d)   Haematopoietic and lymphoreticular cancer

The occupational statements on the death records of 1549 white males of 25 years or more who died in upstate New York between 1940-1953 or between 1957-1964 were compared with controls matched for age, sex, race, month of death and county of residence. Seventy cases of Hodgkin's disease occurred in woodworkers *versus* 31 in controls;   RR = 2.3. Specifically, there were 14 lumber workers and sawmill workers among the cases *versus* 5 in the control group; RR = 2.8 (Milham & Hesser, 1967).

In the paper by Milham (1974) (see above), lumber workers and sawmill workers showed a slightly increased SMR for leukaemia/lymphoma group cancers: SMR = 121 based on 27 deaths, as compared with low SMRs for all cancers and for lung cancer (<80). Millmen also showed a slight increase, with a SMR of 117 for leukaemia, based on 10 deaths, and a SMR of 159 for multiple myeloma, based on 4 deaths.

Of 123 cases of mixed-cell type Hodgkin's disease, 5.7% had worked in 'afforestation or lumbering' *versus* 2.4% of controls (RR = 2.3) (Abramson *et al.*, 1978). (See also monograph on carpentry and joinery, p. 153 .)

Three related Swedish studies (Eriksson *et al.*, 1979; Hardell, 1979; Hardell & Sandström, 1979) were designed to test the association between exposures to phenoxy herbicides and to chlorophenols and the development of soft-tissue sarcomas and histiocytic lymphomas. A 6.6-fold increased risk of these cancers was associated with chlorophenol exposures. Although no data are provided to assess risks by occupations, industrial hygiene surveys indicate that most chlorophenol use in Sweden occurs in the sawmill industry.

No data were available to the Working Group on the occurrence of cancer in workers in the cork industry.

5. SUMMARY OF DATA AND EVALUATION

5.1 Summary of data

Information on the occurrence of cancer in lumber and sawmill workers is limited, and there are no cohort or detailed case-control studies involving sizeable numbers of cases in these specific occupations. The available epidemiological data are primarily from surveys of statements of occupation on death certificates.

The possibility that an increased risk of nasal tumours may exist for lumber or sawmill workers was suggested by British occupational mortality statistics, and in two case-control series using death certificate data in the US. A study in Australia found a higher frequency of lumber and sawmill employees among patients with adenocarcinomas than among patients with other nasal cancers. Each of these studies was based on small numbers of cases (five or less) with lumber-sawmill jobs; in none were detailed occupational histories obtained and in none was employment classification verified, so that the possibility of employment in the furniture-making industry at some time could not be excluded.

Lung cancer mortality was found to be low among lumber and sawmill workers in statistics from the US and England & Wales. Similar results were found in a study of lumber and sawmill workers who were members of an American carpenters' union. A death certificate review showed a three-fold excess of lung cancer among lumber, sawmill and forestry employees in rural, but not urban, areas of coastal Georgia in the US. None of these surveys took smoking habits into consideration.

A nearly three-fold increased risk of Hodgkin's disease was found among lumber and sawmill workers in a case-control comparison of statements of occupation on death certificates from upstate New York. No overall increased risk of Hodgkin's disease among persons occupationally exposed to 'wood and trees' was reported in a case-control study in Israel; however, an increased risk for the mixed-cellularity type of Hodgkin's disease was reported for afforestation and lumber workers. Another review of death certificates for patients with Hodgkin's disease in the US showed a 40% excess risk for all woodworkers, including lumber-sawmill workers. A 20% elevated risk for all lymphproliferative and haematopoetic cancers combined was reported for lumber and sawmill workers who were members of the US carpenters' union. The mortality statistics for Washington state do not show elevated mortality ratios for Hodgkin's disease among sawyers or among miscellaneous woodworkers (including sawmill workers). In none of the above studies were more than 15 cases of Hodgkin's disease found among persons with lumber-sawmill jobs.

A suggestion of an increase in incidence of stomach cancer arises from the general trend of elevated mortality ratios for sawyers, lumbermen, loggers and related woodworking trades in the state and national occupational mortality series. The increases were in the order of 10-50%.

Increased risks of about six-fold of both histiocytic lymphomas and soft-tissue sarcomas associated with exposures to chlorophenols have been reported in Sweden. Although data relating risks to occupation were unavailable, most use of chlorophenols is in the sawmill industry.

The confusion between the two occupational groups - lumber and sawmill workers - might be a reason for the discrepancies among the epidemiological findings for different cancers in different countries at different times.

Definition of the occupational groups in the future should take into account that lumber and sawmill occupations are quite different from the point of view of exposure to dust and to chemicals. The description of the industrial processes given in the text shows that some of the chemicals used are those for which there is sufficient evidence of carcinogenicity in humans and/or in experimental animals (see Appendix 4). Some of these chemicals are no longer used; however, some are still in use.

5.2   Evaluation

The epidemiological data are not sufficient to make a definite assessment of the carcinogenic risks of employment in the lumber and sawmill industries. Some studies suggest that the incidences of nasal cancers and Hodgkin's disease may be increased. It is not known whether some nasal cancer patients described as working in lumber and sawmill industries may have worked in furniture manufacturing. The hypothesized link to Hodgkin's disease is not adequately supported. Soft-tissue sarcomas and histiocytic lymphomas have been reported following exposures to chlorophenols; although the risk to sawmill and lumber workers was not quantified directly, the use pattern of chlorophenols suggests that sawmill workers in this study were at increased risk for both of these malignancies. Stomach cancer is slightly elevated among these occupational groups in six mortality series; however, this might be related to nonoccupational factors.

6. REFERENCES

Abramson, J.H., Pridan, H., Sacks, M.I., Avitzour, M. & Peritz, E. (1978) A case-control study of Hodgkin's disease in Israel. *J. natl Cancer Inst., 61*, 307-314

American Conference of Governmental Industrial Hygienists (1979) *Threshold Limit Values for Chemical Substances in Workroom Air Adopted by ACGIH for 1979*, Cincinnati, OH, p. 30

Arbetarskyddsstyrelsen (1978) *Hygieniska gränsvärden [Hygienic Limit Values] (Arbetarskyddsstyrelsens Regulation no. 100)*, Stockholm, Liberförlag, p. 20

Arsenault, R.D. (1976) Pentachlorophenol and contained chlorinated dibenzodioxins in the environment. A study of environmental fate, stability, and significance when used in wood preservation. *Am. Wood-Preserv. Assoc., 72*, 122-148

Avila, R. (1972) Some aspects of suberosis: respiratory disease in cork workers. *Bronches, 22*, 121-128

Ball, M.J. (1967) Nasal cancer and occupation in Canada. *Lancet, ii*, 1089-1090

Ball, M.J. (1968) Nasal cancer in woodworkers. *Br. med. J., ii*, 253

Belin, L. (1978) Wood trimmers' disease - an allergic reaction to molds in Swedish sawmills (Abstract no. 106). *J. Allergy clin. Immunol., 61*, 160

Belin, L. (1980) Clinical and immunological data on 'wood trimmers' disease' in Sweden. *Eur. J. resp. Dis., 61 (Suppl. 107)*, 169

Blaser, W.W., Bredeweg, R.A., Shadoff, L.A. & Stehl, R.H. (1976) Determination of chlorinated dibenzo-*p*-dioxins in pentachlorophenol by gas chromatography-mass spectrometry. *Anal. Chem., 48*, 984-986

Blot, W.J. & Fraumeni, J.F., Jr (1976) Geographic patterns of lung cancer: industrial correlations. *Am. J. Epidemiol., 103*, 539-550

Brinton, L.A., Blot, W.J., Stone, B.J. & Fraumeni, J.F., Jr (1977) A death certificate analysis of nasal cancer among furniture workers in North Carolina. *Cancer Res., 37*, 3473-3474

Buser, H.R. (1976) Preparation of qualitative standard mixtures of polychlorinated dibenzo-*p*-dioxins and dibenzofurans by ultra-violet and γ-irradiation of the octachloro compounds. *J. Chromatogr., 129*, 303-307

Buser, H.R. (1978) *Polychlorinated Dibenzo-p-dioxins and Dibenzofurans: Formation, Occurrence and Analysis of Environmentally Hazardous Compounds*, Thesis, University of Umeå, Sweden

Buser, H.R. & Bosshardt, H.-P. (1976) Determination of polychlorinated dibenzo-*p*-dioxins and dibenzofurans in commercial pentachlorophenols by combined gas chromatography-mass spectrometry. *J. Assoc. off. anal. Chem., 59*, 562-569

Buser, H.R. & Rappe, C. (1978) Identification of substitution patterns in polychlorinated dibenzo-*p*-dioxins (PCDDs) by mass spectrometry. *Chemosphere, 7,* 199-211

Buser, H.R., Bosshardt, H.-P. & Rappe, C. (1978a) Identification of polychlorinated dibenzo-*p*-dioxin isomers found in fly ash. *Chemosphere, 7,* 165-172

Buser, H.R., Bosshardt, H.-P , Rappe, C. & Lindahl, R. (1978b) Identification of polychlorinated dibenzo-furan isomers in fly ash and PCB pyrolyses. *Chemosphere, 7,* 419-429

Cirelli, D.P. (1978) *Patterns of pentachlorophenol usage in the United States of America - an overview.* In: Ranga Rao, K., ed., *Pentachlorophenol, Chemistry, Pharmacology and Environmental Toxicology,* New York, Plenum, pp. 13-18

Cohen, H.I., Merigan, T.C., Kosek, J.C. & Eldridge, F. (1967) Sequoiosis: a granulomatous pneumonitis associated with red-wood sawdust inhalation. *Am. J. Med., 43,* 785-794

Crosby, D.G. & Wong, A.S. (1976) Photochemical generation of chlorinated dioxins. *Chemosphere, 5,* 327-332

De Carbalho Cancella, L. (1963) Suberosis: a pneumoconiosis due to cork dust. The present stage of the problem. *Ind. Med. Surg., 32,* 435-445

Dougherty, R.C. (1978) *Human exposure to pentachlorophenol.* In: Rao, K.R., ed., *Pentachlorophenol, Chemistry, Pharmacology and Environmental Toxicology,* New York, Plenum, pp. 351-361

Dow Chemicals (1978) *The Trace Chemistries of Fire*, Memo, November, Midland, MI

Emanuel, D.A., Lawton, B.R. & Wenzel, F.J. (1962) Maple-bark disease. Pneumonitis due to *Coniosporium corticale. New Engl. J. Med., 266,* 333-337

Emanuel, D.A., Wenzel, F.J. & Lawton, B.R. (1966) Pneumonitis due to *Cryptostroma corticale* (maple-bark disease). *New Engl. J. Med., 274,* 1413-1418

Eriksson, M., Berg, N.O., Hardell, L., Möller, T. & Axelson, O. (1979) Case-control study on malignant mesenchymal tumours of the soft tissues and exposure to chemical substances (Swed.). *Läkartidningen, 76,* 3872-3875

Firestone, D. (1977)   Determination of polychlorodibenzo-*p*-dioxins and polychlorodibenzofurans in commercial gelatins by gas-liquid chromatography. *J. Agric. Food Chem., 25,* 1274-1280

Firestone, D., Ress, J., Brown, N.L., Barron, R.P. & Damico, J.N. (1972) Determination of polychloro-dibenzo-*p*-dioxins and related compounds in commercial chlorophenols. *J. Assoc. off. anal. Chem., 55,* 85-92

Food & Agricultural Organization (1979) *Yearbook of Forest Products, 1977,* Rome

Gell, P.G. & Coombs, R.R. (1963) *Clinical Aspects of Immunology*, Oxford, Blackwell, p. 317

Haahtela, T., Riihimäki, M., Mönkàre, S., Vilkka, V. & Vaara, S. (1979)   Allergic alveolitis caused by mouldy wood dust (Finn.). *Duodecim, 95*, 851-854

Haguenauer, J.P., Romanet, P., Duclos, J.C. & Guinchard, R. (1977)   Occupational cancers of the ethmoid (Fr.). *Arch. Mal. prof., 38*, 819-823

Hardell, L. (1979)   Malignant lymphoma of histiocytic type and exposure to phenoxyacetic acids or chlorophenols. *Lancet, i*, 55-56

Hardell, L. & Sandstrom, A. (1979)   Case-control study: soft-tissue sarcomas and exposure to phenoxyacetic acids or chlorophenols. *Br. J. Cancer, 39*, 711-717

Harrington, J.M., Blot, W.J., Hoover, R.N., Housworth, W.J., Heath, C.A. & Fraumeni, J.F., Jr (1978)   Lung cancer in coastal Georgia: a death certificate analysis of occupation: brief communication. *J. natl Cancer Inst., 60*, 295-298

Hay, A. (1979)   Dispute over Dow Chemicals' theory of dioxin traces. *Nature, 251*, 619-620

Hoos, R.A.W. (1978)   *Patterns of pentachlorophenol usage in Canada - an overview.*   In: Rao, K.R., ed., *Pentachlorophenol, Chemistry, Pharmacology and Environmental Toxicology*, New York, Plenum, pp. 3-11

IARC (1978)   Long-Term Hazards of Polychlorinated Dibenzodioxins and Polychlorinated Dibenzofurans. *IARC intern. tech. Rep. No. 78/001*

IARC (1979)   *IARC Monographs on the Evaluation of the Carcinogenic Risk of Chemicals to Humans,* Vol. 20, *Some Halogenated Hydrocarbons,* Lyon, pp. 303-325, 349-367

International Labour Office (1976)   *Occupational Health and Safety,* Vol. 1, 5th ed., Geneva, pp. 335-336

International Labour Office (1977)   *Occupational Exposure Limits for Airborne Toxic Substances (Occupational Safety and Health Series No. 37)*, Geneva

Ironside, P. & Matthews, J. (1975)   Adenocarcinoma of the nose and paranasal sinuses in woodworkers in the State of Victoria, Australia. *Cancer, 36*, 1115-1121

Kauppinen, T., Lindroos, L. & Makinen, R. (1979)   *Wood dust in a sawmill in eastern Finland* (Swed.) (Abstract).   In: *28:e nordiska yrkeshygieniska möte i Sverige 22-24 okt 1979, Resumèer [28th Meeting of the Scandinavian Occupational Hygiene Group, 1979, Abstracts] Solna,* Arbetarskyddsstyrelsen,   pp. 8:21-8:22

Kettner, H. (1979)   Maximal concentrations in the work environment in 1978 - USSR. Basis of standardization (Ger.). *Staub-Reinhalt. Luft, 39*, 56-62

Lacey, J. (1973)   The air spora of a Portuguese cork factory. *Ann. occup. Hyg., 16*, 223-230

Lamberton, J., Griffin, D., Arbogast, B., Inman, R. & Deinzer, M. (1979)   The determination of polychlorodibenzo-*p*-dioxins in pentachlorophenol and wood treatment solutions. *Am. ind. Hyg. Assoc. J., 40*, 816-823

Le Coulant, P., Texier, L., Maleville, J., Geniaux, M., Tamisier, J.-M. & Bancons, F. (1966) *Frullaria* allergy: its role in 'oak wood dermatitis' (Fr.). *Bull. Soc. fr. Dermatol. Syphil., 73*, 440-443

Levin, J.-O. (1978) *Exposition för sågàngor. Identifiering odh kvantifiering av terpenkomponenter [Exposure to Sawing Vapours. Identification and Quantification of Terpene Components] (Undersöknings-rapport 1978:36)*, Stockholm, Arbetarskyddsstyrelesen

Levin, J.-O., Rappe, C. & Nilsson, C.-A. (1976) Use of chlorophenols as fungicides in sawmills. *Scand J. Work Environ. Health, 2*, 71-81

McConnell, E.E., Moore, J.A., Haseman, J.K. & Harris, M.W. (1978) The comparative toxicity of chlorinated dibenzo-*p*-dioxins in mice and guinea-pigs. *J. Toxicol. appl. Pharmacol., 44*, 335-356

McKenzie, W.M. (1967) *The basic wood cutting process.* In: Dost, W.A., ed., *Woodmachining Seminar, Proceedings,* Richmond, CA, University of California, Forest Products Laboratory, pp. 3-8

Milham, S., Jr (1974) *A Study of the Mortality Experience of the AFL-CIO United Brotherhood of Carpenters and Joiners of America, 1969-1970 (DHEW Publ. No. (NIOSH) 74-129),* Springfield, VA, National Technical Information Service

Milham, S., Jr & Hesser, J.E. (1967) Hodgkin's disease in woodworkers. *Lancet, ii,* 136-137

Mitchell, J.C. (1965) Allergy to lichens. *Arch. Dermatol., 92,* 142

Mitchell, J.C. & Chan-Yeung, M. (1974) Contact allergy from *Frullaria* and respiratory allergy from *Thuja. Can. med. Assoc. J., 16,* 653

Moore, J.A., McConnell, E.E., Dalgard, D.W. & Harris, M.W. (1979) Comparative toxicity of three halogenated dibenzofurans in guinea-pigs, mice and rhesus monkeys. *Ann. N.Y. Acad. Sci., 320,* 151-163

Mosbech, J. & Acheson, E.D. (1971) Nasal cancer in furniture-makers in Denmark. *Dan. med. Bull., 18,* 34-35

Nicholson, W.J. & Moore, J.A., eds (1979) Health Effects of Halogenated Aromatic Hydrocarbons. *Ann. N.Y. Acad. Sci., 320,* 1-730

Nilsson, C.-A., Andersson, K., Rappe, C. & Westermark, S.-O. (1974) Chromatographic evidence for the formation of chlorodioxins from chloro-2-phenoxyphenols. *J. Chromatogr., 96,* 137-147

Nilsson, C.-A., Norström, Å., Andersson, K. & Rappe, C. (1978) *Impurities in commercial products related to pentachlorophenol.* In: Rao, K.R., ed., *Pentachlorophenol, Chemistry, Pharmacology and Environmental Toxicology,* New York, Plenum, pp. 313-324

Olie, K., Vermeulen, P.L. & Hutzinger, O. (1977) Chlorinated-*p*-dioxins and chlorodibenzofurans are trace components of fly ash and flue gas of some municipal incinerators in The Netherlands. *Chemosphere, 8,* 455-459

Pfeiffer, C.D., Nestrick, T.J. & Kocher, C.W. (1978) Determination of chlorinated dibenzo-*p*-dioxins in purified pentachlorophenol by liquid chromatography. *Anal. Chem., 50,* 800-804

Poland, A. & Glover, E. (1973) Chlorinated dibenzo-*p*-dioxins: potent inducers of δ-aminolevulinic acid synthetase and aryl hydrocarbon hydroxylase. II. A study of the structure-activity relationship. *Mol. Pharmacol., 9*, 736-747

Poland, A., Greenlee, W.F. & Kende, A.S. (1979) Studies on the mechanism of action of the chlorinated dibenzo-*p*-dioxins and related compounds. *Ann. N.Y. Acad. Sci., 320*, 214-230

Ramel, C., ed. (1978) Chlorinated Phenoxy Acids and their Dioxins: Mode of Action, Health Risks and Environmental Effects. *Ecol. Bull. (Stockh.), 27*, 1-302

Rao, K.R., ed. (1978) *Pentachlorophenol, Chemistry, Pharmacology and Environmental Toxicology*, New York, Plenum

Rappe, C. & Levin, J.-O. (1976) *Kemiska Hälsorisker i Sågverksindustrin [Chemical Health Risks in the Sawmill Industry] (ASF - Project 74/102, Final Report)*, Umeå

Rappe, C. & Nilsson, C.-A. (1972) An artifact in the gas chromatographic determination of impurities in pentachlorophenol. *J. Chromatogr., 67*, 247-253

Rappe, C., Garå, A. & Buser, H.R. (1978a) Identification of polychlorinated dibenzofurans (PCDFs) in commercial chlorophenol formulations. *Chemosphere, 7*, 981-991

Rappe, C., Marklund, S., Buser, H.R. & Bosshardt, H.-P. (1978b) Formation of polychlorinated dibenzo-*p*-dioxins (PCDDs) and dibenzofurans (PCDFs) by burning or heating chlorophenates. *Chemosphere, 7*, 269-281

Reineke, L.H. (1966) *Wood Flour (Research Note FPL-0113, Jan.)*, Madison, WI, US Department of Agriculture, Forest Service, Forest Products Laboratory

Roush, G.C., Meigs, J.W., Kelly, J., Flannery, J.T. & Burdo, H. (1980) Sinonasal cancer and occupation: a case-control study. *Am. J. Epidemiol., 111*, 183-193

Smith, R.J. (1978) Dioxins have been present since the advent of fire, says Dow. *Science, 202*, 1166-1167

Söderqvist, A. & Ager, B. (1975) *The physical environment (Swed.)*. In: Ager, B. *et al.*, eds, *Arbetsmiljön i sågverk - en tvärvetenskaplig undersökning [Work Environment in the Sawmill - A Scientific Investigation] (Undersokningsrapport AM 101/75)*, Stockholm, Arbetarskyddsstyrelsen, pp. IV:29-IV:42

Sosiaali- Ja Tereveysministeriö (1975) *Työpaikan ilman epäpuhtauksien enimmäispitoisuudet [Maximal Values for Air Pollution in Work Places] (Teknilliset turvallisuusohjeet n:o 11)*, Helsinki, Tyoterveyslaitos, p. 26

Terho, E.O., Husman, K., Kotimaa, M. & Sjoblom, T. (1979) Extrinsic allergic alveolitis in a sawmill worker (Finn.). *Duodecim, 95*, 843-850

US Federal Supply Service (1974a) Wood preservatives: water-repellent. *Fed. Spec.,* TT-W-546

US Federal Supply Service (1974b) Wood preservatives. *Fed. Spec.,* TT-W-549

US Federal Supply Service (1974c) Wood preservatives. *Fed. Spec.,* TT-W-550

US Forest Products Laboratory (1974)   *Wood Handbook: Wood as an Engineering Material (Agriculture Handbook No. 72)*, Forest Service, US Department of Agriculture, Washington DC, US Government Printing Office

Villanueva, E., Burse, V.W. & Jennings, R.W. (1973) Chlorodibenzo-*p*-dioxin contamination of two commercially available pentachlorophenols. *J. agric. Food Chem., 21*, 739-740

Vorreiter, L. (1953) Fundamental properties of sawdust **(Ger.).**   *HolzZentralblatt, 79*, 1127-1128

Vorreiter, L. (1960) Wood flour, its properties, manufacture and uses (Ger.). *HolzZentralblatt, 86* 1734-1736, 1791-1794, 1828-1829

Wimander, K. & Belin, L. (1980) Recognition of allergic alveolitis in the trimming department of a Swedish sawmill. *Eur. J. resp. Dis., 61 (Suppl. 107),* 163

Woods, B. & Calnan, C.D. (1976) Toxic woods. *Br. J. Dermatol., 94 (Suppl. 13),* 1-97

Wyllie, J.A., Gabica, J., Benson, W.W. & Yoder, J. (1975) Exposure and contamination of the air and employees of a pentachlorophenol plant, Idaho - 1972. *Pestic. Monit. J., 9*, 150-153

THE FURNITURE AND CABINET-MAKING INDUSTRY

1. HISTORICAL OVERVIEW OF THE INDUSTRY

Wood is man's oldest and one of his most useful natural resources. It has been used from earliest times to fulfill many of his needs, including the fabrication of furniture and cabinets (a term used to describe all the varied pieces of furniture whose chief function is storage). The simple shape of these objects, and the trend to mechanization with the expansion of supply and demand are at the root of the changes in work methods in this industry.

During the Renaissance, the method of building furniture required the use of solid hardwood, in particular walnut, which is easily worked from an artistic point of view. In the 1700s, a surface made by moulding and glueing together many strips of wood, including softwoods, in double curves was prevalent.

In the 'cartellature' method, developed during the 1800s, a skeletal system was introduced into furniture, which was finished with softwood on the outside. During the first ten years of this century, furniture was characterized by straight lines and flat planes, by a framework constructed of softwood, by the disappearance of solid wood and by the introduction of exotic woods, panels and plywood.

Until the industrial revolution, most woodworking was done with hand tools. The mechanization of the furniture industry, and of woodworking in general, followed that of the metal industry and others: until a few decades ago, all the steps of fabrication were carried out by craftsmen and by hand, although a circular saw had been produced in The Netherlands as early as 1777, and a planing machine was patented in England at about the same time (Encyclopaedia Britannica Inc., 1964).

Mechanization in this area was most intense and extensive in the period around the First World War. In particular, machine tools (circular saws, bandsaws, planers, lathes) were developed which make possible a high percentage of 'work' and 'feed' because of the increased ease with which wood can be cut. Some of the results of this new situation are: an increase in work accidents, especially at advanced stages; an increase in noise; and an extraordinary increase in dust in the entire working environment. For several decades, and especially during the period immediately after the Second World War, such machines continued to be produced, used and kept running for many hours of the day with no system for extracting or precipitating the dust (Acheson *et al.*, 1968; Leroux-Robert, 1974); and the dust pollution already present in the furniture factories increased with the introduction of power-driven sanders at about that time. Especially during mass-production, such machines are often used by only one or a few workers. This situation continued during the 1960s, changing slowly and in different ways in different countries.

Other factors have contributed to the evolution of this industry: the use of preservatives, such as creosote, which dates back to the 1800s in the US and to the 1900s in Canada (Hoos, 1978); the more rational and intensive use of wood in terms of quality and quantity; after the Second World War, the massive use of exotic and precious woods, and, later on, of softwoods; from the 1940s, the use of synthetic resin glues (formaldehyde -urea, formalde-hyde-melamine, formaldehyde-resorcinol); greater access to power-driven tools, such as trimmers and edge-bonding machines, mortisers for making hollows, grooves and notches, tenoners for making joints. Over the last 10 or 20 years, the methods for carrying out the various stages of varnishing and finishing furniture have also changed considerably: during the 1930s the technique of spray varnishing was borrowed from the automobile industry; during the 1950s film varnishing was employed; more recently, electrostatic varnishing has been introduced.

The technological development of varnishes (first based on cellulose and then on polyester and polyurethane) and of other surface treatments, along with the equipment for applying them made it possible, in some cases, to automate the processes for finishing furniture surfaces.

However, in many areas, traditional methods are still used to carry out the individual phases of fabrication (production of panels, parts or accessories, varnishing, finishing, assembly). In such cases, the environmental health conditions cannot but vary and must be established for each individual production unit.

2. DESCRIPTION OF THE INDUSTRY

2.1 Processes used previously and changes over time

Until the 1930s and 1940s, the woods used most widely in the furniture industry were the hard and semi-hard woods that grow in Europe (birch, box, chestnut, cherry, beech, walnut, olive, pear, oak, bay, etc.). Subsquently, exotic woods began to be used more and more (sycamore, ebony, mahogany, Brazilian rosewood, pitch pine, teak, Western red cedar, cedar, Douglas fir, sequoia, avodire, ekki, iroko, makore, mansonia, obeche, ramin, etc.). The European woods that are still used are fir, larch, pine, sycamore, birch, box, beech, oak, ash and poplar; however, in general, solid wood is being replaced more and more by panels, plywood and veneer. With increased production and the introduction during the first decade of the 1900s of power-driven tools for sawing, planing and squaring, there was an increase in the dust pollution of working areas. The introduction of control devices came later: in European countries generally in the 1950s.

Sanders with orbital movements and a horizontal belt were introduced widely in the years preceding the Second World War; and these are one source of dust pollution that in most factories is not yet completely controlled, because of the diameters and physico-chemical characteristics of the dusts involved.

In order to preserve lumber and to make it more resistant to parasites and to atmospheric conditions, various materials have been used. At the beginning of the 1900s, coal-tar oil and creosote were employed. Since the 1930s, substances such as pentachlorophenol and its alkali salts, technical hexachlorocyclohexane, lindane, fluoro and arsenic compounds, copper sulphate, etc. have been used more often. The persistence of these compounds in treated wood varies. That of pentachlorophenol may vary from a few weeks to a few years, depending on conditions such as temperature, humidity, etc. (See also p. 76 .)

The various chemical techniques available in 1700 for preserving and bettering wood had been largely replaced by 1800 by the processes of staining with mineral salts (cobalt sulphate, ferrous sulphate, potassium hexacyanoferrate, etc.), natural organic stains and mordants. Synthetic colouring substances derived from coal-tar were first used over 60 years ago. Up to the 1930s, varnishes were made from a base of natural and solvent oils which had been known since ancient times.

Water-based fillers, which are now obsolete, were prepared from hydrated alumina, kaolin, talc, pipe-clay (loam or ball clay), magnesium carbonate, barium sulphate, zinc oxide, calcium phosphate, bone powder or powdered pumice. Other fillers are oil-based (from varnish), jelly-like (with strong glue) or alcohol-based.

Plasters and putties have become virtually superfluous with the use of power-buffers. Water-based plasters and putties were made with strong glue (extracted from skins and bones), with the addition of naphthol, benzaldehyde or eucalyptus oil. Fast colours were made by adding calcium carbonate, pipe-clay, casein, starch, dextrin and barium sulphate. Plasters and putties soluble in oil or varnish were made of zinc oxide, ochre-coloured kaolin, and at least 10% barium sulphate. To obtain putty, cooked linseed oil was added; to obtain plaster, oil, turpentine, petrol or other petroleum products were added. Hard and adhesive putties were made similarly, except that a flat varnish, diluted with turpentine and containing a certain quantity of white lead $[Pb(OH_2)(CO_3)_2]$, was used. Subsequently, cellulose plasters and putties were largely adopted, in which cellulose and nitrocellulose are mixed with ester gum, copal, maleic resins modified with rosin or alkyd resins containing zinc stearate; the solvents used were esters, ketones and higher alcohols. To this were added fillers (slate, talc), covering pigments [lithopone, barium sulphate, red lead (Pb_3O_4)] and supporting pigments (zinc oxide, white lead). Shellac, which was also used as a hard putty, is prepared by adding small quantities of other resins (dammar, rosin) or wax and colouring powders.

From 1930 on, the traditional glues were replaced by synthetic ones: urea-formalde-hyde resins, phenol-formaldehyde resins, melamine-formaldehyde resins, resorcinol-for-maldehyde resins and mixtures of these. Previously, animal or strong glues were made by prolonged boiling of animal tissues (hide scraps, cartilage, tendons, bones); vegetable glues were made from wheat flour, potato starch, cassava flour or soya beans; other glues were made of dried blood, egg white, casein or sodium silicate.

The use of chromic mordants (potassium dichromate, sodium dichromate, chromium fluoride, chromic acid anhydride, chromium aluminium sulphate) and mordants based on tannins has decreased over the past 40 years.

Since the 1940s, the natural organic colouring substances (logwood, turmeric, 'herba guada', 'fustello giovane', natural indigo, yellow wood, red wood, 'orcanetto', oriana, 'orchil', 'guercitrone' and cochineal) have been used less and less. Many of the synthetic stains (and in particular those based on aniline) introduced during the first part of this century have been substituted by others.

By the Second World War, the nitrocellulose varnishes, and later those with a synthetic resin base, had already superseded the natural resin varnishes (shellac, copal, rosin, dammar, elemi, sandarac, acaroid, benzoin) and the modified or hardened natural resins (metallic and esterified). Also now of secondary importance are varnish thinners such as mineral turpentine, kerosene, pine oils, butyl alcohol, naphtha, benzene and paraffin oil, which occurred almost invariably in devarnishing products.

2.2 Processes used currently

The sequence of industrial furniture production in recent years can be broken down into the following phases:

(a) Wood preservation
(b) Sawing
(c) Seasoning and artificial drying
(d) Veneering
(e) Panel-making
(f) Mechanical work
(g) Sanding
(h) Plastering, puttying and insulating
(i) Degreasing
(j) Bleaching
(k) Staining
(l) Buffing or varnishing and sanding
(m) Assembling and finishing

In practice, it is very rare that the entire sequence is carried out in a single workshop, although it is more frequent in the US, Canada and the Scandinavian countries. In Mediterranean countries, it is more common that one factory carries out phases *(a)* to *(e)* and another phases *(f)* to *(m)*; and many factories in that area work on only one phase - *(b)*, *(e)* or *(I)*, and, less commonly, phases *(f)* or *(g)*.

Many workshops (in Italy and Spain, for example) produce traditional furniture or furniture that resembles antiques; these work places are characterized by the use of a large number of manual operations.

(a) Wood preservation (See also p. 77.)

Wood may undergo a preservation treatment, depending on the species being used or on the particular use forseen. Logs and sawn wood can be preserved in two ways; physically (by drying) or chemically (Table 1). Chemical protection can be applied by brush, spraying (in tunnels), dipping, osmosis, injection, under pressure or in retorts. Occupational risks may result either from the techniques employed or from the nature of the chemical substances used.

Commercial wood preservatives contain:
- diluting agents (benzene, ketones, fuel oil, anthracene oil, aliphatic hydrocarbons, aromatic hydrocarbons, halogenated hydrocarbons, polyglycols)
- 'fixative' agents (dehydroabietylamine, linseed oil)
- water-repellent agents (paraffins, abietic resins, chlorinated resins, coumarin resins, epoxy resins, glycerophthalic or alkyd resins)
- dispersing agents, wetting agents.

Salts of chlorophenols are used as fungicides (See p. 63.), and are applied as aqueous solutions containing approximately 1% of the potassium or sodium salt; however, fungicides are rarely used in furniture making. The textile industry uses pentachlorophenol, sodium pentachlorophenol or pentachlorophenol laurate to protect canvas and other textiles for outdoor use, as well as on rope binder twine and cable covering for protection against mildew. Most of these outdoor textiles are used in the furniture industry.

(b) Sawing

In some factories, wood is purchased as logs. Sawing is a highly mechanized phase, and the essential machinery consists of:
- a machine to even up the ends of the trunks: this is usually a very large chain saw;
- one or more saws to reduce the trunks to squared boards; and
- an end-trimmer and edge-trimming machine: this consists of a circular saw for levelling the rough lateral edges of the boards which come from the long saw.

Table 1. Partial list of active fungicidal and insecticidal products used alone or in commercial wood preservatives

Compound	Purpose	Mode of application
Arsenicals (alone or mixed)	insecticides	low-pressure injection, osmosis, by pressure
Borates, polyborates, boric acid (alone or mixed)	fungicides, insecticides, flame retardants	soaking, low-pressure injection, by pressure
Alkaline chromates and dichromates (alone or mixed)	fungicide, insecticide	soaking, low-pressure injection, by pressure
Copper sulphate	insecticide	low-pressure injection
Alkali fluorides, complex fluorides, fluorosilicates (alone or mixed)	insecticide	by brush, spraying, soaking
Mercury dichloride	fungicide, insecticide	soaking
Chlorinated cresols	fungicide	by brush, spraying, soaking
Dinitrophenols (in mixtures)	fungicide	by brush, spraying, soaking, injection under pressure
Alkali pentachlorophenates	fungicide, insecticide	by brush, spraying, soaking
Alkali phosphates (alone or mixed)	fungicide, insecticide, flame retardant	by brush, spraying, soaking
Zinc chloride	fungicide, insecticide	by brush, spraying, soaking
Aldrin (in mixtures)	insecticide	by brush, spraying, soaking
Phenol	fungicide, insecticide	by brush, soaking, under pressure, in retorts

Table 1 (contd)

Compound	Purpose	Mode of application
Chlorobenzenes (in mixtures)	insecticide	by brush, soaking
Creosote (from coal-tar)	fungicide	by brush, soaking, injection under pressure, retorts
DDT (in mixtures)	insecticide	by brush, spraying, soaking
Dieldrin (in mixtures)	insecticide	by brush, spraying, soaking
Hexachlorocyclohexane or lindane (in mixtures)	insecticide	by brush, spraying, soaking, injection under pressure

The main working risks are represented by sawdust and by saw flour, which is finer than sawdust .(See p. 59 .) In addition, the working environment is usually very noisy, and fires and explosions may occur, since the finer sawdust can explode in the presence of a spark. Traumas and injuries are frequent in this phase (International Labour Office, 1967). In addition, pyrolysis may take place during sawing; under these conditions, polynuclear aromatics like benzo[a]pyrene might be formed. However, no data were available concerning the nature of the pyrolysis products formed, although it is important that the hypothesis be substantiated.

(c) Veneering

In this phase, very thin sheets of wood, called veneers, are glued to supporting panels to make plywoods and products such as boxes, shelves, fancy goods, etc.

Veneers are now obtained by either slicing or peeling, using a blade and press-bar. In slicing, the log, after initial squaring, is held against a blade which is slightly longer than the log. In peeling, the log is rotated in claws while the blade moves horizontally against it; the setting of the blade governs the thickness of the veneer, while its width depends on the length of the log.

The main work risks in this phase are represented by dust (usually not abundant), by noise, by the energy sources, and by trauma and injury. In addition, during the veneering process, fumes may develop, especially from resinous and biologically active and irritating woods, which are for the most part the exotic ones. The preheating of the wood and the friction of the veneering blade produce a kind of distilled resin. The volatile fraction of this resin is released into the environment, while the remaining components are deposited on the wood surface, where they can be seen in the form of a whitish film.

(d) Seasoning and artificial drying

Natural seasoning is effected by stacking the cut wood in a well-ventilated area with 'stickers' between the boards so as to ensure proper aeration. This is a relatively long procedure (about three months) and cannot reduce the moisture content below 15-20%.

Artificial drying is more widespread, since the precentage of moisture is reduced below that of the open air within 5-10 days. Of the many processes available, the most prevalent is exposure to hot air in compartment kilns (static) or progressive kilns (in which stacks move progressively). The air in such drying areas may be polluted by toxic and irritating vapours from woods of resinous and exotic species.

The main working risks in this phase are represented by noise, adverse microclimate, energy sources and traumas.

(e) Panel-making

In comparison with boards, panels have greater surface area, less dimensional variation with moisture and a more homogeneous character. A wide range of adhesives is used in the bonding of man-made panels, depending on the characteristics required in the finished products (Table 2), although the most widely used are the synthetic resins. In some countries adhesives are heat-cured by high-frequency electric fields (Alberti, 1976).

(i) *Plywood*: Plywood has been made on an industrial scale since just before the Second World War. It is made up of relatively thin layers, or plies, in an odd number, glued together with the grains of adjacent layers at an angle of 90°. Special plywoods are made also, including one in which the inside is made up of wooden slats laid one beside another, and another in which the two external panels contain a hairline insulating space filled with a trellis work made up of either wood or plastic materials.

When the sheets have been dried in tunnels, a veneer spread with glue on both sides is inserted between two unglued sheets, and the panel is transferred into a hot press.

Phenol-resin adhesives are widely used to produce softwood plywood for severe service conditions; urea-resin adhesives, used extensively in producing hardwood plywood for furniture and interior panelling, are often fortified with melamine resin.

(ii) *Wood-base fibre and particle panel materials*: Chip, particle and shavings panel materials are all reconstituted wood, in that the wood (conifer, poplar and other softwoods) is first reduced to small fractions and then bonded together again with synthetic resins

Table 2. Composition of adhesives used in the furniture industry

Glue	Composition		Mode of application
Sodium silicate	dry matter: solvent:	sodium silicate water	cold, in aqueous solutions
Amylased glues	dry matter: solvent: bactericide: fluidifier:	starchy foodstuffs (manioc, potatoes, etc.), flours (wheat, maize, bean, vetch, etc.) water chlorocresol sodium hydroxide	cold, in aqueous solution
Vegetable glues	dry matter: solvent: adjuvants: antiseptics:	soya flour water sodium hydroxide, lime, sodium silicate pentachlorophenol, *ortho-*phenylphenol	hot or cold, in aqueous solution
Gelatine glues	dry matter: solvent: bactericides: adjuvants:	gelatine water sodium trichlorophenates, formaldehyde tannins, aluminium sulphate, alkali dichromates	cold, in aqueous solution
Blood glues	dry matter: solvent: solubilizer: bactericide:	powdered blood water lime, sodium or ammonium hydroxide formaldehyde	hot or cold, in aqueous solution
Fish glues	dry matter: solvent:	fish gelatine water	cold, in aqueous solution
Casein glues	dry matter: solvent: solubilizer: bactericide: adjuvants: retarders:	milk casein water lime or sodium hydroxide formaldehyde copper chloride, sodium fluoride, sodium silicate alkali fluorides	hot or cold, in aqueous solution

Table 2 (contd)

Glue	Composition		Mode of application
Urea-formaldehyde	dry matter:	urea and formaldehyde resins, partially condensed	hot or cold, in aqueous solution
	solvent:	water	
	fillers:	leguminous or cereal flours, casein, lime sulphate, colloid clay, diatomite, etc.	
	hardeners:	hydrochloric acid, phosphoric acid, ammonia	
Melamine-formaldehyde	dry matter:	melamine and formaldehyde resins, partially condensed	hot or cold, in aqueous solution
	solvent:	water	
	fillers:	bean, soya, rye flours, starch, kaolin, gypsum, asbestos, barium sulphate	
	hardeners:	salts of ammonia, organic acids (acetic acid)	
Resorcinol-formaldehyde	dry matter:	resorcinol and formaldehyde resins, partially condensed	hot or cold, in aqeuous solution
	solvents:	water, alcohol	
	fillers:	phenolic resins, flours	
	hardeners:	formaldehyde, paraformal-dehyde	
	catalyst:	formaldehyde	
Vinylic glues	dry matter:	polyvinyl acetate and butyrate	cold, in aqueous emulsion
	solvent:	water	
	dry matter:	polyvinyl acetate and butyrate	hot, in organic solvents
	solvents:	toluene, xylene, acetone, methyl ethyl ketone, cyclo-hexanone, dichloromethane, methanol, ethanol, etc.	
Cellulose glues	dry matter:	cellulose acetate	cold, in organic solvents
	solvents:	amyl acetate, ethyl acetate, etc.	
Chlorinated rubber glues	dry matter:	chlorinated rubber	cold, in organic solvents
	solvents:	toluene, xylene, etc.	
	softening agents:	chloronaphthalenes	

Table 2 (contd)

Glue	Composition		Mode of application
Neoprene glues	dry matter:	neoprene	cold, in organic solvents
	solvents:	toluene, xylene, acetone, methyl ethyl ketone, cyclo- hexanone, cyclohexane, amyl acetate, ethyl acetate, etc.	
Formaldehyde	dry matter:	phenolic and formaldehyde resins, partially condensed	water, alcohol or aqueous alcohol solution, hot
	solvents:	water, methanol	or cold
	fillers:	wood flour, nutshell flour, crushed bark, blood albumin	
	hardeners:	acids or bases	
Formol cresol	dry matter:	cresol and formaldehyde resins, partially condensed	water, alcohol or aqueous alcohol solution, hot or
	solvents:	water, methanol, ethanol	cold
	fillers:	wood flour, nutshell flour, crushed bark, blood albumin	
	hardeners:	acids or bases	

(phenolic and urea-formaldehyde resins) in the presence of heat and pressure, to produce panels of 3-25 mm thickness. In another procedure, wood (fir, poplar, willow) is reduced to long strips 2-4 mm wide and 1 mm thick, which are dipped into fast-bonding adhesives (phenolic, vinylic or urea-formaldehyde resins) and hot-pressed together.

(f) Mechanical wood preparation

The power-driven equipment is extremely complex and differs in every production unit. It includes planing machines, sanders, buffers, milling machines, mortisers, tenoners and more complex equipment in which a group of machines automatically finishes the pieces ready for assemblage.

The main working risks are represented by dust, noise, power sources and trauma.

(g) Sanding

Sanding serves to smooth the surface of the wood. This process is based on the use of abrasives and can be done manually or, more often, by machine. The abrasives used are of various types, including carborundum, emery, glass or pumice. In some countries turpentine is used for pumice sanding.

Power sanding is very noisy and presents risks related to the energy sources. More importantly, this is the phase of furniture-making in which the most respirable dust is generated.

(h) Plastering, puttying and insulating

(i) *Plastering and puttying:* Plasters and putties are used to cover raw wood, usually by hand, and are made up from an active soluble principle that is hard when dry (usually a polyvinyl acetate resin), a solvent (often ketones or esters) and fillers (slate, talc, etc.).

(ii) *Insulating:* This process is often carried out before buffing and consists of the application, usually by spraying, of an insulating varnish which is usually made of synthetic resins (glycerophthalic, glyceromaleic, etc.), desiccating oils (from flax, tung or aticyca) and semidesiccating oils (from poppies, grape pips, walnuts or soya beans).

The main risks of these procedures are linked to the materials themselves.

(i) Degreasing

Degreasing is a preparatory step before dyeing or bleaching and, for resinous wood, before covering with transparent varnish. It is usually carried out by hand and involves the application of a solvent (methanol, ethanol, acetone or esters), alone or with successive hot applications of sodium or ammonium carbonate.

(j) Bleaching

Bleaching is used to obtain white wood from darker wood or to prepare woods for painting with light colours. This process is also usually done by hand, and involves application of solutions of reducing or oxidizing agents (sulphuric acid, sulphurous acid, sodium bisulphite, alkali hyposulphite, hydrogen peroxide, alkali persulphates).

(k) Staining

Staining makes it possible to obtain colours other than the natural one, to give a better appearance, to hide surface defects, to join woods of different colours together and to imitate other, more precious woods without masking the aesthetic aspects and certain characteristics of the wood (grain, texture, veining, marbling).

Rough wood can be treated with penetrating stains; however, staining is usually super-ficial and applied to small finished or partially finished objects, which are often sprayed or dipped. Stains used currently are usually synthetic compounds dissolved in a volatile solvent (esters, alcohols, ketones). The list of these substances is very long; and the fact that many are mixtures with trade names makes their identification difficult. The following is a practical classification:

(i) *Acid stains* (croceine, Ponceaux 3R, SX and MX, rosaniline, acid fuchsine, resorcinol, nitrosine, induline) are applied with an acid (acetic or sulphuric acid) or with aluminium sulphate in an aqueous solution.

(ii) *Reducing or shaft stains* (indigo, by-products of anthracene production)

(iii) *Sulphur stains* (blacks, browns, light blues, greens): benzyl violet 4B, brilliant blue FCF (diammonium salt), guinea green B, rhodamine B, from aromatic bases (2,4-diaminotoluene, dihydrothiotoluidine, benzidine) or from *para*-oxydiphenylamine or dinitrophenol

(iv) *Oxidizing stains* (pyrogallic acid, *para*-phenylenediamine, Sudan dyes)

The latter group of stains and many of the others are applied to surfaces previously treated with mordants, which both stabilize and increase resistance to light. The most commonly used mordants are copper acetate and bismuth, titanium and manganese salts.

A partial list of dyes known to be used in the furniture and cabinet-making industry is given in Appendix 6.

(l) Buffing or varnishing

Wood buffing consists in covering the surface of a product with a transparent finish. In the wood industry, the word 'varnishing' is used for the application of paints, enamels or lacquers (Table 3).

(i) *Nitrocellulose varnishes* are now used to only a small extent and primarily for rapid finishing touches. They have a cellulose polymer base, which, with the rapid evapora-tion of the solvent, leaves a covering film; they are usually applied by spraying.

The main risks of use of these varnishes is related to the solvents used (esters and ketones).

(ii) *Hardening acid varnishes* are used for coating wooden floors and external panelling. They consist of a base of melamine resin dissolved in a butanol-isobutanol-xylene-toluene mixture. Hardening is obtained by the addition, at the moment of application, of an acid (*para*-toluenesulphonic acid, hydrochloric acid or phosphoric acid).

(iii) *Varnish mixtures* are basically enamels based on alkyd or acrylic resins or modified natural oils. The alkyd resins are polymerization products of a polyalcohol (usually glycerine) with dicarboxylic acids (adipic acid, terephthalic acid) or anhydrides (usually phthalic anhydride) and with fatty acids (extracted from linseed oil, soya bean oil, castor oil, coconut oil). When combined with other resins (melamine, epoxide, phenol), they assume plastic properties and can be sprayed. The most commonly used solvent is Cellosolve (hydroxy-ether). The acrylic-base enamels, which are dissolved in toluene, xylene or Cellosolve, are primarily used domestically.

(iv) *Polyester varnishes:* The series of varnishes with an unsaturated polyester resin base are polycondensed products with a modified alkyd base (such as polyalcohols, certain glycols, glycerol, trihydroxymethylpropane and dicarboxylic acids) dissolved in a solvent (almost always styrene), which polymerizes with the resin. Catalysts (cobalt naphthenate and hexanoate) are also present in the mixture; and at the moment of use, an organic peroxide (butyl or benzoyl) is added to start the resin-styrene polymerization.

The risks of applying these varnishes, which are always sprayed, are irritation of the eyes and respiratory tract, mostly due to the presence of styrene in air, but also to the peroxides. Sanding or polishing of these varnishes disperses polymer particles into the air; these contain substances like cobalt salts, which have an allergic effect on the mucous membranes and on the skin.

(v) *Polyurethane varnishes* are typical two-component polymers formed from a polyhydroxylate and a diisocyanate. The base may consist of glycols, acrylic resins, alkyd resins, polyamide resins, glycerophthalic resins, vinyl resins or saturated polyesters. The diisocyanates usually used are toluene diisocyanate (TDI) and hexamethylene diisocyanate (HDI). In the furniture industry, polyurethane varnishes are prepared just before use. They are used increasingly as insulators, mats and lustres and are applied by spraying, coating, dipping and electrostatic varnishing. After varnishing, buffing may be carried out.

The hazard from polyurethane varnishes derives primarily from the diisocyanates, which are known to be very strong irritants and sensitizing agents.

(vi) *Varnish removal:* Varnish removers are usually found in small workshops and are applied by hand; they consist of a strong base (sodium hydroxide, potassium carbonate, caustic lime) in an aqueous emulsion with cyclohexanol, dichloromethane, tetralin, carbon tetrachloride, acetone, cyclohexanone, etc.

Table 3. Composition of varnishes

Varnish	Composition		Mode of application and process of drying
Varnishes containing volatile solubilizers	binders: solvents:	natural gums ethanol or toluene	pad dries by evaporation of solvents
Cellulose varnishes	binders: plasticizers: solvents: diluents:	nitrocellulose resins maleic resins, alkyd resins, natural resins, adipates, phthalates, tricresyl phosphate acetone, cyclohexanone, ethyl, butyl and amyl acetate, ethanol, cyclohexanol toluene, xylene	spray-gun; varnishing machine with screen dries by evaporation of solvents
Vinyl varnishes	binder: dispersion medium: emulsifiers:	polyvinyl acetate water arylalkyl sulphonate, alkyl phenols	brush, roller, spray-gun; varnishing machine with drum (perforated nozzle for priming) dries by evaporation of solvents
Oil varnishes	binders: solvents: desiccants:	natural or synthetic resins, linseed oil, stand oil oil of turpentine, white spirit lead or cobalt salts	brush, roller, spray-gun dries by evaporation of solvents and oxidation
Glycerophthalic varnishes	binders: solvents: dessicants:	alkyl resins, linseed or soya oil white spirit, toluene, xylene lead or cobalt salts	brush, roller, spray-gun dries by evaporation of solvents
Urea-formaldehyde varnishes in organic solution	binder: solvents: catalysts:	aminoplast ethanol, butanol, toluene, xylene hydrochloric acid, phosphoric acid	brush, roller, varnishing machines dries by evaporation of solvents and polycondensation

Table 3 (contd)

Varnish	Composition		Mode of application and process of drying
Epoxide varnishes	binders:	epoxide resins	brush, spray-gun; varnishing machine with screen dries by evaporation of solvents and polycondensation
	solvents:	methyl ethyl ketone, diacetone alcohol, ethyl glycol, ethyl glycol acetate	
	diluents:	toluene, xylene, iso-propanol and butanol	
	catalysts:	ethylene diamine, di-ethylene triamine, tri-ethylene tetramine	
Polyurethane varnishes with two components	binders:	(1) polyesters containing free hydroxyls; (2) polyisocyanates	brush, dipping, spray-gun; varnishing machine with screen dries by evaporation of solvents and poly-condensation
	solvents:	ethyl acetate, butyl acetate, ethyl glycol acetate, methyl ethyl ketone, cyclohexanone, dichloromethane	
	diluents:	toluene, xylene	
Polyurethane varnishes with single component	binders:	polyesters containing free hydroxyls and polyisocyanates	dipping dries by evaporation of solvents and polycondensation
	solvents:	xylene, toluene, acetates	
	hardener:	moisture in air	
Polyester varnishes	binder:	unsaturated polyester resin	double-feed spray-gun; varnishing machine with screen and two heads
	monomers:	styrene-dichlorostyrene, allyl phthalate, triallyl cyanurate, methyl methacrylate	
	catalysts:	cyclohexanone peroxide, methyl ethyl ketone peroxide, benzoyl peroxide	dries by copoly-merization
	accelerators:	cobalt naphthenate or octoate, lead salts	

A good varnished surface can only be obtained by following a complex varnishing cycle, in which each step requires use of a different varnishing product, depending on the technique of application, the shape of the object, the kind of wood used, and the designated purpose of the object.

Chairs are dyed by dipping or spraying (in Italy, usually with polyurethane varnishes) and then dried in a hot-air tunnel. Finished furniture may also be spray-dyed (usually by 'airless' or 'electrostatric' processes) in varnishing booths (dry, water curtain or pressurized) and air- or tunnel-dried. When the first layer is dry, it is sanded by hand or with orbital vibrating tools.

(m) Assembling and finishing

These phases may be part of an assembly line, isolated or situated next to other work. In the latter case the workers have a mixed exposure.

2.3 Qualitative and quantitative data on exposures (See also Appendix 4.)

(a) Dust levels

Very few reliable studies of occupational health aspects of the furniture industry are available. Hanslian & Kadlec (1964) showed that during the manufacture of furniture a concentration of wood dust as high as 200 mg/m^3 of air may develop; the average level of 40 mg/m^3 that they found was far above the maximum level which they stated should be allowed (10 mg/m^3; recommended average levels, 1 mg/m^3). These authors also found that in high concentrations of wood dust, 90% of the particles were smaller than 5 μm. Clinical studies performed by these authors allowed them to differentiate wood into three categories: (1) woods with 'low toxicity' (relatively nontoxic), e.g., oak, beech, maple, ash, birch, lime; (2) woods with 'high toxicity', e.g., pine, larch, ebony, mahogany; and (3) strongly allergenic woods, e.g., yew, box, mansonia. [The Working Group assumed that these authors were referring only to short-term toxicity in forming these categories.]

Salamone *et al.* (1969) established that during the working of mansonia wood, dust levels are remarkable, particularly in the sawing and veneering phases: the dust level measured 3 m from a work surface was 500 particles/m^3 and that at 50 cm 1000 particles/m^3. In the trimming workshop, and especially at the sanding stage where the machines have no exhaust system, the dust level after four working hours was 100 particles/m^3. Size distribution analysis showed that 31% of the dust particles had a diameter of less than 5 μm.

In the German Democratic Republic, Ruppe (1973) correlated the lung diseases of workers in a woodworking factory using exotic woods with the levels of dust to which they were exposed (<5 to >20 mg/m^3). He concluded that 5 mg/m^3 should be adopted as the limit value for exposure to exotic woods.

Otto (1973) reported dust levels ranging from 2-151 mg/m^3 in the vicinity of belt sanders.

Hounam & Williams (1974) studied five furniture factories located in and around High Wycombe, UK, selected to give a range of sizes and products. The machine operations covered (which were well ventilated by extraction systems) included:

- sawing planks with either band or circular saws,
- evening wood with either planers or a four-cutter,
- using a router plane,
- using a spindle moulder, and
- sanding shaped wood.

The results of the study can be summarized as follows:

(i) The distribution of sample weights taken with personal air samplers in the breathing zones of operators of various woodworking machines appeared to be approximately log-normal, with a median value of 4.6 mg/m^3 (representing the concentration most probably found in a random sample) (Table 4).

Table 4. Concentrations of airborne dust (mg/m^3), measured with a personal air sampler, at five furniture factories in the UK[a]

| Factory | Sample | Operation | | | | | | |
		Bandsawing	Planing	Routing	Spindle moulding	Sanding	Assembly	Turning
A	Day 1	20.0[b]	2.0	1.8	5.8	2.4	25.5[d]	—
	Day 2	7.3[b]	2.4	3.8	6.3	3.6	2.1	—
B	Day 1	5.0	8.5	8.6	6.5	8.2	3.5	—
	Day 2	7.3	9.1	3.7	8.4	3.2	4.4	—
C	Day 1	1.0	1.8	3.5	1.5	2.0	3.7	—
	Day 2	1.8	2.8	3.3	4.4	2.4	4.5	—
D	Day 1	12.5[b,c]	3.1	94.6[b]	—	25.2[b]	5.9	—
	Day 2	9.2[b]	6.3[b]	8.2[b]	—	22.6	7.6	—
E	Day 1	6.5	10.9	—	3.2	7.9	8.2	4.6
	Day 2	4.1	4.1	—	4.4	12.2	9.8	12.5

[a] From Hounam & Williams (1974)
[b] Sample contained 'inertials' in addition to fine dusts
[c] Includes circular as well as bandsawing
[d] This operator was sanding table tops before assembly.

(ii) The median value obtained with the cascade impactor (4.2 mg/m^3) was similar to that obtained with the personal air samplers. Although the TLV was exceeded frequently, 90% of the measurements were less than 10 mg/m^3. The mass median equivalent diameters ranged from about 5-11 μm. The coarsest dust was produced during sawing operations and the finest during sanding and assembly (which frequently involves sanding) (Table 5).

It was concluded on the basis of the particulate distribution, that a relatively low percentage of the dust was sufficiently fine to penetrate the alveolar region of the respiratory tract. Most particles had dimensions greater than 5 μm and appeared to be either fibrous or flaky in character. Dust with these dimensions would be effectively trapped in the nasal passages.

Table 5. Concentrations and mass median equivalent diameters of airborne dust measured with the cascade impactor in five UK furniture factories[a]

Operation	No. of measurements	Dust concentration (mg/m^3)		Mass median equivalent diameter (μm)
		Range	Mean	
Band/circular sawing	7	0.8 - 100	20.1	11.5
Planing	5	1.7 - 9.4	3.6	9.2
Routing	4	2.5 - 11.3	5.5	10.0
Spindle moulding	6	2.0 - 36.3	17.0	10.0
Sanding	8	0.5 - 34.3	8.0	8.4
Assembly	6	1.3 - 5.3	3.4	7.6
Turning	1	—	9.0	11.5
Shaping	1	—	7.2	8.8
Cyclone shed	1	—	15.2	5.6
Near bag filters	1	—	1.4	6.4

[a] From Hounam & Williams (1974)

The dust involved is equivalent to a fine wood flour and fits the description of a dust that would be formed from dense, dry hardwood lumber. Sanding and high-speed machining operations should rupture the wood cells and probably delaminate the cell wall giving rise to plate-like rather than fibrous residues. The woods that were being machined, beech and oak, do contain very broad multiserial rays. The manner in which such rays may fragment under the conditions noted could give rise to very fine fibre fragments. Moreover, fragmentation of these cells could release inclusions and extractive materials.

Andersen *et al*. (1977) determined the dust levels in work rooms in eight furniture factories in Åarhus, Denmark. They found that 63% of measurements with personal samplers were above 5 mg/m³ and 28% were above 10 mg/m³. Dust measurements with stationary equipment gave almost identical results. The distribution of particle sizes was: 33% <5 μm, 41% <6-10 μm, 11% <11-15 μm and 15% >16 μm. [It was unclear to the Working Group if these percentages were based upon particle count or mass.] Average dust concentrations during machine and hand sanding were 14.3 mg/m³, and those during work such as drilling, planing or sawing, 5.3 mg/m³.

According to Chiesura (1978), the usual conditions in the Italian furniture industry are represented by the following dust levels (Table 6), measured in 10 factories with good ventilation by an extraction system:

Table 6. Dust levels in 10 Italian furniture factories[a]

Total dust (mg/m³)	No. of samples	%
<1	42	52.5
1 - 3	21	26.2
3 - 5	10	12.5
>5	7	8.7

[a] From Chiesura (1978)

In a furniture factory in Mantova in 1979, dust control devices were installed near employees in the hand-sanding and resin application departments. These consisted of a grille in the bench and a suction system in front of the work being done. The efficiency of the system, in terms of total dust and respirable dust, was evaluated with and without suction by stationary dust sampling. The results (Table 7) show that this system reduced the dust exposure during work by about half.

Other dusts may occur in the workplace that could have an adjunctive effect. Garnet sandpaper, for example, is traditionally used as a high quality abrasive (Connelly, 1971). It is a silicate mineral that wears by the loss of small crystal attrition. The loss of such particles leaves the parent crystal in a resharpened state. Similarly, the fine crystals that leave as dust have sharp edges.

Table 7. Stationary dust sampling in the workplace of a furniture factory
in Mantova, Italy, 1979

Position of sampler	Sample	Dust (mg/m^3)
Sanding (without suction)	total dust	3.15
Sanding (without suction)	respirable dust	0.70
Sanding (with suction)	total dust	1.25
Sanding (with suction)	respirable dust	0.35
Hand-sanding (without suction)	total dust	5.06
In the middle of the work-place	total dust	0.50

(b)   Solvents (See also monograph on carpentry and joinery, p.148 .)

The varnish solvents that evaporate most rapidly are the ketones (methyl ethyl ketone, methyl isobutyl ketone, acetone) and other esters (ethyl acetate, butyl acetate and, less frequently, methyl acetate). Those with medium and low volatilities are Cellosolve and the aromatic solvents (toluene, xylene, ethyl benzene). The use of varnishes containing predominantly aromatic solvents has been strictly regulated in Italy since 1963. The use of benzene is subject to legislation in many other countries.

Another group of solvents are the alcohols (propanol, isopropanol, butanol, isobutanol), which are used to adjust the stickiness of varnishes.

In a survey of the concentration of solvent vapours in the varnishing department of a wood factory in Mantova, Italy, a varnishing booth, closed on three sides and provided with both a vapour suction system and a water film to carry away the mist from the sprayed varnishes was set up and samples were taken using two personal pumps. The results are summarized in Table 8.

Table 8. Solvent vapours in a furniture factory in Mantova, Italy, 1979

Position of sampler	Solvent vapours (mg/m^3)						
	Acetone	Methyl ethyl ketone	Ethyl acetate	Isobutyl acetate	Butyl acetate	Toluene	Xylene
Preparation of varnishes	80	9	5	34	27	101	48
Spray-varnishing	45	7	5	24	20	80	37

(c) Isocyanates

The most frequently used isocyanates are toluene diisocyanate (TDI) and hexamethylene diisocyanate (HDI). The levels of TDI measured in three areas in a woodworking factory in the district of Veneto, Italy, were as follows: (1) near the varnishing booth with an air suction system, 0.043 mg/m^3; (2) near a booth equipped with an air extractive device and with a system to carry away the mist by means of a water film, 0.056 mg/m^3 (mean of 8 samples; range, 0.015-0.122); and (3) near the drying rooms, 0.056 mg/m^3.

2.4 Biological factors

Many insects carry out their biological cycles in wood - parasitic insects in standing trees and saphrophytic insects in fallen trees or those used in construction. Of particular importance are *Cossus cossus* and *Saperda carcharias* in poplar, *Cerambix cerdus* in oak, and various wood ants *(Camponotus* spp.) which attack old coniferous trees. Wood-wasps *(Sirex* spp.) mature in fallen oak trees; house borers *(Hylotrupes bajulus)* attack coniferous wood; and termites *(Calotermes* and *Reticulitermes* spp.) attack many kinds of wood. *Lyctus* beetles attack tropical woods, broad-leaf woods, softwoods, various eucalyptus woods and oak sapwood. Woodworm is very common. However, certain woods, e.g., Canadian balsam and cedar, are naturally toxic to insects and higher vertebrates.

Fungi may also install themselves on wood, using its components for their own growth (Sharp, 1975). Various Ascomycetes, Deuteromycetes, and Basidiomycetes are responsible for wood destruction. Specific xylophagic fungi, which attack rotting wood, are *Stereum purpureum, Polyporus* and *Polystictus* spp. and *Lenzites sepiaria*. Lumber stored in damp places may be attacked by *Merulius lacrymans, Coniophora cerebella* or *Poria* spp. The most common of the chromogenic fungi, which stain wood, is *Ceratostomella pilifera*.

2.5 Current regulations and recommendations on exposures

See 'General Remarks on Wood, Leather and Some Associated Industries', p. 23.

2.6 Number of workers involved

See 'General Remarks on Wood, Leather and Some Associated Industries', p. 19.

In Italy, the 1971 census showed that wood and furniture workers totalled 400,000. Almost 90% of the businesses were craftsmen's workshops, and these employed half of the total number of workers.

When the Italian situation is compared with that in other countries (Fig. 1), it is evident that the number of workers in this sector of the manufacturing industries decreases with an

Fig. 1. Percentage of woodworkers among the total number of workers in manufacturing industries in relation to the average size of factories in some producer countries[a]

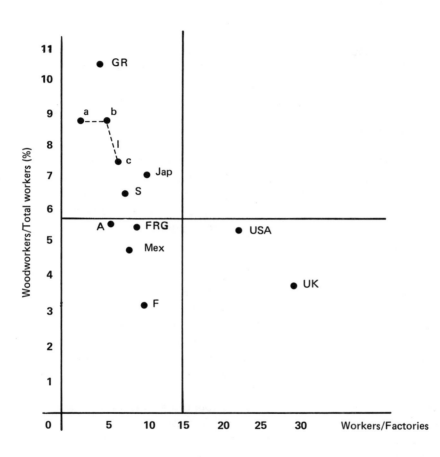

[a]GR - Greece, 1963; I - Italy (a) 1951, (b) 1961, (c) 1971; Jap - Japan, 1969; S - Switzerland, 1965; A - Argentina, 1964; FRG - Federal Republic of Germany, 1967; Mex - Mexico, 1966; F - France, 1966; USA - USA, 1967; UK - United Kingdom, 1968

increase in the average dimension of the production unit, i.e., as it passes from a predominantly craft situation to a predominantly industrial situation. Thus, during the 1950s, the percentage that this section represented of the total manufacturing industries remained the same, although the average dimensions of the premises rose. During the 1960s, however, there was a sizeable reduction in the number of units (Filca-Cisl del Veneto, 1979).

3. TOXIC, INFLAMMATORY AND ALLERGIC EFFECTS IN HUMANS

Toxic effects attributed to a particular wood are described below in relation to the occupation with which they have been associated most frequently or most conspicuously. However, it may be expected that whenever the same type of wood is used in other occupations, similar adverse effects could occur.

3.1 Respiratory diseases (other than cancer)

Ruppe (1973) analysed discomfort emanating from the respiratory tract in furniture workers in the German Democratic Republic and found a correlation between the incidence of sinusitis, sneezing, watery nasal discharge, nasal mucosal irritation and cough and wood dust concentration in the working place. In his study, 14 persons were exposed to a dust concentration below 5 mg/m^3, 15 to between 5 and 9 mg/m^3, 36 to between 10 and 19 mg/m^3, and 36 to 20 mg/m^3 or more.

Diseases of the respiratory airways among Danish woodworkers were studied by Solgaard & Andersen (1975) in relation to wood dust concentrations, whether below or above 5 mg/m^3. Middle-ear inflammation was significantly more common among those exposed to higher concentrations of wood dust. Other diseases, like sinusitis, long-term upper respiratory infections, asthma and epistaxis were also more common (although not statistically significantly so) among those exposed to higher concentrations. Spirometric investigations showed no difference between these two groups.

In a Swedish investigation (Ager, 1976), it was found that discomfort due to exposure to wood dust occurred among 38% of the workers. However, this percentage was lower than the incidence of discomfort caused by other kinds of dust occurring in the furniture industry. In another Swedish investigation, comprising 723 furniture workers, nasal obstruction was found in 36% and chronic nasal discharge, possibly due to allergy, in 16% (Drettner & Wilhelmsson, 1980).

Among 226 workers in a woodworking enterprise in the German Democratic Republic, chronic rhinolaryngological changes were observed in 63%. The changes were of varying degrees of severity and occurred mainly in the mucous membranes of the nose (Werner, 1979).

Occupational asthma has been described in people working with mansonia wood (Bourne, 1956; Gaffuri *et al.*, 1968), Western red cedar and iroko (Gandevia & Milne, 1970; Pickering *et al.*, 1972; Chan-Yeung *et al.*, 1973), oak and mahogany (Sosman *et al.*, 1969), cedar of Lebanon (Greenberg, 1972), kejaat, amboyna, box, obeche, teak (Woods & Calnan, 1976; Belli *et al.*, 1979), and less often with a number of other woods such as abiruana (Booth *et al.*, 1976), zebra wood (Bush *et al.*, 1978) and sawdust from Californian redwood (Chan-Yeung & Abboud, 1976; doPico, 1978).

Chen-Yeung & Abboud (1976) suggested that phenolic extractives (sugiresinol, hydroxy-sugiresinol and isosequiric acid) in the redwood were the agents responsible for the reactions. Besides tannin, dyes, pitch, resin and lignins, Western red cedar contains plicatic acid; this occurs as a major fraction among the water-soluble components. It is probably a causative agent of asthma, since it has been found to produce the same bronchial reaction as crude dust extract in provocation tests on affected individuals (Chan-Yeung *et al.,* 1973).

Allergenic woods are listed in Table 9.

Table 9. **Some common wood varieties that have been reported to be allergenic**

Genus	Species	Common name
Apocynaceae	Gonioma kamassi	Kamassi, knysna, boxwood
	Nerium oleander	Oleander
	Rauwolfia pentaphilla	Muirajussara rana
Bignoniaceae	Tabebuia spp.	Ipe, lapachol, etc.
	Paratecoma peroba	White peroba
Buxaceae	Buxus sempervirens	European, Iranian, Turkish boxwood
Combretaceae	Terminalia alata	Indian laurel
Cupressaceae	Thuja plicata	Western red cedar
Ebenaceae	Diospyros celebica	Macassar ebony
	Diospyros ebenum	Ceylon ebony
	Diospyros crassiflora	African ebony
Fagaceae	Fagus sylvatica	Beech
	Quercus rubra	Northern red oak
Plindersiaceae	Chloroxylon swietenia	Ceylon satinwood

Table 9 (contd)

Genus	Species	Common name
Leguminosae, Caesalpinioideae	*Peltogyne densiflora*	Purpleheart
Leguminosae, Papilionoideae	*Andira inermis*	Angelin, kuraru, cochenilla
	Andira coriacea	Red cabbage tree, mocha colorado
	Brya ebenus	Crocuswood, green ebony
	Bowdichia nitida	Sucupira, black sucupira
	Diplotropis purpurea	Sucupira assu, supupira
	Dalbergia retusa	Cocobolo, granadillo
	Dalbergia nigra	Brazilian rosewood, palisander
	Dalbergia latifolia	Indian rosewood
	Dalbergia sissoo	Sissoo, shishan
	Dalbergia oliveri	Brazilian tulipwood
	Dalbergia graveana	Madagascar rosewood
	Dalbergia cochinchi- *nensis*	Thailand rosewood
Meliaceae	*Dalbergia melanoxylon*	African blackwood
	Machaerium scleroxy- *lon*	Caviuna, pao ferro
	Pterocarpus spp.	Amboyna, muninga, African padauk
	Khaya anthotheca	African mahogany
	Swietenia mahogani	Hondura, Tabasco, Cuban, Spanish and West Indian mahogany, baywood
	Toona sureni *(Cedrella tooni)*	Burma cedar
Moraceae	*Chlorophora excelsa*	Iroko, kambala, African teak
Pinaceae	*Pinus sylvestris*	Scots pine, northern redwood
	Pinus pinaster	Maritime pine
	Pinus palustris	Pitch pine
	Abies alba	Silver fir
	Pseudotsuga menziesii	Douglas fir
Rutaceae	*Fagara flava*	West Indian satinwood
Salicaceae	*Populus albus*	White poplar
Sapolaceae	*Mimusops* spp.	Makore, moabi, mukulungu
Simaroubaceae	*Quassia amara*	Quassia, bitter wood
Sterculiaceae	*Mansonia altissima*	Mansonia, bėtė, aprono, koul
	Triplochiton scler- *oxylon*	Obeche, abachi, samba, wawa

Table 9 (contd)

Genus	Species	Common name
Taxaceae	*Taxus baccata*	Yew
Thymelaeaceae	*Gonystylus bancanus*	Ramin, melawis
Verbenaceae	*Tectona grandis*	Teak, teck, djati

3.2 Irritating effects

Primary irritating effects include skin symptoms, conjunctival irritation with inflammation and keratitis, irritation of the mucosa of the respiratory tract and epistaxis, chronic rhinitis and bronchitis. These effects are common in woodworkers, particularly when they work with certain woods, e.g., sequoia, Western red cedar, sabicu, dahoma, sneezewood, scented guarea, mansonia, makore, opepe, stavewood (Woods & Calnan, 1976).

Headache, salivation, thirst and nausea in woodworkers are sometimes too severe to be explained by simple mucosal irritation. Giddiness, drowsiness, visual disturbances, colic, muscle cramps and cardiac arrhythmia suggest the effects of alkaloids or glycosides absorbed through the respiratory or alimentary tracts, or occasionally through skin abrasions (Sandermann & Barghoorn, 1956; Woods & Calnan, 1976).

3.3 Skin effects

The common picture is that of sensitization contact dermatitis. Mild cases have only erythema and slight irritation, but there are often papular or vesicular lesions which may progress to chronic eczema after repeated exposure. Dermatitis arises from a variety of exotic woods. Newly introduced woods, when handled by workers for the first time, have also been associated with dermatitis (Woods & Calnan, 1976).

Contact urticaria is characteristic following exposure to obeche (Oehling, 1963); however, urticarial reactions have been reported with other types of wood, such as larch (Hanslian & Kadlec, 1964) and iroko (Woods & Calnan, 1976).

One epidemiological investigation from Norway revealed true teak *(Tectona grandis)* as a frequent cause of allergic contact eczema in 20.5% of workers in a furniture factory. Patch tests showed that lapachol (a derivative of naphthoquinone) was the sensitizing agent in teak wood as well as in jacaranda wood (Krogh, 1962, 1964).

Dalbergia rosewood, rengas and obeche are reported to be strongly allergenic. These woods can sensitize even on simple contact. The allergens of Dalbergia rosewoods have been identified as quinones not unlike primin, a very common contact allergen from the plant *Primula obconica*, and cross-reactivity has been observed. In Anacardiaceae, as well as in Moraceae, Urticaceae, Euphorbiaceae and Apocynaceae, the sap or latex is highly irritant and often also contains sensitizers. One of the most potent botanical contact allergens known is urushiol, a pentadecylcatechol produced by *Rhus toxicodendron*, a member of the family Anacardiaceae (Woods & Calnan, 1976).

A list of chemical allergens that may be found in wood dust is given in Table 10.

Table 10. Certain naturally occuring chemical allergens found in wood dust and specific response

Chemical allergen	Botanical and common name of wood	Symptom or response
Lapachol	*Tectona grandis* - teak	contact allergic eczema
A sesquiterpene lactone	*Frullania* - liverworts and lichens on bark	contact dermatitis
Turpentine Colophony (?)	*Pinus palustris* - conifers	sensitizers to contact dermatitis
Usnic acid	*Thuja plicata* - Western red cedar	epidermal sensitization
Pentadecylcatechol	*Rhus toxicodendron, Ana cardiaceae* ?	contact allergen
Oleoresins	*Tectona grandis* - teak *Khaya ivorensis* - mahogany	dermatitis; mucosal irritation
Sugiresinol, hydroxysugiresinol isosequiric acid	*Sequoia sempivirens* - redwood	bronchial asthma
Plicatic acid	*Thuja plicata* - Western red cedar	bronchial asthma

4. CARCINOGENICITY DATA[1]

(a) Nasal cancer

The first report dealing with woodworkers and tumours of the nasal sinus that was available to the Working Group is that of Macbeth (1965). He described two groups of patients with this cancer - 40 diagnosed between 1951 and 1959 and 28 diagnosed from 1960 on. Twenty of the patients came from High Wycombe, UK, where the principal industry for many years has been chair-making, and 15 of them (75%) were employed in the furniture industry.

Acheson *et al*. (1967), in a preliminary communication, reported on 85 incident cases of carcinoma of the nose, nasal cavities, middle ear and accessory sinuses (ICD 160) first diagnosed during the decade 1956-1965 in a defined area of the UK, i.e., the Oxford Hospital Region, comprising Buckinghamshire, Oxfordshire and Berkshire. Seventeen of the 59 males (29%) were woodworkers and another 6 were affiliated with woodworking trades. Among the approximately 12,000 male woodworkers in the study area, 1 tumour would have been expected on the basis of age- and sex-standardized incidence rates, whereas 17 were observed. Of these 17 tumours observed among woodworkers 13 were adeno-carcinomas (76%), and of the 6 tumours observed among men affiliated with woodworking 4 were adenocarcinomas, while only 6 of 36 tumours in men employed in other occupations (16%) were adenocarcinomas. No cases were described in either joiners or carpenters, although these occupations comprised about half of the woodworkers in the area.

Acheson *et al*. (1968) restricted their study to two groups of incident cases of carcinoma of the nasal cavity and accessory sinuses in the defined area of the UK described above. Group 1 consisted of 83 patients, 56 men and 27 women, identified during 1956-1965. Group 2 consisted of 65 patients, 42 men and 23 women, identified either before 1 January 1956 or after 31 December 1965. Of the men in Group 1, 42 were employed at the time of their diagnosis, and 16 of these (38%) were woodworkers (14 cabinet- or chair-makers or wood-machinists in the furniture industry, 1 crate maker and 1 cooper), compared with 3.3% of the total population so employed. In Group 1, 23 male patients had adeno-carcinomas: 14 were currently woodworkers in the furniture industry, 1 was a yard labourer in a furniture factory and 5 were ex-workers in the furniture industry (2 cabinet-makers, 2 wood-machinists and 1 French polisher). In Group 2, 10 of the 42 male patients had adenocarcinomas: 3 were woodworkers in the furniture industry, 1 was a French polisher, 1 was a yard labourer in a furniture factory and 1 had been a clerk in the furniture industry. No cases were reported as carpenters or joiners, although these occupations comprised about half of the woodworkers in the area.

---

[1] This section should be read in conjunction with Appendices 1 and 2, pp. **295 and 301.**

Ball (1967, 1968) identified death certificates from Canada for the period 1956-1965 which listed cancers of all histological types of the nose, nasal sinuses or maxillary sinuses (ICD 160) as an underlying cause of death. Controls were the next certificate in sequence that was similar in respect of province of death, sex and year of death. Age was matched within 2 years for 96% of the case-control pairs. No increase specific to furniture makers was apparent (2 cases and 1 control). The author pointed out that hardwood furniture manufacture comprises only a small part of the Canadian wood industry.

Debois (1969) reported that among 30 cases of nasal sinus tumours diagnosed between 1958 and 1968 in Belgium, 19 (63%) worked in the furniture industry. Twenty of the cases were adenocarcinomas, and 14 of these (70%) were in persons who worked in the furniture industry.

Delemarre & Themans (1971) reported on 16 adenocarcinomas diagnosed in The Netherlands during the period 1944-1967; 11 (69%) occurred in people working in the furniture industry. These were compared with 33 cases of other carcinomas of the nasal sinus, among which 3 (9%) were found in workers in the furniture industry.

Acheson et al. (1972) identified all cases of adenocarcinoma 'registered in recent years' (mostly covering the years 1961-1966) with all the cancer registries in England and Wales (excluding Oxford). Controls were patients with other nasal cancers similarly ascertained, matched for age (within 5 years), sex, year of death and area of registry. A total of 145 adenocarcinomas and 133 other nasal cancers (controls) were ascertained; slides of 107 adenocarcinomas and 98 controls were analysed; and histological confirmation by a pathologist was carried out for 74 adenocarcinoma cases and 94 controls. Nineteen of 80 men with adenocarcinomas (24%) had been mainly employed as furniture workers, compared with 5 of 85 (6%) men with other nasal cancers. About 0.2 cases of adenocarcinoma would have been expected in this group on the basis of incidence figures for England and Wales, giving an SMR of 9500. Nine of the 80 men with adenocarcinomas (11%) were employed in other woodworking professions, compared with 4 of 85 controls with other nasal cancers (5%); 1.9 cases would have been expected, giving an SMR of 474. Interestingly, the risk of other nasal cancers in individuals in woodworking trades is also higher than would be expected by chance (P<0.001), suggesting that wood exposures may contribute to these cancers as well.

Andersen (1975) and Andersen et al. (1976, 1977) described 157 patients with cancer of the nose and paranasal sinuses treated at one hospital in Denmark between 1964 and 1974. Seventeen of the tumours were classified as adenocarcinomas, and 12 of the men who had them (71%) had been exposed to wood dust (10 furniture makers, 1 coach builder and 1 'turner'): thus, 17 adenocarcinomas occurred among the 157 men (11%) in all occupations combined, compared with 12 adenocarcinomas among the 22 men (55%) who were woodworkers. Although snuff has been suggested as a contributing factor to these tumours (see Acheson, 1976), none of the woodworkers in this series were reported to have used snuff.

Acheson (1976) reviewed the association between furniture occupations and nasal cancer. He estimated that the incidence of adenocarcinoma in High Wycombe cabinet- and chair-makers was 0.7 per 1000 per year during the decade 1956-1965, i.e., about 500 times the risk in the general male population of southern England. Twenty-eight of the 34 nasal tumours (82%) were adenocarcinomas, compared with 4 of 52 nasal tumours (8%) in men reporting other lines of work; and 22 of the 28 adenocarcinomas occurred in woodworkers in the furniture industry and in other workers in that industry. While almost half of all other nasal tumours occurred after the age of 65, the average age of adenocarcinoma patients is in general 10 years lower than that of patients with cancers of other cell types. The average period between commencement of employment and diagnosis was 43 years (range, 27-69 years); however, adenocarcinomas developed after exposures as short as 4, 5 and 7 years, and Acheson quotes Hadfield (1970), who reported a patient whose period of exposure to dust within the furniture industry was only 18 months. There was no significant difference between the mean latent period for men who left the industry prior to diagnosis of their tumour and that for those who were still employed when diagnosed. Acheson also suggested that the factors that were responsible for the increase were at least present in the furniture industry between about 1920 and 1940. In the UK, no person who entered the industry after the Second World War is known to have developed a nasal adenocarcinoma. In France, however, 1 of 2 furniture makers with adenocarcinoma started work in 1941 (Fombeur, 1972). Acheson suggested that beech (almost certainly) and oak (probably) are associated with the disease; however, the evidence does not rule out the possibility that a carcinogenic factor is also present in other woods. Cancer risks were highest for men in jobs with exposure to wood dust (turners, machinists, sanders) rather than in jobs with exposure to polishes, varnishes, etc. Men working in the wood industries in fact smoke less than other workers, since they are forbidden to smoke during working hours; for this reason snuff-taking had been a traditional habit among these workers. However, only 3 of 17 furniture workers with adenocarcinoma for whom it was possible to obtain information had ever taken snuff, and while snuff-taking cannot explain the association, the habit cannot be ruled out as a possible contributing factor.

Brinton et al. (1976) performed a correlation study comparing cancer mortality rates in US counties in which more than 1% of the population was employed in making furniture and fixtures with those in socio-economically similar control counties in which there was no significant amount of furniture manufacture. A 19% excess of deaths from nasal cancer was seen in counties with furniture industries.

Brinton *et al*. (1977) identified 37 death certificates listing nasal cancers (ICD 160) as an underlying cause of death from counties in North Carolina, USA, where more than 1% of the work force was employed in furniture and fixtures manufacture. Two controls were selected for each case and matched for sex, race, county of death, age at death (±2 years) and year of death. Eight of 37 people (22%) who had died from nasal cancer had worked in the furniture industry, compared with 5 of 73 controls (7%), a relative risk of 4.4 (95% confidence limits, 1.3-15.4).

Haguenauer *et al*. (1977) found 27 furniture workers among 115 French cases of ethmoid cancer. Of 32 woodworkers with nasal ethmoid carcinomas, 1 was a plywood worker and 1 a shipboard worker. All but two of the furniture workers had adeno-carcinomas; 60% of all the adenocarcinomas seen occurred in woodworkers. This corres-ponds well with studies from other parts of France (Luboinski & Marandas, 1975; Curtes *et al*., 1977) in which, respectively, 21 of 43 adenocarcinoma cases (49%) were in furniture/cabinet-makers and 15 of 21 adenocarcinomas (71%) were in woodworkers, most of whom were furniture workers.

Gignoux & Bernard (1969) observed that all 17 woodworkers (16 with adenocarcinomas and 1 with a reticulosarcoma) among 53 cases of malignant ethmoid cancer were under 58 years of age and that these tumours appeared in the woodworkers some 10 years earlier than did other nasal sinus tumours. Fifteen of the 17 woodworkers in this study were cabinet-makers. Desnos & Martin (1973) reported that of 7 woodworkers with adenocarcinoma (5 furniture workers), 3 (2 furniture workers) were between 37 and 42 years of age.

In a study in the German Democratic Republic (Löbe & Ehrhardt, 1978) of 428 cases of malignant nasal and paranasal sinus tumours diagnosed between 1931 and 1977, a question-naire concerning occupational history was distributed and returned by 179 (43%) of the cases. Thirteen of 18 patients with adenocarcinoma (78%) had been working in the furni-ture industry; 10% of all the nasal tumours were adenocarcinomas, while 35% of the nasal tumours in woodworkers were adenocarcinomas. Thirty-seven cases (20.8%) out of the total number of tumours, regardless of cell type, occurred among woodworkers; this incidence was reported to be far higher than that in the population engaged in this type of work.

Engzell *et al*. (1978) identified cases of carcinoma of the nose and paranasal sinuses from the cancer registry of the National Board of Health and Welfare of Sweden: adenocar-cinomas registered between 1961 and 1971 and squamous-cell and poorly differentiated carcinomas registered between 1965 and 1971. Occupation was then ascertained for each case by a questionnaire completed either by the patient or by a close relative. Nineteen of the 36 patients with adenocarcinomas (53%) were classified as 'joiners'; 12 of these were further described as cabinet-makers. [The Working Group noted that in Swedish it is not possible to distinguish between joiners and furniture/cabinet-makers.] Among 127 men with other nasal tumours, 5 (4%) were joiners in wood-related industries. Nineteen of the 32 woodworkers (59%) had adenocarcinomas compared with 17 of 131 patients (13%) who reported other occupations. The average age of men with adenocarcinomas was 62 years, compared with 64 years for men with other nasal cancers. The incidence of smoking and snuff-taking among patients who completed the questionnaire was similar to that of the general population. When cases of adenocarcinoma were traced up to 1972, Engzell (1979) found that 3 out of the 8 new cases were in joiners. The latent period averaged 45 years (range, 22-70 years) for 21 joiners. Two workers employed in oak parquet flooring factories developed adenocarcinomas after only 8 and 9 years' duration of employment.

Olsen & Sabroe (1979) conducted a prospective study on mortality between 1971 and 1976 among 40,000 active and retired members of the Danish Carpenter/Cabinet Makers' Trade Union. Only the number of deaths due to nasal cancer was significantly higher in woodworkers compared with national rates (SMR = 467; 95% confidence limits, 253-679; based on only 4 cases). Data on the actual work exposures of the subjects were not available, but the authors reported a higher risk among men trained as cabinet-makers than among men trained as carpenters (3 of the 4 cases were cabinet-makers). [The short period of follow-up and the fact that only limited data were available on retired workers may account for the fact that the SMR is lower than those reported in previous studies.]

Mosbech & Acheson (1971) reported 4 cases of nasal adenocarcinoma in Danish cabinet-makers.

(b)   Respiratory cancers other than of the nose

Brinton *et al*. (1976) reported age-adjusted rate ratios of 0.87 for both cancers of the larynx and cancers of the lung. [Refer to section *(a)*, p.129, for discussion of methods.]

Wolf (1978) discussed the distribution of occupations among 46 patients with laryngeal carcinomas diagnosed in 3 districts of the German Democratic Republic from 1969 to 1976, and compared them with a general occupational distribution. Furniture workers were at increased risk: 1.44% of the patients were furniture workers, but they had 10.87% of the laryngeal carcinomas.

Esping & Axelson (1980) examined death and burial registers for the years 1963-1977 and identified 25 men who had died of respiratory cancer (ICD 160-163, which includes nasal cancers), as well as 70 men who had died of gastrointestinal cancer (ICD 140-159) [See section *(f)*, p. 132 for results on gastrointestinal cancers.] in a small Swedish town with a prominent woodworking industry specializing in furniture production. Controls comprised both the preceding and the following male entry in the register. No cases of nasal cancer were found. Five of the 23 (22%) lung and 1 of 2 laryngeal cancer cases (in all, 24%) were employed as woodworkers, compared with 28 of 370 (8%) controls. The relative risk, controlling for age, was 4.1 (95% confidence limits, 1.6-10.6). Four of the woodworkers with lung cancer were described as furniture makers, compared with 12 of the controls, giving a crude risk ratio of 6.0; 2 of the cases with other wood-related jobs and 16 of the controls had lung cancer, giving a crude risk ratio of 2.3. This suggests that the furniture makers were at a higher risk of lung cancer than were other woodworkers. [The smoking habits of the workers were not known.]

(c)   Bladder cancer

Henry *et al*. (1931), in a study of death certificates in England and Wales between 1921 and 1928, reported 19 bladder cancers observed, whereas 18.3 were expected (relative risk, 1.04), in cabinet-makers.

(d)   Haematopoietic and lymphoreticular cancer

In a case-control study of Hodgkin's disease in the US (Milham & Hesser, 1967), 2 furniture workers appeared in the case group and none among the controls. [See also monograph on carpentry and joinery, p. 152.]

Acheson (1967) studied the occupations of patients with Hodgkin's disease registered in the Oxford area of England and found 3 woodworkers among the patients, compared with an expected number of 4, a relative risk of 0.8 (95% confidence limits, 0.2-2.2).

Brinton *et al*. (1976) studied patients from US counties where more than 1% of the population was employed in furniture making, and found an excess risk for multiple myeloma (risk ratio, 1.09) but not for Hodgkin's disease (RR = 0.98), other lymphomas (RR = 0.98) or leukaemias (RR = 0.99). [Refer to section *(a)*, p. 129, for discussion of methods.]

(f)   Other cancers not previously specified

Henry *et al*. (1931) found 16 cases of prostate cancer whereas 19.7 were expected (relative risk, 0.81) among cabinet-makers. [See also section *(c)*, above.]

Esping & Axelson (1980) found a relative risk of 1.2 (95% confidence limits, 0.5-2.9) for gastrointestinal cancer in furniture workers. [Refer to section *(b)*, p.131 , for discussion of methods.]

5. SUMMARY OF DATA AND EVALUATION

5.1 Summary of data

A number of studies are available on the relationship between nasal cancer, in particular nasal adenocarcinoma, and occupational exposure in the furniture and cabinet-making industry. An initial clinical report, pointing out the high frequency of furniture workers among nasal adenocarcinoma cases from High Wycombe (near Oxford), in England, has been followed by three epidemiological studies from the same country. In the first, an approximately twenty-fold increase in the incidence of nasal cancer has been observed in the southern part of the Oxford Hospital region, with three-quarters of the cases being represented by adenocarcinomas. In the second study, based on complete ascertainment of all cases of nasal cancer that occurred in a defined area around Oxford during a decade, a ten-fold excess risk of nasal cancer was observed for furniture workers, with 90% of the cases being adenocarcinomas (against about 10% among other occupations). The third study comprises all cases of nasal cancer registered in the whole of England and Wales (excluding the Oxford region) during a defined period, and shows an increased incidence of nasal adenocarcinoma (relative risk, about 100) among furniture workers. A smaller but still significant increase in relative risk was also found for nasal cancers other than adenocarcinomas.

Studies in other countries also show excesses of nasal cancers in furniture workers.

Less information is available with respect to other cancer risks. A death certificate survey in England and Wales showed a 30% increased incidence of lung cancer among cabinet-makers; this survey showed a decrease of a similar size for patternmakers. A SMR of 84 was seen in US mortality statistics for furniture-fixture occupations. A case-control study (involving interviews with next-of-kin of dead people) from Sweden reported a six-fold increased risk of lung cancer for furniture makers (based on four cases with the relevant exposure). The same study found a small, non-significantly increased risk for gastrointestinal cancers.

Of three studies (two from the US, one from England), which have examined the association between Hodgkin's disease and occupation in the furniture industry, none has shown an association.

There is evidence of a link between the occurrence of nasal cancers in furniture workers and the introduction of mechanized operations that produce high levels of wood dust. The English epidemiological study strongly suggests a linkage of these cancers with exposure to hardwood dusts. Nevertheless, case reports from France also relate to exposures that began in the 1950s when softwoods and exotic hardwoods came into use. One report suggests a linkage with exposure to plywood dust for some cases.

The description of the industrial process indicates the use of chemicals for which there is evidence of carcinogenicity in humans and/or experimental animals (see Appendix 4). Some of these chemicals are no longer used, but others still are.

5.2 Evaluation

There is *sufficient evidence* that nasal adenocarcinomas have been caused by employment in the furniture-making industry. The excess risk occurs mainly among those exposed to wood dust. Although adenocarcinomas predominate, an increased risk of other nasal cancers among furniture workers is also suggested. One study showed an increased relative risk for lung cancer (based on four cases from one factory); however, mortality statistics have in general shown no increase in lung cancer. No evaluation of the risk of lung cancer is possible.

6. REFERENCES

Acheson, E.D. (1967) Hodgkin's disease in woodworkers. *Lancet, ii*, 988-989

Acheson, E.D. (1976) Nasal cancer in the furniture and boot and shoe manufacturing industries. *Prev. Med., 5*, 295-315

Acheson, E.D., Hadfield, E.H. & Macbeth, R.G. (1967) Carcinoma of the nasal cavity and accessory sinuses in woodworkers. *Lancet, i,* 311-312

Acheson, E.D. Cowdell, R.H., Hadfield, E. & Macbeth, R.G. (1968) Nasal cancer in woodworkers in the furniture industry. *Br. med. J., i*, 587-596

Acheson, E.D., Cowdell, R.H. & Rang, E. (1972) Adenocarcinoma of the nasal cavity and sinuses in England and Wales. *Br. J. ind. Med., 29*, 21-30

Ager, B. (1976) Health effects in workers in the wood industry (Swed.). *Särtrvek Träindustrin, 1*

Alberti, S. (1976) Risks and resulting injuries from occupational exposure to high-frequency electromagnetic fields (Ital.). *Securitas, 61,* 27-35

Andersen, H.C. (1975) Exogenous causes of cancer of the nasal cavities (Dan.). *Ugeskr. Laeg., 137*, 2567-2571

Andersen, H.C., Solgaard, J. & Andersen, I. (1976) Nasal cancer and nasal mucus-transport rates in woodworkers. *Acta otolaryngol., 82*, 263-265

Andersen, H.C., Andersen, I. & Solgaard, J. (1977) Nasal cancers, symptoms and upper airway function in woodworkers. *Br. J. ind. Med., 34*, 201-207

Ball, M.J. (1967) Nasal cancer and occupation in Canada. *Lancet, ii,* 1089-1090

Ball, M.J. (1968) Nasal cancer in woodworkers. *Br. med. J., ii*, 253

Belli, S., Bracci, C., Comba, P. & Settimi, L. (1979) Wood dust (Ital.). *Med. Lav., 61*, 409-418

Booth, B.H., LeFoldt, R.H. & Moffitt, E.M. (1976) Wood dust hypersensitivity. *J. Allergy clin. Immunol., 57,* 352-357

Bourne, L.B. (1956) Dermatitis from mansonia wood. *Br. J. ind. Med., 13,* 55-58

Brinton, L.A., Stone, B.J., Blot, W.J. & Fraumeni, J.F., Jr (1976) Nasal cancer in US furniture industry counties. *Lancet, ii*, 628

Brinton, L.A., Blot, W.J., Stone, B.J. & Fraumeni, J.F., Jr (1977) A death certificate analysis of nasal cancer among furniture workers in North Carolina. *Cancer Res., 37*, 3473-3474

Bush, R.K., Yunginger, J.W. & Reed, C.E. (1978) Asthma due to African zebrawood *(Microberlinia)* dust. *Am. Rev. resp. Dis., 117,* 601-603

Chan-Yeung, M. & Abboud, R. (1976) Occupational asthma due to California redwood *(Sequoia semper-virens)* dusts. *Am. Rev. resp. Dis., 114,* 1027-1031

Chan-Yeung, M., Barton, G.M., McLean, L. & Grzybowski, S. (1973) Occupational asthma and rhinitis due to Western red cedar *(Thuja plicata). Am. Rev. resp. Dis., 108,* 1094-1102

Chiesura, P. (1978) *Exotic wood dusts* (Ital.). In: *Le Broncopneumopatie Professionali con Particolare Riferimento a Quelle di Nuova Tabellazione [Occupational Bronchopneumopathies with Particular Reference to Newly Tabulated Ones]*, Roma, Istituto Italiano di Medicina Sociale, pp. 53-54

Connelly, H.H. (1971) *Abrasive planing equipment and practices.* In: Dost, W.A., ed., *Wood Machining Seminar, University of California*, Richmond, CA, Forest Products Laboratory

Curtes, J.-P., Trotel, E. & Bourdiniere, J. (1977) Adenocarcinomas of the ethmoid in woodworkers (Fr.). *Arch. Mal. prof., 38,* 773-786

Debois, J.M. (1969) Tumours of the nasal cavities among woodworkers (Flem.). *Tijdschr. v. Geneeskd. 2,* 92-93

Delemarre, J.F.M. & Themans, H.H. (1971) Adenocarcinoma of the nasal cavities (Dutch). *Ned. T. Geneeskd., 115,* 688-690

Desnos, J. & Martin, A. (1973) Adenocarcinomas of the ethmoid in woodworking (Fr.). *Cah. Otorino-laryngol., 8,* 367-374

Drettner, B. & Wilhelmsson, B. (1981) *Epidemiological and experimental animal studies of the effects of various wood dust on the mucosis of the upper and lower respiratory tract* (Swed.). *Proc. Swed. Otolaryngol. Soc.* (in press)

Encyclopaedia Britannica, Inc. (1964) *Woodworking machinery.* In: *Encyclopaedia Britannica*, Vol. 23, Chicago, W. Benton, p. 726

Engzell, U. (1979) Occupational etiology and nasal cancer. *Acta otolaryngol., Suppl. 360,* 126-128

Engzell, U., Englund, A. & Westerholm, P. (1978) Nasal cancer associated with occupational exposure to organic dust. *Acta otolaryngol., 86,* 437-442

Esping, B. & Axelson, O. (1980) A pilot study of respiratory and digestive tract cancer among wood-workers. *Scand. J. Work Environ. Health* (in press)

Filca-Cisl del Veneto (1979) *L'Industria del Mobile e del Legno [The Furniture and Wood Industries]* Venezia, Arsenale Cooperativa Editrice, p. 13

Fombeur, J.-P. (1972) Recent cases of ethmoido-maxillary tumours in woodworkers (Fr.). *Arch. Mal. prof., 33,* 454-455

Gaffuri, E., Bonino, R., Terribile, P.M. & Reggiani, A. (1968) Occupational pathology due to mansonia wood (Ital.). *Folia med, 51,* 569-579

Gandevia, B. & Milne, J. (1970) Occupational asthma and rhinitis due to Western red cedar *(Thuja plicata)* with special reference to bronchial reactivity. *Br. J. ind. Med., 27,* 235-244

Gignoux, M. & Bernard, P. (1969) Malignant tumours of the ethmoid in woodworkers (Fr.). *J. Méd. Lyon, 50,* 731-736

Greenberg, M. (1972) Respiratory symptoms following brief exposure to cedar of Lebanon *(Cedra libani)* dust. *Clin. Allergy, 2,* 219-224

Hadfield, E.H. (1970) A study of adenocarcinoma of the paranasal sinuses in woodworkers in the furniture industry. *Ann. R. Coll. Surg. (UK), 46,* 301-319

Haguenauer, J.P., Romanet, P., Duclos, J.C. & Guinchard, R. (1977) Occupational cancers of the ethmoid (Fr.). *Arch. Mal. prof., 38,* 819-823

Hanslian, L. & Kadlec, K. (1964) Timber and timber dust (Czech.). *Prac. Lèk., 16,* 276-282

Henry, S.A., Kennaway, N.M. & Kennaway, E.L. (1931) The incidence of cancer of the bladder and prostate in certain occupations. *J. Hyg., 31,* 125-137

Hoos, R.A.W. (1978) *Patterns of pentachlorophenol usage in Canada - an overview.* In: Rao, K.R., ed., *Pentachlorophenol, Chemistry, Pharmacology, and Environmental Toxicology,* New York, Plenum, pp. 3-11

Hounam, R.F. & Williams, J. (1974) Levels of airborne dust in furniture making factories in the High Wycombe area. *Br. J. ind. Med., 31,* 1-9

International Labour Office (1967) *Tripartite Technical Meeting for the Woodworking Industries,* Report III, *Occupational Safety, Health and Welfare in the Woodworking Industries,* Geneva

Krogh, H.K. (1962) Contact eczema caused by true teak *(Tectona grandis).* An epidemiological investigation in a furniture factory. *Br. J. ind. Med., 19,* 42-46

Krogh, H.K. (1964) Contact eczema caused by true teak *(Tectona grandis).* A followup study of a previous epidemiological investigation, and a study into the sensitizing effect of various teak extracts. *Br. J. ind. Med., 21,* 65-68

Leroux-Robert, J. (1974) Cancers of the ethmoid in woodworkers (Fr.). *Cah. Otorinolaryngol., 9,* 585-594

Löbe, L.-P. & Ehrhardt, H.-P. (1978) Adenocarcinoma of the nose and paranasal sinuses - an occupational disease in workers in the wood industry (Ger.). *Dtsch. Gesundheitswes., 33,* 1037-1040

Luboinski, B. & Marandas, P. (1975) Cancer of the ethmoid: occupational etiology (Fr.). *Arch. Mal. prof., 36,* 477-487

Macbeth, R. (1965) Malignant disease of the paranasal sinuses. *J. Laryngol., 79,* 592-612

Milham, S., Jr & Hesser, J.E. (1967) Hodgkin's disease in woodworkers. *Lancet, ii,* 136-137

Mosbech, J. & Acheson, E.D. (1971) Nasal cancer in furniture-makers in Denmark. *Dan. med. Bull., 18,* 34-35

Oehling, A. (1963) Occupational allergy in the wood industry (Ger.). *Allerg. Asthma, 9,* 312-322

Olsen, J. & Sabroe, S. (1979) A follow-up study of non-retired and retired members of the Danish Carpenter/Cabinet Makers' Trade Union. *Int. J. Epidemiol., 8,* 375-382

Otto, J. (1973) Gravimetric measurements of dust levels near belt sanding of exotic wood for furniture (Ger.). *Z. ges. Hyg., 19,* 266-269

Pickering, C.A.C., Batten, J.C. & Pepys, J. (1972) Asthma due to inhaled wood dusts - Western red cedar and iroko. *Clin. Allergy, 2,* 213-218

doPico, G.A. (1978) Asthma due to dust from redwood *(Sequoia sempervirens). Chest, 73,* 424-425

Ruppe, K. (1973) Diseases and functional disturbances of the respiratory tract in workers in the wood-working industry (Ger.). *Z. ges. Hyg., 19,* 261-264

Salamone, L., Di Blasi, S. & Coniglio, L. (1969) Remarks on the pathology of mansonia wood (Ital.). *Folia med., 52,* 427-449

Sandermann, W. & Barghoorn, A.-W. (1956) Toxic types of wood (Ger.). *Z. Holz. Roh-Werkstoff., 14,* 37-40

Sharp, R.F. (1975) The microbial colonization of some woods of small dimensions buried in soil. *Can. J. Microbiol., 21,* 784-793

Solgaard, J. & Andersen, I. (1975) Airway function and symptoms in woodworkers (Dan.). *Ugeskr. Laeg., 137,* 2593-2599

Sosman, A.J., Schlueter, D.P., Fink, J.N. & Barboriak, J.H. (1969) Hypersensitivity to wood dust. *New Engl. J. Med., 281,* 977-980

Werner, U. (1979) On the effects of wood dust and irritant gases on the upper respiratory tract (Ger.). *Z. ges. Hyg., 25,* 290-293

Wolf, O. (1978) Occupational and nonoccupational factors involved in laryngeal cancer (Ger.). *Z. ges. Hyg., 24,* 174-177

Woods, B. & Calnan, C.D. (1976) Toxic woods. *Br. J. Dermatol., 94 (Suppl. 13),* 1-97

CARPENTRY AND JOINERY

1. HISTORICAL OVERVIEW OF THE INDUSTRY

The origins of the carpentry trade are lost in time, since wood was the first material used, even in prehistoric times, to build shelters and boats. As shelters evolved from primitive huts to the wooden houses and other constructions that we know today, the woodworking trades became increasingly more complex. Jobs that could be performed by anyone - and in the case of farm buildings, for instance, that was true even at the beginning of the century - have become specialized occupations.

A thousand or more years ago, when people began to draw together in urban and trading centres, and when stone began to compete with wood as a structural material, artisans with similar woodworking crafts banded together in professional associations, or guilds. In France, those who built habitations were distinguished by the kind of work they did into 'big felling-axe' or 'mature stand' carpenters, and 'small' or 'small felling-axe' carpenters. The latter were the ancestors of joiners. The word 'menuiserie', or joinery, was used for the first time in the sense known today in 1371. In Sweden, guilds began to be formed in the late fourteenth century. By the end of the nineteenth century, when mechanization had become widespread throughout Europe, wooden houses were built on a large scale, especially in countries with a large production of sawn timber.

In some areas of the world, woodworkers in the building industry are divided roughly into 'carpenters' and 'joiners', the carpenters being those who put up the shell of a building, make the forms for casting concrete and generally do the heavier types of work, and the joiners being those who deal with all interior details, with windows, doors, cupboards, mould-ings, panels, etc. In reality, however, there is no hard and fast division between the jobs performed, and in most parts of the world, this division is not made.

2. DESCRIPTION OF THE INDUSTRY

2.1 Processes used previously and changes over time

Originally, logs were simply jointed at either end to form corners and placed one on top of another to make a house. Later, planks were sawn - by hand - from logs. The mechanization of the sawmill industry (*vide supra*)   over the last two centuries has made it unnecessary for carpenters to prepare their own timber, and it is now usually ordered from lumber merchants.

The evolution of woodworking in the building industry has followed very much the same pattern as that of the furniture and cabinet-making industry, since many of the same materials and tools are used. However, since carpentry and some aspects of joinery are usually carried out at building sites, hand tools are still used extensively.

Until about 1930, the health problems experienced by woodworkers appear to have derived largely from the handling of wood tar and resinous wood. In the years following the Second World War, a succession of new materials were introduced on building sites. Wooden mouldings have in some cases been replaced by plastic products, and some surfaces that were previously painted have been replaced by laminated panels. Particle boards and plaster boards have replaced wood cladding; mineral wood has replaced shavings and other insulating materials.

2.2 Processes used currently

The building and public works industries require woodwork in a wide variety of applications, e.g.,
- structures exposed to water: wharfs, sluice gates, bridge sections, concrete forms
- open-air structures: pylons, railway ties, scaffolding
- covered structures: structural members and roof timbers
- closed, heated buildings: floorboards, staircases, joinery.

In France in 1978, the census showed 107,000 woodworkers in the building sector, who were employed by 20,000 employers; thus, most of the firms were craft industries. Although certain firms specialize in carpentry or in joinery, most are obliged to carry out nearly all types of woodwork required in the construction industry, with perhaps a prevalence for one or the other, depending on the training of the head of the firm.

Certain large or medium-sized firms in the construction industry own sophisticated, highly mechanized equipment with which they can carry out all operations from sawing to end product; however, such firms are rare and highly specialized, e.g., in the fabrication and installation of modern glued-laminated structural members.

The carpenter's task is to prepare, trim and assemble the various pieces of wood that make up the structure of a building, and to carry out various other aspects of construction. The structure comprises all weight-bearing members, including the roof timbers, beams, floor joists, wall sections, staircases and supports.

New techniques make wood competitive with metal and reinforced concrete, even in large constructions. Examples are toenailed jointing, triangular structures, and, most recently, due to progress in glue technology, glued-laminated structures which are particularly resistant to weight. These are made almost exclusively from northern wood.

The adhesives used in chipboard are also occasionally found in other prefabricated units used in building.

(e) Plaster (gypsum)

Inner walls and ceilings are now often constructed of plaster panels with cardboard on both sides. The dust that arises from sawing these panels is inert, but it dessicates the skin.

(f) Mineral wool

Walls and ceilings are often insulated with mineral wool. Handling of this wool releases large fibres ($>$ 0.005 mm) which may enter the skin. Finer fibres ($<$ 0.003 mm) may also be released, and these can accompany inhaled air through the respiratory tract down to the finest bronchioles.

(g) Asbestos

Although in some countries asbestos is no longer used in the construction of new buildings, it has been used widely, both alone and in the form of asbestos-cement boards and piping. Woodworkers saw and drill such boards when cladding rooms, garages and sometimes entire buildings. Almost pure asbestos may be used to plug into concrete when putting up shelves, etc.

Asbestos spraying is usually carried out by specialized companies. Since it is done at the same time as the erection of inside walls and the installation of interior fittings, however, many woodworkers are or have been exposed to asbestos or asbestos-cement dust.

Even in countries such as Sweden, where use of asbestos in new buildings has been banned since 1975, exposure to asbestos is not a thing of the past: in demolition, conversions and repairs, workers may be exposed to asbestos dust for many years to come.

(h) Acoustic boards

To improve the acoustics of completed buildings, boards made, for example, of wood-wool, pressed mineral wool or asbestos are sometimes installed. Dust containing fibres is produced when these are drilled and mounted. Wood-wool slabs consist of long wood shavings with a cementing material, which have been processed with a cement wash; the dust produced from working this material thus also contains cement.

(i)   Plastic materials

Plastic materials are used in many places on the building site; e.g., plastic foil is sometimes used to prevent diffusion in the insulation of outer walls; laminated plastic boards are installed over sinks and wash-basins; and various mouldings are made of plastic.

(j)   Polyurethane materials

Polyurethane foam was introduced into the building industry in the early 1970s. It originally appeared as a two-part product, and the resin and the curing agent were mixed in the nozzle of the spray. This material was used to fill interior walls for insulation, in place of mineral wool. It was also used on a large scale for sealing joints around windows, doors, partition walls, etc. The standard practice today is to use a pre-reacted material, called 'one-part sealing foam'. It has also proved to be a useful adhesive. When mounting the studs for interior walls, for example, a layer of polyurethane foam may be applied to the ceiling and walls before the studs are fastened. Nailing of the studs may cause splashes of foam, producing extensive skin contact with the polyurethane.

The incorrect use of polyurethane, particularly in one-part polyurethane containers, can also lead to the release of large quantities of isocyanate into the respiratory zone of workers, which may cause allergic reactions in the respiratory tract. Contact with polyurethane products before they have hardened can cause skin disorders such as eczema.

(k) Adhesives

Adhesives used in woodworking are listed in the monograph on furniture and cabinet-making, p. 107 . In some countries, such as Sweden, there is now a general requirement that adhesives containing solvents should be avoided. They are still used for the installation of, for example, laminated plastic panels; and large quantities of such adhesives have been and are still used. Many carpenters and joiners have thus been exposed to petroleum ether, toluene, xylene and benzene.

In Sweden, there are also regulations to limit the use of products containing epoxy and polyurethane compounds whenever possible. Currently, aqueous dispersion adhesives containing polyvinyl acetate or acrylate are used widely. These adhesives may contain conserving agents such as formaldehyde.

(l)   Nails and screws

The nails and screws used on building sites are sometimes polluted with the oil used during their manufacture. Nickel-plated screws are often used in work on interiors: the handling of such screws, and particularly the habit of holding them in the mouth, results in exposure to nickel.

(m) Oil on formworks

When formworks are used, personnel come into contact with the oil that is sprayed to prevent the concrete from burning. The oils in general use for this purpose contain no ingredients known to cause persistent injury to the skin. Formerly, however, waste oil was occasionally used for this purpose.

(n) Varnishes

One category of woodworkers rubs down and varnishes parquet floors. During the rubbing down, a dust is generated that consists of old varnish and wood dust.

The varnishes used in woodworking are listed in the monograph on furniture and cabinet-making, p. 113. Those used on floors contain urea resins, with formaldehyde as the curing agent, and solvents such as ethanol, butanol and ethylene glycol. When ambient concentrations have been measured during the varnishing of parquet floors in Sweden, levels of up to four times the threshold limit value have been recorded for individual solvents.

Window frames are generally varnished in the workshop. However, in certain cases, when the varnish is to be applied after installation, a light application of some antifungal material may be made in the workshop. Window frames are often given a first coat of varnish by dipping or flow-coating, then sanded and sprayed one or more times with finishing coats. They may be dried in a hot-air tunnel. Alkyd varnishes are usually used for dipping, and alkyd or polyurethane varnishes for the spray finish.

Panels, such as doors, are often varnished using the belt system, consisting of the following steps:

- sanding
- roller application of stain
- infra-red drying
- roller application of the first coat of varnish
- drying by high-intensity ultra-violet radiation
- roller application of the second coat of varnish
- drying by high-intensity ultra-violet radiation
- sanding
- last coat of varnish
- hot-air drying.

The varnishing products commonly used in this process are stains containing poly-acrylate, polyvinyl acetate or nitrocellulose in Cellosolve, polyester-allylic varnishes in styrene, and polyurethane varnishes for finishing coats.

A partial list of dyes known to be used in joinery is given in Appendix 6.

2.3 Qualitative and quantitative data on exposures (See also monograph on the furniture and cabinet-making industry, p. 115 and Appendix 4.)

Concentrations of solvents were measured in the air of three joinery workshops in France. Maximum allowable concentrations (MAC) in the US over an 8-hour working day were cited for purposes of comparison.

Samples from the first workshop were analysed for toluene. In those obtained by suction pump, 187.5 mg/m^3 (50 ppm) toluene were detected. In samples taken in the breathing zone of a worker and analysed by ultraviolet absorption spectrometry-gas chromatography, 257 mg/m^3 (67 ppm) toluene were found in those taken while the worker was spreading glue, and 157 mg/m^3 (41 ppm) in those taken a few minutes later. The US MAC for toluene is 375 mg/m^3 (100 ppm).

In the second workshop, the levels of various solvents were determined in samples taken by sampling tube during the spraying of varnish (Table 1).

Table 1. Levels of solvents in the air during varnish spraying

Solvent	Concentration (mg/m^3)	US MAC (mg/m^3)
xylene	6	435
toluene	92	375
ethyl benzene	3	435
ethyl acetate	45	1400
butyl acetate	39	710
methyl isobutyl ketone	133	410

In the third workshop, samples were taken in the area of gluing operations. In direct samples taken with an air sampling pump, no solvents were detected, due to the limits of detection of the method. In samples taken at two working positions with personal samplers fitted with activated charcoal tubes, the following levels were observed (Table 2):

Table 2. Levels of solvents in the air near gluing operations

Position	Solvent	Concentration (mg/m^3)	US MAC (mg/m^3)
1	cyclohexane	137	1050
	methyl isobutyl ketone	3.97	410
	toluene	44	375
	ethyl benzene	6.68	435
	meta- + *para*-xylene	20.09	435
2	cyclohexane	186	1050
	toluene	3.2	375
	meta- + *para*-xylene and ethyl benzene	4.2	435
	ortho-xylene	0.3	435

In the same study, determinations were also made of total dust in the air of several joinery workshops employing 2-10 workers using woodworking machines intermittently. In addition, two samples were taken in the breathing zone of workers operating circular saws (Table 3). No size distribution analyses were carried out.

Table 3. Total dust levels in six joinery workshops

Workshop	Total dust (mg/m^3 of air)	
	General air	Breathing zone
1	3.4	23.4
2	4.5	
3	2.4	
4	39.8	
5	9.1	
6[a]	72.7	547.8

[a] This was the only workshop in which there were no ventilation-extraction systems fitted at the sources of wood dust.

2.4   Biological factors

The insects and fungi found in all untreated wood are described in the monograph on the lumber and sawmill industries, p. 81 , and in the monograph on the furniture and cabinet-making industry, p. 120 .

2.5   Current regulations and recommendations on exposures

See 'General Remarks on Wood, Leather and Some Associated Industries', p. 23.

2.6   Number of workers involved

See 'General Remarks on Wood, Leather and Some Associated Industries', p. 19.

3. TOXIC, INFLAMMATORY AND ALLERGIC EFFECTS IN HUMANS

No data specific to carpentry and joinery were available. See, however, the monographs on the lumber and sawmill industries, p.   84   , and on the furniture and cabinet-making industry, p. 122 .

4. CARCINOGENICITY DATA [1]

(a)   Nasal cancer

In two Canadian studies (Ball, 1967, 1968), no excess proportion of carpenters was reported among nasal cancer (no histological type given) deaths, when deaths from nasal cancer at all sites were compared with deaths due to other causes, after controlling for year of death, age (within 2 years),and sex. [See also monograph on the furniture and cabinet-making industry, p. 128 .]

In a study covering the southern part of the Oxford Hospital Region and including an estimated subpopulation of about 7000 carpenters and joiners, complete ascertainment was attempted of cases of nasal cancer for the period 1956-1965; no case was reported for carpenters (whereas among 2000 cabinet- and chair-makers and wood machinists, 21 cases were observed) (Acheson *et al.*, 1968). [See also monograph on the furniture and cabinet-making industry, p. 127   .]

---

[1] This section should be read in conjunction with Appendices 1 and 2, pp. 295   and   301.

In a case-control study comparing cases of adenocarcinoma of the nasal cavity and sinuses with controls composed of cases of other nasal cancers in England & Wales (excluding the Oxford region), 9 cases in the series of adenocarcinomas were observed among carpenters and joiners, whereas 1.9 were expected on the basis of the occupational distribution of the one-to-one series of controls, who were matched for age (within 5 years) and who had been registered in the same region in the same year. Two of the 9 patients with adenocarcinoma had worked for only a short (unspecified) time as carpenters, and the working histories of another 2 were somewhat uncertain (Acheson et al., 1972).

In a study carried out in the state of Victoria, Australia (Ironside & Matthews, 1975), 'carpenter' was given as the occupation in 3 of 19 cases of adenocarcinoma of the nose and paranasal sinuses (16%), as compared with 2 out of 80 cases of other nasal cancers (2.5%). In the Victoria census, carpenters were included in a group of 'Carpenters, joiners, cabinet-makers and related workers'.

Andersen (1975) and Andersen et al. (1976, 1977) found no adenocarcinomas of the nose or paranasal sinuses among carpenters. [See monograph on the furniture and cabinet-making industry, p. 128, for details.]

In a study of carcinoma of the nose and paranasal sinuses carried out in Sweden (Engzell et al., 1978), 19 men out of 36 with nasal adenocarcinoma were reported to be joiners (12 of these were cabinet-makers), whereas there were 5 joiners among 127 men with squamous-cell or poorly differentiated carcinomas.

A mortality cohort study (Olsen & Sabroe, 1979) of active and retired members of the Danish Carpenter/Cabinet Makers' Trade Union showed a statistically significant elevation in the SMR for nasal cancer deaths from all histological types combined (4.67, based on 4 deaths) for the two occupational categories taken together, as compared with the general population; 1 of the 4 deaths was in a carpenter. [See also monograph on the furniture and cabinet-making industry, p. 131.]

In a case-control study in Finland comparing 45 cases of cancer of the nose and para-nasal sinuses (of which 2 were adenocarcinomas) with age- and sex-matched controls (with cancers other than of the respiratory tract), no excess of carpenters or of joiners was found among the cases. There was 1 joiner among the adenocarcinoma cases and 1 carpenter among the controls (Tola et al., 1980).

Milham (1974) found a SMR for nasal cancer of 50.4 (based on 7 deaths) in a study of members of the US Carpenters' Union. [See monograph on the lumber and sawmill industries, p. 88, for details of method.]

Seven cases of histologically confirmed nasal carcinomas, 5 in men and 2 in women, were recorded as occurring in 'woodworkers' in the Danish death registry between 1956 and 1966. The 2 women were wives of carpenters and had undifferentiated carcinomas; the tumours in the men were 4 adenocarcinomas and 1 squamous-cell carcinoma (Mosbech & Acheson, 1971).

One carpenter was mentioned in a group of 7 cases of nasal adenocarcinomas observed in one French endoscopy service between 1964 and 1972 (Desnos & Martin, 1973).

(b)   Lung cancer

Milham (1974) found an excess of tumours of the bronchus and lung (SMR = 106.7) in carpenters and joiners, based on 1218 deaths observed *versus* 1141 deaths expected; the SMR for all causes was 80.4. [See monograph on the lumber and sawmill industries, p. 88 , for details of method.]

A 3-fold increase in lung cancer was associated with wood- and paper-related occupations among rural but not urban residents in a death certificate survey in coastal Georgia (Harrington *et al.*, 1978). Although no data were presented for specific wood-working trades, the authors stated that an excess was seen among carpenters. [No data were given on smoking habits.]

A general survey of the occupations of cancer patients was undertaken at Roswell Park Memorial Institute, New York State, between 1956 and 1965 as a hypothesis-generating study. Case-control analyses were performed for patients diagnosed with one of many different cancer sites, the controls being patients diagnosed with non-neoplastic diseases. One of many results showed a relative risk of 0.87 for lung cancer among men who had worked for five or more years as carpenters, based on 31 cases (relative risk adjusted for differences in smoking habits, 1.22; not significant) (Decouflé *et al.*, 1977; Bross *et al.*, 1978).

(c)   Bladder cancer

In an early study of the incidence of bladder cancer in people in various occupations, no deviation from the expected numbers was observed among carpenters (observed deaths, 134; expected deaths standardized for age, 123.6; RR, 1.08) (Henry *et al.*, 1931).

(d)   Haemotopoietic and lymphoreticular cancer

A case-control investigation using the death certificates of 1549 white males, aged 25 years or more, who had died of Hodgkin's disease in upstate New York in the years 1940-1953 and 1957-1964 showed an excess of carpenters (33 cases *versus* 22 controls) as compared with control deaths matched by age (within 5 years), sex, race, county of residence and month of death (Milham & Hesser, 1967).

In a matched case-control study of all cases of Hodgkin's disease diagnosed in Israeli residents in the years 1960-1972, Abramson *et al.* (1978) found no overall association with occupational exposures to wood. For men who worked with 'wood or trees' the relative risk was 1.1 based on 37 cases and 34 controls. Of the 123 cases of histological subtype 'mixed cellularity', 13% were in men who worked with wood, 'predominantly in carpentry', *versus* 2.4% in controls. The relative risk for working with wood or trees for men with tumours of this cell type was 5.2 (P = 0.0005) based on 21 cases and 4 controls.

Milham (1974) found a SMR of 177 for Hodgkin's disease, based on 25 deaths, among carpenters and joiners over 60 years of age. [See monograph on the lumber and sawmill industries, p. 88   , for details of method.]

Grufferman *et al.* (1976) carried out an incidence survey of Hodgkin's disease in the Boston Standard Metropolitan Statistical Area for 1959-1973. Information on affected persons, 20-64 years old, was related to the 1960 and 1970 US decennial censuses to evaluate the rates of Hodgkin's disease in several occupational groups. Fifteen woodworkers had Hodgkin's disease (12 carpenters, 2 cabinet-makers and 1 furniture finisher), with 9.1 expected; a relative risk of 1.6 (95% confidence limits, 0.9-2.6).

(e)   Other cancers not previously specified

In the reports of Decouflé *et al.* (1977) and Bross *et al.* (1978) described above, men who had worked as carpenters for 5 years or more showed a relative risk of 1.64 (P > 0.05) for stomach cancer, based on 9 cases.

Henry *et al.* (1931) observed no increase in the incidence of prostatic cancer among carpenters (observed deaths, 114; expected deaths, 133; RR, 0.86).

5. SUMMARY OF DATA AND EVALUATION

5.1 Summary of data

An increased proportion of carpenters and joiners among nasal adenocarcinoma patients is reported from a case-control study from the UK comparing nasal adenocarcinoma with other types of nasal cancers and from two studies, one from Australia and one from Sweden, comparing series of cases of nasal adenocarcinoma with cases of other nasal cancers. In a cohort mortality study from Denmark, an increased risk for nasal cancer (any type) is reported for carpenters and cabinet-makers taken together; three of the four observed deaths occurred in workers in the latter category. No carpenter was recorded in a large Danish clinical series of patients with nasal adenocarcinomas. No cases of nasal cancer were observed among carpenters in an incidence study in the UK, which revealed a substantial number of nasal adenocarcinomas in furniture workers. No excess risk of nasal cancer (all types) for carpenters could be shown in two case-control studies, one from Canada and one from Finland.

A small elevation of relative risk for lung cancer among carpenters and joiners has been reported in one analysis of death certificates in the US, and in each of the three decennial analyses of occupational mortality reports in England and Wales. Two of these surveys also indicated an increased mortality for bladder cancer among carpenters and joiners. Four case-control studies (three from the US, one from Israel) on Hodgkin's disease show an increased risk for carpenters, limited in one study to one subcategory of the cases. An elevated risk is also reported in one analysis of occupational mortality from the US, but not in a similar study from England and Wales.

An increased risk for stomach cancer was observed in a Washington State occupational mortality analysis, but not in the data from England and Wales.

The term 'carpenter' is applied to completely different kinds of jobs in different countries: carpenters can be employed in occupations such as building, shipbuilding, metal factories and mining. Therefore, the exposure of this group of workers to chemicals and other materials varies widely and comprises a wide range of substances, for some of which there is evidence of carcinogenicity in humans and/or experimental animals (see Appendix 4).

5.2 Evaluation

The epidemiological data are not sufficient to make a definitive assessment of the carcinogenic risks of employment as a carpenter or joiner. A number of studies, however, raise the possibility of an increased risk of Hodgkin's disease. There is conflicting evidence about an association between nasal adenocarcinoma and work as a carpenter. The highest level of relative risk reported is much lower than that for cabinet-makers and other wood-workers in the furniture industry, and much of the evidence is anecdotal; the possibility that the reported cases of nasal cancer had worked in these industries could not be ruled out. The evidence suggesting increased risks of lung, bladder and stomach cancer comes from large population-based occupational mortality statistical studies and is inadequate to allow an evaluation of risks for these tumours.

6. REFERENCES

Abramson, J.H., Pridan, H., Sacks, M.I., Avitzour, M. & Peritz, E. (1978) A case-control study of Hodgkin's disease in Israel. *J. natl Cancer Inst., 61,* 307-314

Acheson, E.D., Cowdell, R.H., Hadfield, E. & Macbeth, R.G. (1968) Nasal cancer in woodworkers in the furniture industry. *Br. med. J., ii,* 587-596

Acheson, E.D., Cowdell, R.H. & Rang, E. (1972) Adenocarcinoma of the nasal cavity and sinuses in England and Wales. *Br. J. ind. Med., 29,* 21-30

Andersen, H.C. (1975) Exogenous causes of cancer of the nasal cavities (Dan.). *Ugeskr. Laeg., 137,* 2567-2571

Andersen, H.C., Solgaard, J. & Andersen, I. (1976) Nasal cancer and nasal mucus-transport rates in woodworkers. *Acta otolaryngol., 82,* 263-265

Andersen, H.C., Andersen, I. & Solgaard, J. (1977) Nasal cancers, symptoms and upper airway function in woodworkers. *Br. J. ind. Med., 34,* 201-207

Ball, M.J. (1967) Nasal cancer and occupation in Canada. *Lancet, ii,* 1089-1090

Ball, M.J. (1968) Nasal cancer in woodworkers. *Br. med. J., ii,* 253

Bross, I.D.J., Viadana, E. & Houten, L. (1978) Occupational cancer in men exposed to dust and other environmental hazards. *Arch. environ. Health, 33,* 300-307

Decouflè, P., Stanislawczyk, K., Houten, L., Bross, I.D.J. & Viadana, E. (1977) *A Retrospective Survey of Cancer in Relation to Occupation (DHEW Publ. No. (NIOSH) 77-178),* Washington DC, US Government Printing Office

Desnos, J. & Martin, A. (1973) Adenocarcinomas of the ethmoid in woodworking (Fr.). *Cah. Otorinolaryngol., 8,* 367-374

Engzell, U., Englund, A. & Westerholm, P. (1978) Nasal cancer associated with occupational exposure to organic dust. *Acta otolaryngol., 86,* 437-442

Grufferman, S., Duong, T. & Cole, P. (1976) Occupation and Hodgkin's disease. *J. natl Cancer Inst., 57,* 1193-1195

Harrington, J.M., Blot, W.J., Hoover, R.N., Housworth, W.J., Heath, C.A. & Fraumeni, J.F., Jr (1978) Lung cancer in coastal Georgia: a death certificate analysis of occupation: brief communication. *J. natl Cancer Inst., 60,* 295-298

Henry, S.A., Kennaway, N.M. & Kennaway, E.L. (1931) The incidence of cancer of the bladder and prostate in certain occupations. *J. Hyg., 31,* 125-137

Ironside, P. & Matthews, J. (1975) Adenocarcinoma of the nose and paranasal sinuses in woodworkers in the State of Victoria, Australia. *Cancer, 36,* 1115-1121

Milham, S., Jr (1974) *A Study of the Mortality Experience of the AFL-CIO United Brotherhood of Carpenters and Joiners of America, 1969-1970 (DHEW Publ. No. (NIOSH) 74-129),* Springfield, VA, National Technical Information Service

Milham, S., Jr & Hesser, J.E. (1967) Hodgkin's disease in woodworkers. *Lancet, ii,* 136-137

Mosbech, J. & Acheson, E.D. (1971) Nasal cancer in furniture-makers in Denmark. *Dan. med. Bull., 18,* 34-35

Olsen, J. & Sabroe, S. (1979) A follow-up study of non-retired and retired members of the Danish Carpenter/Cabinet Makers' Trade Union. *Int. J. Epidemiol., 8,* 375-382

Tola, S., Hernberg, S., Collan, Y., Linderborg, H. & Korkala, M.-L. (1980) A case-control study of the etiology of nasal cancer in Finland. *Int. Arch. occup. environ. Health, 46,* 79-85

THE PULP AND PAPER INDUSTRY

1. HISTORICAL OVERVIEW OF THE INDUSTRY

'Paper' is a term generally used to describe sheet materials made up of small fibres bonded together. Most commonly, the fibres are cellulose and are formed into a sheet from a water suspension. Paper derives its name from papyrus, which was used in Egypt as early as 3500 BC. Papyrus itself, however, cannot be considered paper.

Unlike many other industries, the origins of papermaking are known with some precision. Paper was invented by Ts'ai Lun, in China, in 105 AD. Using bark from the mulberry tree, bamboo, old rags and fishing nets of ramie he succeeded in producing a writing material in sheet form. The method consisted of retting, liming and pounding the raw material in a mortar and, finally, dispersion in water and straining on a bamboo sieve. The earliest surviving manuscript on paper dates back to 150 AD (Carey, 1969). The first use of paper was as a writing medium; however, writing paper now comprises less than 5% of US production (Häggblom & Ranta, 1977).

The Chinese kept their secret for over 600 years. Then the knowledge spread to the Arabs of Baghdad, where a paper-mill began operating in 793 AD. The earliest piece of paper to reach Europe was a message of congratulations from Caliph Haroun el Raschid to Charlemagne on the occasion of the latter's coronation as Emperor in 800 AD. The skills of paper making spread from Mesopotamia to Egypt and from there to the Moors of Spain. From Spain it spread through France, Italy and Germany, just in time for the invention of printing by Gutenberg in 1440, then through Holland to England. In both Russia and in the territory of the present USA, the first paper-mill was started in 1690. The founding dates of the first paper-mills are listed in Table 1.

Some discoveries indicate that the Mayans of Mexico were making paper from fig wood about 2000 years ago, before Ts'ai Lun. The details of the method are not known, however. In any event, the tradition of paper making in America was lost before the arrival of the Spaniards (Carey, 1969).

Up until the 1800s, paper was made by hand, sheet by sheet. Essentially, the method was to reduce vegetable matter by beating or pounding into individual fibres, to suspend these in a lot of water, and to pick up a charge of this suspension on a rectangular 'mould' or sieve, allowing the water to drain through, leaving the fibres as a matted web of 'paper'.

Table 1. Founding dates of first paper-mills[a]

COUNTRY	YEAR AD
China	105
Arabia	c. 750
Egypt	c. 850
Morocco	c. 1100
Spain (Xativa)	1150
France (Herault)	1189
Italy (Fabriano)	1260
Germany (Nuremberg)	1389
Switzerland (Marly)	1400
Belgium	1407
Holland (Gennep)	1428
Great Britain (Hertfordshire)	1490
Sweden (Motala)	1532
Denmark	1540
Russia (Moscow)	1690
USA (Germanstown, PA)	1690
Norway (Oslo)	1698

[a]From Carey (1969)

The mould was originally made up of thin strips of bamboo, later of a wire cloth. While the sheet was draining, the paper maker (the 'vatman') worked the mould by a special shaking action which interlocked the fibres into a strong sheet. Finally, the paper was hung up to dry. The vatman's 'shake' was a much prized accomplishment; vatmen would occasionally 'go off their shake'; for instance, having one shoulder higher than the other was an occupational hazard (Carey, 1969).

With the spread of printing, the demand for paper grew enormously, and thousands of small paper mills were established in Europe in the 1600s and 1700s (Jensen, 1968).

The first big jump in technology was the development of the paper machine. In 1798, a paper maker by the name of Louis Robert had the idea of making paper continuously. When he moved to Britain, he was backed financially by the brothers Fourdrinier, whose name has survived as the name of the machine itself. The attempts of Robert and the Fourdriniers ended in bankruptcy; but soon after that the first machine that really worked was built by the English engineer Bryan Donkin (1813). Cylindrical drying cans were patented in 1809, and by that time the machine began to take on the aspect it has today. Already in 1813, twelve continuous 'Fourdriniers' built by Donkin were in operation in Europe. In close succession, drying cylinders (1820), dandy rolls (1825) and suction boxes (1826) were added to the paper making process. The early 19th century also saw the introduction of mineral fillers (1823) and of mineral coatings (1827). The entire process could now be carried to completion in one operation. A major breakthrough in machine speeds was made possible by the invention of the suction couch roll in 1909 (Wrist, 1970).

In the times of handmade paper, the raw materials were almost exclusively rags of cotton and linen. Prior to the discovery of chlorine in 1774, the only way to make paper white was to start with white rags (Carey, 1969). The groundwood pulping process was invented in 1840. After that, in 1851, Burgess in the US and Watt in England obtained a patent for an alkaline process, the so-called 'soda process', in which birch was digested in a sodium hydroxide solution under pressure. Mills using this process were subsequently founded at different sites in Europe. In 1879, Dahl in Germany discovered that the base lost in the soda process could be made up with Glauber's salt (sodium sulphate) (Wrist, 1970). Soon after that most of the soda mills changed their processes to this new so-called 'sulphate process'.

In 1865, the Tilghman brothers in the US succeeded on a laboratory scale in removing lignin from wood using acidic solutions of bisulphite and sulphurous acid as the cooking liquor. Ekman in Sweden developed this method to a plant scale by adding an extra amount of magnesium bisulphite and sulphuric acid to the cooking liquor. The first mill to use this process was started up in 1874 in Sweden.

As calcium was cheaper than magnesium and magnesium could not be recovered, Mitscherlich in Germany developed a process which involved use of a solution of acidic calcium bisulphite as the cooking liquor. This was the origin of the sulphite process.

At first, pulp was made for paper making only. Later on, methods were developed which enabled pulp to be used in other chemical processes (Jensen, 1968). Now, pulp production has developed into an important industry. In 1974, world production of pulp, semichemical pulp and groundwood was 123 million tonnes in all. The US had by far the greatest production, with about 44 million tonnes. The other large producers were Canada, 19.5 million tonnes, Japan, 10.0 million tonnes, Sweden, 9.8 million tonnes and Finland, 6.6 million tonnes. Daily world production of pulp today is about 100 million tonnes (Anon., 1980).

Pulp is used mainly for paper and paperboard products, of which the following are a few: bag and wrapping paper, printing paper, paper for newsprint, various household papers, cartons and corrugated paperboards. The next greatest use for pulp is in various synthetic fibres (Häggblom & Ranta, 1977).

Until recently, paper of the most demanding standards, such as for banknotes and legal documents, was made from rags; but the situation is changing rapidly. The best wood papers can last for 300 or 400 years. Nowadays, 85-90% of paper is made from wood, and there are over 5000 different types of paper (Carey, 1969).

2. DESCRIPTION OF THE INDUSTRY

2.1 Processes used previously and changes over time

(a) Pulp industry

The components of wood are not mixed homogeneously: cellulose makes up the main framework of the cell walls of the wood fibres, and lignin serves as the adhesive material of wood, cementing the fibres and other cells together. Lignin can be removed from the wood, leaving the separated cellulosic fibres in the form of a pulp. In addition to the cell wall substance, wood also contains other materials in the cavities of the cells. The following methods have been used to separate wood fibres (Häggblom & Ranta, 1977):

(i)   mechanical pulping,
(ii) chemical pulping, and
(iii) combinations of chemical and mechanical pulping.

During the 1920s many technical developments were made in the utilization of ground-wood. Synthetic grindstones, introduced in 1920, permitted larger units, and the process could be changed from an intermittent one to a continuous one. Coupled horsepower rose from a record of 1000 hp in 1920 to 6700 hp by 1929. Such achievements were accomplished, however, without a significant increase in the understanding of the process itself, and therefore little improvement was made in reducing the large variation in pulp quality (Wrist, 1970).

The basic mechanisms of the grinding process began to emerge by the 1950s, as a result of work by scientists in Canada and the Federal Republic of Germany. The process was shown to consist of two steps: during the first the fibre is released, and in the second the separated fibres are strengthened. The use of two stages in making groundwood has replaced the traditional grindstones. The result is better strength and greater fibre length. Mechanical treatment alone has proven satisfactory only on softwoods and on soft hardwoods such as aspen. Combinations of very mild chemical systems with mechanical defibrating have been used with limited success to produce very high-yield hardwood pulps (Wrist, 1970).

The most successful high yield chemical/mechanical pulping system has been the Neutral Sulphite Semichemical (NSSC) process, which was developed in 1925 in the US. A mild digestion in a neutral liquor removes a major portion of the lignin, and the loss of hemicelluloses is low. A high yield (65-85%) of pulp results after mechanical defibration. Engineering developments in the 1930s greatly increased the use of NSSC pulping. Today, unbleached NSSC hardwood pulp is used extensively for the manufacture of fluting medium. Bleached NSSC pulp is also used to a limited degree in making fine papers. In the past two or three decades, recovery systems have been developed for NSSC (Wrist, 1970).

The fastest growing sector in pulping has been the sulphate (kraft) process. This process is suitable for various wood species, and the strength of the fibres produced is high. Chemical recovery systems have also been an area of remarkable development. In recent years, major advances have been made in the field of continuous digesters; several designs have been developed. The most widely installed digester for kraft has been the Kamyr digester. Units with capacities of up to 1000 tonnes/day have been built, and many of them are being operated under computer control. Batch digesters have been developed, and the result has been pulp of much better quality. Reduction of process volume and of cooking time are current objectives in the development of continuous processes (Wrist, 1970).

Over the past 60 years, several modifications have been made in the sulphite process, although as a whole this process has experienced very limited growth. Changes in base from calcium to sodium, ammonium or magnesium and to multistage procedures have permitted a wider range of woods to be pulped by this method and have facilitated evaporation and combustion of the waste liquor; in a few instances, these changes have aided chemical recovery.

The total number of uses for the sulphite waste liquor has increased notably. Many mills utilize the sugar in waste liquor to produce alcohol, another use is in the production of protein-rich products. For example, some mills in Finland produce the so-called Pekilo protein and Torula yeast from waste liquor. Vanillin is another by-product and is used as a raw material for spices and pharmaceuticals (Wrist, 1970; Häggblom & Ranta, 1977).

(b) Paper industry

(i)   *Raw materials:* Table 2 illustrates the changes that have occurred over the last century in the raw materials used in Germany.

Table 2. Raw materials used in the paper industry in Germany, in percentages[a]

year	rags	cellulose	wood pulp	waste paper
1870	40	48	12	-
1900	10	44	37	9
1914	6	43	40	11
1937	2	37	33	28
1950	4	40	25	31
1965	2	34	17	47

[a]From Brecht (1970)

In 1880, the amount of straw cellulose used was as high as 40%, compared with 1.3% in 1968 (Brecht, 1970).

(ii)   *Beating and refining:*   Before the Second World War, three important development stages in the mechanical treatment of raw pulp coming into the paper mill had taken place: batch hollander → continuous hollander (in 1925) → hydropulper (in 1939).

The change from hollander to hydropulper also meant a change from treatment of a comparatively dry material to a material with a high water content which could be pumped. The new technique made it possible to use waste paper as a raw material. The flotation method, developed in 1956, for removing printing ink from waste paper was an important contributing factor. Development of the hydropulper also meant an essential changeover in the machinery of pulp treatment: the result was a hydropulper-sorting-refiner system (Brecht, 1970).

In the early 1950s, several high velocity vortex cleaners were developed for removing dirt and bark. Around 1960, pressurized screens using hydrodynamic pulsations to clean the slotted plate appeared. The role of air bubbles in promoting flocculation was recognized, and vacuum chambers are now used to increase the rate of drainage from the paper machine. On the basis of research done in the early 1950s, fibre length distribution is now controlled by precision disc refiners (Wrist, 1970).

(iii) *Paper and paper board machines:* The capacity of paper machines has grown enormously over the last 100 years (Tables 3 and 4).

Table 3. **Development of the rotation press paper machine**[a]

year	screen width (m)	speed (m/min)	production (tonnes/24 hr)
1866	1.5 - 1.6	5 - 30	∿ 2.5
1880	1.80	5 - 30	∿ 4.0
1881	2.35	4 - 34	6.3
1890	2.00	60 - 80	9.0
1904	2.70	120	23.0
1919	5.90	300	130.0
1924	6.00	300	130.0
1929	7.72	300	175.0
1937	3.60	450	110.0
1956	8.68	650	∿ 350.0
1961	8.35	650 - 700	∿ 350.0
1967	9.00	750 - 800	550.0
1967	8.50	915	580.0
1970	9.855	920	650.0

[a] From Brecht (1970)

The increase in speed has been most marked in the production of tissue paper and related products, which are now made at a speed of 1500 m/min. During the last 100 years the capacity of the flat sieve paper machine has increased 150-fold and that of the cylinder sieve paper board machine 50-60 fold (Brecht, 1970).

The emphasis in machine design during the 1920s and 1930s was to exploit the drilled suction roll, particularly in the press section. Other developments before 1950 were Grewin cross ventilation, the Minton and Yankee dryers and air hoods (Wrist, 1970). By 1940, the change from use of the Siphon headbox to the use of pressurized air was complete (Brecht, 1970).

Table 4. Development of the cylinder screen paper board machine[a]

year	screen width (m)	speed (m/min)	production (tonnes/24 hr)
1875	1.5 - 2	10 - 15	1.5 - 2
1905	1.5 - 2	10 - 15	10
1917	3	60 - 80	90 - 110
1935	3.0 - 4.5	100 - 110	120 - 180
1957	6.0	200	400 - 600
1970	3.0 - 5.5	100 - 200	120 - 250
1970	5.5	350	over 300

[a]From Brecht (1970)

By 1950, top newsprint speeds were around 550 m/min, and tissue machine speeds about 750 m/min; in 1970, top speeds for newsprint were about 900 m/min. This was a result of many developments in machine design, e.g., the modern pressure headbox with its cross-flow manifold and the vacuum pickup press section (Wrist, 1970).

During the 1970s attempts were made to find technical solutions different from the classical Fourdrinier machine. It can be anticipated that the supremacy Fourdrinier has enjoyed for 170 years will be severely challenged within the near future. Instead of an open wire sieve, for instance, several 'enclosed formation' approaches have been presented for both flat papers and tissues (Wrist, 1970).

The breakthrough in machine roll coating came in the 1930s. The second important development in the conversion product field resulted in a blade coating process that is prevalent today. Other features of the new paper conversion technology are, e.g., incorporation of noncellulosic fibres, and combinations with plastics either in coatings, by impregnation or by chemical reactions (Wrist, 1970).

(iv)   *Additives and slime controlling substances:* Sizes, fillers and colouring matters were brought into use in the 1800s. Nowadays, about 90% of all paper and paper board contain additives. New chemicals come onto the market every year, and, in fact, production of paper additives is increasing more rapidly than is that of paper itself.

Originally, the term 'size' was applied to compounds that made paper more or less water-repellent. It is now extended to other substances which are used to improve not only resistance to liquid penetration but also many other quality factors (Freeman, 1969).

Aniline dyestuffs were discovered in the late 1800s; now practically all of the dyestuffs used in the paper industry belong to this class of compounds, traditionally obtained by the distillation of coal-tar (Freeman, 1969).

Originally, mercury compounds and other toxic substances were used for controlling slime growth in the paper process (Ball, 1972). In the late 1950s and the 1960s, pentachlorophenol and/or its sodium salt began to be used as slimicides and defoaming agents in the manufacture of paper and paper board. Pulp and finished paper products are protected against mildew, rot and termites by the addition of sodium pentachlorophenol. Now there is a great selection of specific chemicals available (Ahlberg, 1976).

2.2 Processes used currently

(a) Pulp industry

Raw materials for the pulp and paper industry can be classified as fibrous and nonfibrous. Wood is the most important fibrous raw material. In some countries the major sources of fibre are linen rags, cotton linters, cereal straws, esparto, hemp, jute, flax, bagasse and bamboo.

Wood is converted into pulp by mechanical, chemical or semichemical processes. The most common chemical processes are the sulphite, sulphate (kraft) and soda processes. Neutral sulphite is the principal semichemical process. Coniferous wood species are the most desirable, but the share of deciduous woods has been growing rapidly and presently constitutes about 25% of the total pulpwood material produced.

Nonfibrous raw materials include the chemicals used for the preparation of pulping liquors and bleaching solutions. These comprise sulphur, lime, limestone, sodium hydroxide, salt cake (sodium sulphate), soda ash, hydrogen peroxide, chlorine, sodium chlorate, magnesium hydroxide and magnesium carbonate.

(i) *Wood preparation:* The bark of trees contains relatively little fibre, and the quality of this fibre is poor; bark also contains much strongly coloured nonfibrous material, which usually appears as dark-coloured specks in the finished paper. Therefore, the bark is removed to produce high-grade pulps, if the finished paper is to appear clean. Debarking must be very thorough in the cases of groundwood and sulphite pulps.

At present, logs are debarked in mills almost exclusively by various types of machines, which can be classified according to their operating principles:

(1) knife debarkers, which cut the bark with knives;
(2) rubbing debarkers, in which bark is removed by the rubbing action of logs against each other and against the walls of the apparatus, either in drum debarkers, in which the logs are in random array, or in pocket debarkers, in which the logs are parallel;
(3) debarkers in which the logs are debarked one by one by rubbing or scraping (for example, the Cambio barker); and
(4) hydraulic debarkers, which use high-pressure water jets.

The recent growth in the use of wood residues has been remarkable. Residues that were formerly burned can now be used to make pulp, and almost one-third of the wood used in the pulp industry can be classified as waste wood.

Wood used in producing groundwood or mechanical pulp requires no further preparation after debarking. Wood used in the chemical processes must first be chipped into small pieces of 15-30 mm in length and about 3-6 mm in thickness. Chipping is accomplished with a machine consisting of a rotating disc with knives. The desired chip geometry may be achieved by changing the number of knives on the discs, the feeding angles of the logs and the knife sizes. Chip size is not uniform, and screens are necessary to separate the oversize chips and sawdust from the acceptable chips.

(ii) *Mechanical pulping:* Mechanical pulping does not involve a chemical process; however, it is one of the more important methods of making pulp: newsprint consists of about 80% mechanical pulp. Groundwood pulp is made by forcing entire logs against the face of a cylindrical abrasive stone rotating at a relatively high speed. The logs are positioned so that their axes are parallel to the axis of the rotating stone. Sufficient water must be applied to the stone to cool it and to carry the pulp away. The quality and coarseness of the grindstone can be varied to produce pulps to fit their desired end use. Pulp characteristics can also be varied by changing the stone surface pattern, the stone speed, the pressure of the logs against the stone and the temperature of the ground-pulp slurry. The type and condition of the wood are also important factors, although groundwood pulps usually come from coniferous or long-fibred species, because deciduous or short-fibred species produce very weak pulps.

One recent development has been the use of trimming residues and sawdust as raw material for mechanical pulping. First, the wood is chipped; then the chips are fed between a rotating disc containing steel plates with fine teeth. This method produces a stronger groundwood and has the additional advantage of allowing some chemical pretreatment of the chips. Thus, a class of pulp called chemimechanical pulp is produced by treating the chips with a dilute solution of sodium hydroxide or sodium sulphite prior to refining. The chips can also be pretreated with water vapour, in which case the pulp is called thermo-mechanical pulp.

Groundwood or mechanical pulp is low in strength compared with the chemical pulps. It is composed of a mixture of individual fibres, broken fibres, fines and bundles of fibres. Papers made from groundwood also lose strength and turn yellow with time. Thus, ground-wood pulps are used only in relatively impermanent papers such as newsprint, catalogues, etc., especially since groundwood papers have excellent printing qualities. It is the cheapest pulp made since it totally utilizes the wood, resulting in a yield of almost 100% (Jahn & Strauss, 1974; Häggblom & Ranta, 1977).

(iii) *Chemical pulping:* In chemical pulping processes, the lignin between the wood fibres is solubilized with the help of certain chemicals so that the fibres separate from each other relatively undamaged. Thus, the strength of the pulp is high. Unfortunately, reactions of cellulose and other components with the cooking liquors cannot be avoided. As a result, chemical processes have a relatively small yield, usually 45-55%.

Wood pulping operations normally proceed as follows: the logs are debarked and chipped; the chips are cooked or digested in a large vessel under high pressure and temperature. It is at this stage of the operation that the reaction occurs between the effective chemicals and lignin. After cooking, the liquor is washed away from the fibres and the impurities are separated. The washed and screened pulp is now ready for bleaching, if desired; then the bleached or unbleached pulp is collected on sheets or used directly for paper making. The spent cooking liquor is evaporated and burned, and, depending on the process used, the recovered chemicals can be reused.

There are two main chemical processes, namely, the alkaline process and the acidic process.

The most important alkaline process is the sulphate or kraft process. The active chemical is a mixture of sodium hydroxide and sodium sulphide. The term 'sulphate process' is misleading, but it is known as such because sodium sulphate is used as the compensation chemical. The German term 'kraft' is used because the process produces the strongest pulp. The process is also called the 'soda process', if the chemical loss is made up by addition of sodium carbonate or soda. The unbleached sulphate pulp is brown and is used to make different kraft papers and packaging paper boards. Almost any kind of wood can be pulped by the kraft process; pine is the wood most commonly used. The pre-hydrolysing process is one modification of the sulphate process.

Acidic processes involve use of bisulphite solutions as the cooking liquor. The oldest and still the most important process makes use of an acidic solution (pH, about 1.5) of calcium bisulphite, containing an excess amount of sulphur dioxide. Calcium may be replaced by magnesium, sodium or ammonium. This process is often used for low-resin woods, e.g., spruce.

In a modification of this process, the cooking liquor consists of a solution of magnesium, ammonium or sodium bisulphite with no excess of sulphur dioxide, and a pH of 4-6. This process has the advantage that the pH of the liquor can be changed: cooking can thus be carried out in two or three stages each of which is at a different pH, making it possible to vary the pulp type obtained.

Acidic processes produce relatively light-coloured pulps, which are suitable for making some printing papers. Many sulphate and sulphite mills bleach their products so that the pulp can be used for printing papers, newsprint and various kinds of paper board.

Alkaline processes

The pulping (cooking) process has traditionally been carried out on a batch basis in a large vessel called a digester. The type of wood being pulped and the desired quality of the end product dictate the cooking conditions used. For example, in typical kraft cooking the pressure is 690-790 kPa, the temperature is 170-175°C and the cooking time varies between 2 and 3 hours. The acting alkali charge ranges from 15 to 25% of the weight of the wood. The liquor to wood ratio is four to one by weight.

Digesters are cylindrical in shape with a dome at the top and a cone at the bottom. The height of a digester may reach 12 m and the diameter 6 m. The largest digesters hold about 35 tonnes of wood chips. The chips are admitted through a large valve at the top. At the end of the cooking they are blown from the bottom through a valve to a large blow tank. During the cooking the liquor is heated by being circulated through a steam-heat exchanger. This method is used to prevent the dilution of the liquor that would occur if steam were injected into it directly.

In recent years continuous digesters have been developed, in which chips are admitted continuously at the top through a special high-pressure feeder, and the cooked pulp is withdrawn continuously from the bottom through a special blow unit. Recent installations may be up to 50 m high and can produce 1000 tonnes of pulp per day. Cooking liquors and conditions are approximately the same as for the batch digesters. These continuous units offer both economy in the production of pulp and a quality advantage as compared with the batch digester. Still, the capital investment needed to install a continuous digester is substantial; therefore, in new mills thoughout the world batch digesters are as common as continuous ones.

Due to the high alkali charge, the chemicals must be recovered and reused, a practice which also helps to alleviate the pollution problem, since the yield of pulp is only about 45% of the original wood weight and these organic residues must be eliminated. After being cooked, the pulp is washed in a countercurrent rotary vacuum washer system using three or four stages. Then the pulp is bleached or is used in papers for such products as grocery bags in which the brown colour is not objectionable.

The separated liquor, which is very dark and is known as 'black liquor', is concentrated in multieffect evaporators until it is 60-65% solid. At this concentration, the quantity of dissolved organic compounds from the wood is sufficient to allow it to be burned in the recovery furnace. The inorganics are collected on the bottom of the furnace as a molten smelt of sodium carbonate and sodium sulphide. Sodium sulphate is added to the liquor as a compensation compound and is reduced to sodium sulphide by carbon. The smelt is dissolved in water, and the mixture (called 'green liquor') is reacted with caustic lime as follows:

$$Na_2CO_3 + Ca(OH)_2 \rightarrow 2NaOH + CaCO_3 \text{ (as a precipitate)}.$$

Since the sodium sulphide does not react with the lime, the resultant mixture of sodium hydroxide and sodium sulphide (called 'white liquor') can be reused to pulp more wood. The calcium carbonate sludge is filtered off, burned in a lime kiln and reused. The chemical system is a closed one, and this minimizes costs and pollution.

In some countries, the kraft process presents a serious air pollution problem due to the production of hydrogen sulphide, mercaptans and other vile-smelling sulphur compounds. Elsewhere, however, the use of various techniques such as liquor oxidation, improved evaporators and furnaces and the control of emissions have improved the situation.

Because the pulp produced by the kraft process is very strong, this method has become the dominant process used throughout the world. When resin-rich woods are pulped, the kraft process yields turpentine and tall oil as valuable by-products.

Sulphite processes

During the last decades, the production of sulphite pulp has remained relatively constant. The rapid growth of kraft pulping has reduced the overall share of sulphite pulp to less than 10% of the chemical pulp produced in the world today. There are several reasons for this. The primary ones are the inability to cook resinous woods such as pine, problems in producing strong pulps from hardwoods; recently of the greatest importance has been the lack of cheap and simple recovery systems such as those employed in the kraft process. However, the sulphite process is used for producing pulps with special qualities.

This process is relatively easy to carry out. It is based on the fact that under acidic conditions lignin reacts with the bisulphite ion (HSO_3^-) to form lignosulphonates that are soluble in water. The pulp produced is of light colour and is therefore easy to bleach. One attractive feature is that the chemicals used are required in fairly limited amounts.

The cation of the cooking base may be calcium, sodium, magnesium or ammonium; the latter three of which can be recovered. Regardless of the base used, the initial step is to burn sulphur to produce sulphur dioxide. The air supply to the burner must be carefully controlled: too much air will enhance the formation of sulphur trioxide and the subsequent production of sulphuric acid, which is undesirable. The gas must also be cooled quickly from 1000°C to below 400°C in order to minimize the formation of sulphur trioxide. After cooling to 20-30°C, the sulphur dioxide gas must be absorbed in water and reacted with a suitable base to form the cooking liquor.

For a calcium-based liquor, the gas is passed through towers packed with limestone with water flowing down through the towers. Because of the limited solubility of calcium bisulphite, the pH of the liquor must be very low, and free sulphurous acid must be present. It is for this reason that the method is called the 'acid sulphite process'.

The so-called soluble bases have certain advantages: with the acid sulphite process cooking times range from 7-10 hours, whereas 4-5 hours are sufficient with bisulphite. Since solutions of sodium, magnesium and ammonium bisulphite are all soluble at pH 4.5, processes using any of these materials are called 'bisulphite pulping'. The sodium base is the easiest to prepare (sodium carbonate or sodium hydroxide is usually used) and yields the highest quality pulp. The recovery processes available for this base are, however, complicated and expensive. The magnesium base (from magnesium hydroxide) is somewhat more difficult to handle, but good recovery systems are available; a majority of the sulphite pulp is now produced from this base. The ammonium base has also been used, but ammonia cannot be recovered.

Batch digesters are usually used in the sulphite process. Cooking temperatures are lower (140-150°C) and the times are longer than in the alkaline processes. Pulp yields are

about the same as in the kraft process.   Spruce and low-resin firs are the preferred species
for cooking, and the product is a relatively strong, light-coloured pulp.   About 20% of
newsprint consists of unbleached pulp of this type.

Vanillin, alcohol and Torula yeast can be produced as by-products.

Other pulping processes

Various combinations of chemical and mechanical treatment can be used to produce
pulp with specific properties.   Mild chemical treatments give partial delignification and
softening.   A mechanical treatment follows in order to complete fibre separation.

The neutral sulphite semichemical (NSSC) process is one in which wood chips, usually
from hardwoods, are cooked with sodium sulphite liquor buffered with either sodium
bicarbonate, sodium carbonate or sodium hydroxide to maintain a slightly alkaline pH
during the cooking.   Unbleached pulp from hardwoods cooked to a yield of about 75% is
widely used as a corrugating medium.   Bleachable pulps require large quantities of bleaching
chemicals, and the waste liquors are difficult to recover.   Many NSSC mills are located
adjacent to kraft mills, so that the liquors can be treated in the same furnace.

(iv)   *Screening and cleaning of wood pulp:*   The desired pulp fibres are usually
between 1-3 mm in length with a diameter of about 0.01-0.03 mm.   Any bundles of fibres
or other impurities would show up as defects in the finished paper and must be screened
out. Wood knots are difficult to pulp and must be removed.

Screening is usually a two-stage process: at first the coarse material is removed by
screens with relatively large perforations, then fine screening ensures the removal of over-
sized impurities.   Screen-size opening diameters depend on the species of wood being
processed and the desired quality of the end product.   The fibres have a tendency to agglo-
merate when suspended in water;   therefore, the fibre content is kept very low (0.5% fibre
and 99.5% water).

Cleaner and cleaner pulps are being demanded.   As a result, the centrifugal cyclone
cleaner has come into almost universal use.   The screened pulp is pumped through these
cleaning units at a low consistency and a high velocity. Sand and other dirt are removed in
this way. When cleaning is done in many stages, the efficiency increases.

(v)   *Bleaching of wood pulp:*   The colour of unbleached sulphite pulp ranges
from cream to tan.   The colour of unbleached sulphate pulp is dark brown.   In each case,
the pulping process has removed 75-90% of the lignin;   the remaining lignin and other
coloured degradation products must be removed or decoloured by bleaching.

It is possible to improve the brightness of the pulp in one stage; however, the achieve-ment of high brightness requires the use of several stages. Current practice involves use of combinations of chlorination with elemental chlorine, alkaline extraction with sodium hydroxide, and various oxidative stages using sodium or calcium hypochlorite, chlorine dioxide or hydrogen peroxide. Chlorine dioxide must be generated at the site using sodium chlorate as the basic chemical. The pulp is washed between stages to remove solubilized impurities. Many combinations are possible: each mill selects the sequence that fits its requirements best. The greater the number of stages, the higher the quality. Sulphite pulp mills usually use three- or four-stage sequences. Kraft pulps require additional stages.

The bleaching sequences are designed to remove lignin, thereby yielding a highly purified fibre consisting only of carbohydrate material. However, in producing ground-wood, lignin is not removed: the improvement in brightness is attained by using only one stage with either peroxide or hyposulphite (dithionite). No yield loss occurs; the action of these chemicals merely decolourizes the pulp but does not remove any impurities.

(vi) *Collecting and drying of wood pulp:* For transportation and long-term storage, the fibres are collected from the slurry, dried into sheets and packed according to certain sizes and weights (Jahn & Strauss, 1974; Häggblom & Ranta, 1977).

(b) Paper industry

(i) *The modern paper making process:* The steps of paper making are as follows: slushing (hydropulping), beating and refining, addition of additives, control of consistency, cleaning, sheet forming, pressing, drying, glazing, cutting, sorting and packing.

Cellulose or other fibre is *slushed* into a fibre mixture or pulp. The machine most generally used for this purpose is the *hydropulper* (Kemppainen, 1978). In the *beating* stage, the fibres are treated mechanically to enhance bond formation between the fibres. This is accomplished in a pulp-water mixture by means of machines operating either on batches or continuously (Ryti, 1974; Kemppainen, 1978).

After this, *additives,* such as size and fillers, are combined with the fibre-water mixture (Freeman, 1969). The composition of these additives is discussed in section 2.3, p. 182 .

Fillers are used at the wet end of the machine in order to improve the properties of the final product, e.g., brightness, smoothness, softness and ink receptivity. All fillers are insoluble in water (Häggblom & Ranta, 1977).

Sizing is the process of adding materials to the paper in order to render the sheet more resistant to penetration by liquids, particularly water. Writing and wrapping papers are typical sized sheets, as contrasted with blotting paper and tissue which are typically unsized.

The agents may be added directly to the stock to give 'internal' or 'engine' sizing, or the dry sheet may be passed through a size solution or over a roll wetted with a size solution. Rosin, which is refined from pine trees or stumps, is a widely used sizing agent. At paper mills, partially saponified rosin paste is diluted to about 3% solids, and this solution is added to the stock with aluminium sulphate, which precipitates the rosin onto the fibres. This process can be accomplished at a pH of 4.5 - 5.5; in recent years, sizing agents capable of producing sizing at pHs of 7.0 - 8.5 have been developed (Häggblom & Ranta, 1977).

The colour of most papers and paperboards, including white sheets, is achieved in part by the addition of dyes, most of which are added to the stock. Water-soluble synthetic and organic dyestuffs are the principal colouring materials used, although some colouring is done with water-insoluble pigments such as carbon black, vat colours, colour lakes and sulphur colours (Freeman, 1969; Häggblom & Ranta, 1977).

Apart from fillers, sizes and colours, many other additives, such as starch added as an adhesive, may be used.

The *consistency* of the pulp slurry must remain constant so that the slurry flows into the machine as a sheet of even thickness. This is controlled by adding water. The pulp is *cleaned* by removing foreign particles and fibre bunches (Kemppainen, 1978).

Sheet forming begins in the headbox, from which the diluted water-fibre mixture flushes through a sluice to the moving wire sieve. Most of the water is removed at this stage, so that the sheet now contains about 20% solids (Kemppainen, 1978). The most important types of wire sieve machines are th plane-sieve machine (the most common), the cylinder-sieve machine and the double-sieve machine.

From the wire sieve the sheet is moved to the couch *press,* where it loses more water so that the solids content increases to 35%. The types of press are the smooth press (both cylinders are smooth), the suction press (lower cylinder drilled), the wire-sieve press (water removed through a drilled plastic sieve) and the channel press (water flows through channels in the lower cylinder).

Final *drying* of the sheet is accomplished by vapourizing over heated cylinders, so that at the dry end of the machine the sheet contains only 5-8% of water. The most common type of drying machine is the multicylinder dryer. The Yankee dryer is also used to some extent; in this machine the sheet is pressed onto the surface of a large iron cylinder.

Paper is *glazed* by conducting the sheet through a multicylinder calender in which the paper is pressed between the cylinders in order to give it a smooth surface. The completed paper sheet is *cut* into narrower rolls, and part is cut by a sheet cutter into separate sheets. Paper to be sold by sheets is *sorted* and inferior qualities removed (Kemppainen, 1978).

Some types of paper require conversion, usually by coating. The coating methods used are blade coating (the coating mixture is applied to the surface of the paper by means of a blade) and air doctor coating (excess coating material is removed by air flow) (Ryti, 1974). Coatings themselves can be divided into pigment coatings (inorganic), which are used principally on printing papers, and barrier coatings (organic) (Häggblom & Ranta, 1977).

Pigment coatings are applied to the base paper in the form of a water suspension. The total solid content may vary from 35 to 70%. Paper may be coated either on equipment which is an integral part of the paper machine or on separate converting equipment. The operation is rapid compared with the speeds of paper machines, and this has resulted in the development of separate coating machines. Coated paper is also supercalendered to improve its surface properties (Häggblom & Ranta, 1977).

A barrier coating may be needed against water, water vapour, oxygen, carbon dioxide, greases, fats and oils and miscellaneous chemicals. The coating material may be applied in a molten condition, in solution, or as an emulsion. Of the materials applied in molten form, paraffin wax has been the most popular: it is easily applied by passing the paper through a molten bath or nip, removing the excess, and chilling. Another material applied in molten form is polyethylene; special arrangements are needed to permit rapid heating of the polymer pellets while maintaining minimum contact with air. Solvent systems permit the formulation of highly sophisticated coatings which incorporate a wide variety of polymers. Disadvantages include the high cost of the solvents or the necessity of having a solvent recovery system (Häggblom & Ranta, 1977).

(ii) *Biphenyl paper:* Biphenyl paper is used mainly for the packing of citrus fruits. Impregnantion of the paper is usually carried out in the paper mill that manufactures the wrapping. The biphenyl is first dissolved in paraffin oil and then applied by a heater roller to the paper while it is still in the machine.

The biphenyl-paraffin oil solution is prepared in a separate room, where the so-called 'oilman' dispenses biphenyl from paper sacks into a mixing container. The mixture is heated to 90°C and pumped into a basin connected to the paper machine. The solution is then spread on silk paper at the dry end of the machine at a temperature of 90°C. Before the equipment is used to make another type of paper, it is cleaned with tetrachloroethylene (Häkkinen *et al.*, 1973).

2.3 Qualitative and quantitative data on exposures

(a) Chemical exposures in the pulp industry

The majority of the studies on exposures in pulping concern gaseous sulphur compounds, chlorine and chlorine dioxide. The gaseous sulphur compounds can be classified as sulphur dioxide and so-called 'vile-smelling' sulphur compounds, which consist of hydrogen sulphide, various organic sulphides and mercaptans. Vapours emanating from pulp may contain turpentine, sodium hydroxide mist, methanol, ethanol, sulphuric acid, furfural, hydroxymethylfurfural, cymene, acetic acid, formic acid, gluconic acid, aldonic acid and hydrogen peroxide. Dusts consisting of lime, sodium sulphate, etc. are also present and pose a potential exposure risk during the chemical recovery process. Compounds used for control of slime and algae also constitute potentially harmful exposures.

Feiner & Marlow (1956a,b) measured sulphur dioxide concentrations in a number of sulphite pulp mills in the US, using a Mine Safety Appliances gas detector. The results ranged between 2-50 ppm; however, since the upper limit of detection of their equipment was 50 ppm, the authors assumed that concentrations may have been much greater than those they recorded.

Maksimov (1957) made measurements in sulphate mills under normal process conditions, although no information about the sampling methods and exact locations were given. Methylmercaptan concentrations were 3.4-13 ppm and hydrogen sulphide concentrations 1.4-4.6 ppm. The measured concentration of sodium hydroxide mist was 1.5 mg/m^3 and that of turpentine below 54 ppm.

Kurkijärvi (undated) used indicator tubes and liquid absorption followed by iodometric titration to study the sulphur dioxide levels in a number of Finnish sulphite pulp mills. At pyrite and sulphur kilns, the concentrations were usually 2-20 ppm, but during disturbances in the process concentrations were higher. Under normal working conditions, with short exposures, the concentrations were 10-35 ppm. During repairs and servicing, the measured concentrations varied from 10 to 110 ppm. In digester plants, the sulphur dioxide concentrations were 40-180 ppm, but exposures were occasional and their duration was short.

In a study on the long-term effects of exposure to sulphur dioxide in 4 pulp mills, Skalpe (1964) measured the concentrations in the acid tower and in digester plants, using indicator tubes, under general working conditions over one day. The measured values ranged between 2 and 36 ppm. Under special conditions the concentrations increased up to 100 ppm, but the duration of these periods was only a few minutes. Nevertheless, at such times the respiratory irritation was so intense that workers had to use protective equipment. Exposure to sulphur dioxide in the pulp mills investigated appeared to have caused a significantly higher incidence of symptoms of respiratory disease in a group of exposed workers than in a comparable control group.

In a study on the prevalence of chronic respiratory disease in workers in pulp and paper industries (Ferris *et al.*, 1967), sulphur dioxide concentrations measured during three years ranged between < 0.1 and 33 ppm. Both sampling methods and indicator tubes were used.

The Institute of Occupational Health in Finland made 124 measurements of sulphur dioxide concentrations in Finnish pulp mills between 1965 and 1972, using both sampling methods and instruments that gave direct readings. Results ranged from 0.1 - 210 ppm; results from 1971-1976 ranged between 0.05 and 25 ppm (Skyttä, 1978).

Kangas & Turunen (1978) measured sulphur dioxide concentrations in the working atmospheres of various sulphite pulp mills, in digester plants, washer departments and near evaporators. The samples were taken in plastic bags, and the amount of sulphur dioxide was measured by gas chromatography with flame-photometric detection. The results of about 200 measurements ranged between < 0.1 and 5.2 ppm.

During the cooking stage of sulphate pulping, hydrogen sulphide is produced, along with some other organic sulphur compounds, all of which have a characteristic, unpleasantly strong smell. The most common of these compounds are methylmercaptan, ethylmercaptan, dimethylsulphide and dimethyldisulphide.

Ferris *et al.* (1967) reported concentrations of 0-7 ppm hydrogen sulphide to which workers were exposed.

Measurements made by the Finnish Institute of Occupational Health, using indicator tubes, absorption in cadmium acetate solution followed by iodometric titration and other direct-reading analytical methods, from 1965-1972 showed concentrations of 1-10 ppm in 49 samples. Measurements taken in pulp mills during the years 1971-1976 showed concentrations of 0.1-8 ppm (Skyttä, 1978).

Kangas (1980) found that exposure to sulphur-containing compounds was greatest in work places near the bottom of the new, continuously operating digesters of sulphate pulp. Here, methylmercaptan was detected in amounts 10-20 times greater than those found at any other stage of the process. The concentration was regularly higher than 0.5 ppm, which is equal to the Finnish threshold limit value; peak concentrations ranged between 10 and 15 ppm. Further along the process line, the relative concentrations of the sulphur compounds decreased. Except for occasional leaks, the concentrations of sulphur compounds were relatively low. No such obvious emission points were found in the batch digester, and the distribution of concentrations was much more uniform than in the continuously operating processes. The highest emissions occurred when opening the digesters. The sulphur compounds emitted most often were methylmercaptan and dimethylsulphide. In washer plants, concentrations of 0.3-2 ppm methylmercaptan were found. At the evaporators, the concentrations of sulphur-containing gaseous compounds were much lower than in the digester plants; hydrogen sulphide typically made up the largest percentage of the sulphur-containing gases. The sampling method employed by Kangas throughout his investigation involved taking samples in plastic bags or gas pipettes and then analysing them with portable gas chromatographic equipment.

The concentrations of methylmercaptan in pulp mills measured by the Finnish Institute of Occupational Health during the years 1965-1972 ranged from < 0.2 up to 22 ppm in a total of 28 measurements. The concentrations measured between 1971 and 1976 were 0.025-1.4 ppm (Skyttä, 1978).

Ferris *et al.* (1967) reported concentrations of 0-64 ppm chlorine and 0-2.0 ppm chlorine dioxide during bleaching operations.

In studies by the Finnish Institute of Occupational Health, 0.1-4.7 ppm chlorine and < 0.1-2.5 ppm chlorine dioxide were measured between 1965 and 1972, and 0.01-0.5 ppm chlorine and 0.001-0.5 ppm chlorine dioxide in 1971-1976 (Skyttä, 1978). Lindroos (unpublished data) found 0.001-0.5 ppm chlorine and 0.001-0.05 chlorine dioxide in another bleaching operation in 1977.

Gautam *et al.* (1979) reported on chlorine concentrations in the bleaching plants of three paper mills in south India (Table 5). Concentrations of chlorine gas, as determined by an *ortho*-tolidine/potassium dichromate colorimetric method, varied from traces to 16.7 ppm, 10-30 ppm and 0.11-1.68 in the three paper mills, respectively. Improvements in chlorine control in one mill produced dramatic reductions in chlorine gas concentrations measured in a second survey six years later. Guatam *et al.* also conducted a comprehensive survey of many other exposures in the three mills (Table 5), including atmospheric levels of wood dust, bamboo dust, mercaptans, hydrogen sulphide, sulphur dioxide, talc dust, lime dust, salt cake (sodium sulphate) and coal dust in the work place.

In many stages of the chemical recovery processes, relatively large amounts of inorganic dust may be produced. Measurements taken by the Finnish Institute of Occupational Health (1971-1976) showed values of 0.7-7.5 mg/m^3 (Skyttä, 1978).

Fregert *et al.* (1972) reported two cases of sensitization to chromium in men who worked in the recovery area of a sulphate pulp factory. In the case in which analyses were made at different stages of the recovery process, it was found that 'chrome-cake' had been added to the system to make up losses of sodium and sulphur from the process. Chrome-cake is a by-product of the manufacture of chromic acid. The highest concentration of chromium [VI] measured was 3300 μg/g and was found in the green liquor form of sodium sulphate.

Table 5. Occupational environment of paper-mill workers in south India[a]

Location	Nature of contaminants	Concentration of contaminants				TLV
		Factory I 1st survey	Factory I 2nd survey	Factory II	Factory III	
Chipper house						
Feeding point of chippers:						
bamboo chipping	Bamboo dust	—	6.2 mg/m³	—	137.9 mg/m³	5 mg/m³
wood chipping	Wood dust	—	3.0 mg/m³	1.2 mg/m³	—	5 mg/m³
Screening of chips:						
bamboo chip screens	Bamboo dust	—	180.0 mg/m³	—	214.0 mg/m³	5 mg/m³
wood chip screens	Wood dust	—	4.5 mg/m³	0.9 mg/m³	15.2 mg/m³	5 mg/m³
Digester house						
Near digester opening	Mercaptans (as methyl mercaptan)	16.2 ppm	—	—	25.5 ppm	0.5 ppm
	Hydrogen sulphide	0.45 ppm	—	—	—	10 ppm
	Wood dust	—	—	6.6 mg/m³	—	5 mg/m³
Near feeding conveyors	Mercaptans (as methyl mercaptan)	14.1 ppm	—	—	—	0.5 ppm
	Hydrogen sulphide	—	—	—	—	10 ppm
	Wood dust	—	—	2.9 mg/m³	—	5 mg/m³
While blowing the digester	Mercaptans (as methyl mercaptan)	23.7 ppm	—	—	39.0 ppm	0.5 ppm
	Hydrogen sulphide	0.4 ppm	—	—	—	10 ppm
After blowing the digester	Mercaptans (as methyl mercaptan)	21.8 ppm	—	—	—	0.5 ppm
	Hydrogen sulphide	0.23 ppm	—	—	—	10 ppm

Table 5 (contd)

Location	Nature of contaminants	Factory I 1st survey	Factory I 2nd survey	Factory II	Factory III	TLV
Bleaching plant						
Chlorine tower	Chlorine	16.7 ppm	4.5 ppm	—	0.11 ppm	1 ppm
Alkali tower	Chlorine[b]	8.5 ppm	Trace	10.0 ppm[c]	—	1 ppm
Hypo tower	Chlorine	4.7 ppm	1.25 ppm	—	1.68 ppm	1 ppm
Chlorine washer	Chlorine	0.42 ppm	Trace	—	0.15 ppm	1 ppm
Alkali washer	Chlorine[b]	0.29 ppm	Trace	30.0 ppm[c]	—	1 ppm
Hypo washer	Chlorine	0.72 ppm	Trace	—	—	1 ppm
Bleach liquor preparation plant						
Alkali chest	Chlorine	1.54 ppm	—	Trace[d]	1.51 ppm	1 ppm
Near mixing tank	Chlorine	0.47 ppm	—	Trace[d]	—	
Near bleach liquor tank	Chlorine	0.56 ppm	—	Trace[d]	0.16 ppm	1 ppm
Near chlorine cylinder	Chlorine	0.35 ppm	—	Trace[d]	0.2 ppm	1 ppm
Talc mixing plant						
Handling of talc bags	Talc dust	—	1540 mg/m^3	2640 mg/m^3	614 mg/m^3	6 mg/m^3
Near the talc mixer	Talc dust	—	2224 mg/m^3	2757 mg/m^3	1064 mg/m^3	6 mg/m^3
Recovery plant						
Near dissolver tank	Sulphur dioxide	—	—	0.3 ppm	Roaster-type recovery	5 ppm
	Hydrogen sulphide	0.12 ppm	—	2.5 ppm	Furnace particulate matter, 49.0 mg/m^3	10 ppm
Near induced draught fan	Sulphur dioxide	1.38 ppm	—	0.3 ppm	(Probably sodium sulphate fumes and soot)	5 ppm
	Hydrogen sulphide	0.59 ppm	—	4.0 ppm	—	10 ppm
	Mercaptans (as methyl mercaptan)	13.0 ppm	—	—	—	0.5 ppm

Table 5 (contd)

Location	Nature of contaminants	Factory I 1st survey	Factory I 2nd survey	Factory II	Factory III	TLV
Operators' floor	Sulphur dioxide	0.43 ppm	—	Trace	—	5 ppm
	Hydrogen sulphide	0.18 ppm	—	Trace	::	10 ppm
Lime handling						
Sorting of lime and loading on lorry (at lime kiln)	Lime dust	—	13.8 mg/m³	—^{e}	—	10 mg/m³
Lime warehouse: unloading from lorries	Lime dust	—	21.0 mg/m³	680 mg/m³	36.8 mg/m³	10 mg/m³
Feeding lime to pulverizer or crusher	Lime dust	—	10.2 mg/m³	1945 mg/m³	36.8 mg/m³	10 mg/m³
Salt-cake handling						
Salt-cake bag handling and feeding to conveyor	Sodium sulphate	—	3.4 mg/m³	—	40.0 mg/m³	10 mg/m³
Boiler house						
Feeding point of coal conveyor	Coal dust	—	11.0 mppcf^f	3 mppcf	—	12 mppcf or 2 mg/m³ respirable dust
Near coal crusher	Coal dust	—	65.0 mppcf	44 mppcf	—	12 mppcf or 2 mg/m³ respirable dust

^{a}From Gautam et al. (1979)

^{b}Alkali towers are situated near chlorine towers, hence the chlorine evolving from these towers diffuses to the alkali tower also.

^{c}Average of levels observed at various places in that area

^{d}Plant started up after a 4-hr shut-down

^{e}Lime kiln is several miles away from the factory

^{f}mppcf - million particles per cubic foot

Table 6. Chemical exposures in Finnish paper mills, 1971-1976

Chemical	Stage of operation	Ratio of concentration/TLV	Finnish TLV (ppm)
ammonia	dosage	1.08	25
	paper machine	0.60	
biphenyl	storage of chemicals	1.14-2.06	0.2
	hydropulpers	0.16-0.65	
	paper machine	0.23-27.0	
	packing, winding	0.28-0.76	
dust, inorganic		0.20-1.90	
dust, inorganic	weighing of chemicals	0.03	
	beating	0.28	
	feeding	0.04	
	paper machine	0.03-0.80	
formaldehyde	mixing of size	0.15-0.50	2
	converting	0.15-0.50	
	laminating	0.32	
	hardening	0.22-0.78	
	packing, winding	1.23	
isocyanates	feeding of chemicals	0.0-0.10	0.02
ozone	printing machine	0.75-11.30	0.1
	laminating	0.27-3.05	
	cleaning of the roller	0.52	
phenol	laminating	0.02	5
	thermal treatment	0.04	
	packing, winding	0.02	
solvents	storage of chemicals	0.69	
	preparation of stock	0.10	
	printing machine	0.08	
	laminating	0.08-1.90	
	thermal treatment	0.20-0.38	
	converting	0.10-0.37	
	cleaning of the machine	0.06-1.98	
	sizing	0.28	
	packing, winding	0.59	

Agents used for slime control in water pipes are another potential hazard in paper making [see also p. 185]; however, no information was available on the levels of possible exposures.

(b)   Chemical exposures in the paper industry (See also Appendix 4.)

(i)   *General exposure determinations:* Quantitative information about exposures in the paper industry is scarce. Table 6 is based on statistics from the Finnish Institute of Occupational Health for the period 1971-1976. Most of the measurements were made in factories producing special papers and plastic laminate papers.

In normal paper production, the agents to which workers are exposed are either additives or slime-controlling substances. However, paper workers may also be exposed to the gaseous products of pulp production. Table 7 gives results obtained in 1979 at a Finnish paper mill.

(ii)   *Additives:* Additives are applied to the process either at the start (the wet end), where the paper is in the form of a slurry, or at the converting stage, where additives are used principally for coating. Generally, considerable exposure may be expected during mixing and feeding of the chemicals.

Additives used in the paper making process are:
- fillers,
- sizes,
- adhesives,
- additives to improve strength, etc., and
- colours.

Paper is sized in order to increase its resistance to penetration by liquids, particularly water, and to improve its printability. The most common sizing system is rosin soap and paper makers' alum (sodium aluminate, aluminium sulphate). Hydrocarbon and natural waxes, starch, sodium silicate, glues, casein, synthetic resins, latexes and various silicones have also been employed as sizing agents. Asphalt emulsions have also been used. Some sizes may contain toxic solvents (Freeman, 1969; Halpern, 1975).

Retention aids are used to retain inorganic fillers, such as clay and titanium dioxide, within the paper sheet during manufacture. Starch derivatives, acryl amide derivatives and reaction products of epichlorohydrin are important groups of retention aids; the latter have a particular effect on the dry strength of the paper. Additives that improve the wet strength of the paper are, e.g., resins based on epichlorohydrin and modified urea-aldehyde or melamine-aldehyde resins (Halpern, 1975).

Table 7. Occupational exposures at a Finnish paper mill, 1979

Exposure	Stage of operation	Concentration
total dust	beating/refining application of talc and kaolin to the silo hydropulper	$1.2 - 1.8 \, mg/m^3$ $180 \, mg/m^3$ $0.49 \, mg/m^3$
sulphur dioxide	beating/refining paper machine/wet end	0.08 ppm 0.004 ppm
hydrogen sulphide	paper machine/wet end	<0.55 ppm
acetic acid	paper machine/application of colour	$0.15 \, mg/m^3$

Filler pigments may comprise from 2-40% of the final sheet weight. Fillers may improve brightness, opacity, softness, smoothness, etc. The most important ones are:
- kaolin (aluminium silicate),
- titanium dioxide (anastase and rutile),
- calcium carbonate,
- zinc sulphide, and
- lithopone (barium-zinc sulphide-sulphate) (Häggblom & Ranta, 1977).

In addition, lubricants, plasticizers and flow modifiers that are employed in coating include:
- soaps,
- sulphated oils,
- wax emulsions,
- amine products, and
- esters (Häggblom & Ranta, 1977).

Additives used to reduce the viscosity of the colour, and humectants and materials used to increase moisture resistance are:
- urea,
- dicyanodiamide,
- urea-formaldehyde and melamine-formaldehyde resins,
- glyoxal, and
- zinc and aluminium salts (Häggblom & Ranta, 1977).

A number of additives are also employed in barrier coating. Workers can, in principle, come into contact with the following substances used in this process:
- paraffin wax,
- polyethylene,
- ethylene-vinyl acetate copolymer,
- cellulose derivatives,
- rubber derivatives,
- butadiene-styrene copolymers,
- polyvinylidene chloride,
- polyamides,
- polyesters, and
- alkyds (Häggblom & Ranta, 1977).

Colours added during the paper making process are mostly synthetic organic dyes, either water-soluble or water-dispersible. [A partial list of dyes used in the wood, leather and associated industries is given in Appendix 6.]

Paper may be converted by use of either pigment coating or barrier coating. The most important coating pigments are as follows:
- kaolin (aluminium silicate),
- muscovite mica,
- attapulgite (an aluminium silicate derivative),
- talc (magnesium silicate hydrate),
- titanium dioxide,
- calcium carbonate,
- aluminium oxide hydrate,
- satin white (calcium sulphoaluminate),
- barium sulphate,
- calcium sulphate, and
- zinc oxide (Häggblom & Ranta, 1977).

Commercial talc may contain minerals such as tremolite asbestos, serpentine and quartz.

Sizes may also be used in conjunction with coating pigments and may be of natural origin (casein, soya bean protein, starch) or latexes or other polymer emulsions. The list of the latter is long and includes products based on styrene-butadiene, polyacrylate and polyvinyl acetate. The pigment is usually dispersed to the pulp slurry by means of polyphosphate. Other additions to pigment coating include the following foam-controlling agents:
- pine oil,
- capryl and tridecyl alcohol,

- fuel oil,
- tributyl citrate and phosphate, and
- silicones (Häggblom & Ranta, 1977).

(iii) *Slime-controlling agents:* Slime-controlling agents are employed in order to prevent the growth of microbes in the paper making process. In modern mills, these agents are applied to the process water by means of automatic dosing equipment. Vaporization of the agent from the open parts of the machine may, however, expose those working nearby. These substances may also be present as a mist in the machine room. No information was available about levels of exposure.

In Sweden alone, about 50 paper mills frequently use slime-controlling agents (Ahlberg, 1976). These usually contain an effective ingredient, a solvent, a wetting or dispersing agent and impurities. Industrial hygienists have been especially interested in products containing ethylene-bis-dithiocarbamate, because this compound is suspected of causing cancer and malformations. Such products are not widely used, however. The following list gives the effective ingredients of a number of slime-controlling agents:
- methylene-bis-thiocyanate
- *N*-methyl dithiocarbamate
- *N,N*-dimethyl dithiocarbamate
- ethylene-bis-dithiocarbamate
- mercaptobenzothiazol
- Dazomet (3,5-dichlorophenoxyacetic acid)
- DMTT (tetrahydro-3,5-dimethyl-2*H*-13,5-thiadiazine-2-thione)
- 2-(thiocyanomethylthio)benzothiazole
- bis-1,4-bromoacetoxy-2-butene
- 2'-bromo-4'-hydroxyacetophenone
- 2-bromo-2-nitropropane-1,3-diol
- *N*-(1-phenyl-2-nitropropyl)piperazine
- *N*-[α-(1-nitroethyl)benzyl] ethylenediamine
- Paraclox (*N*,4-dihydroxy-α-oxo-benzeneethanimidoyl chloride)

The following compounds can be present in the solvent fraction:
- dimethylformamide,
- ethylenediamine,
- 1,1,1-trichloroethane,
- isopropanol, and
- ethylene glycol.

The wetting agents are not considered to represent any significant hazard (Ahlberg, 1976).

(iv) *Special papers:* Biphenyl-impregnated paper has been used to wrap citrus fruits for many years. Formerly, only low concentrations of biphenyl were found in the working atmosphere of mills producing this paper. In a Finnish factory in which intoxications were reported, concentrations of 4.4 - 128 mg/m^3 were measured (Table 8).

Table 8. Measurements of biphenyl in a Finnish paper mill[a]

Sampling location	Average concentration (mg/m^3)	
	June 1959	January 1970
paper machine hall		
in front of paper reel	17.9	7.2
behind impregnating roller	128.0	64.0
near paper machine	7.2	1.5
near rolling machine	4.4	0.6
oil room		
near measuring container	19.5	3.5
near mixing container		15.5
during addition of biphenyl to mixing container		74.5
above measuring container (lid open)		123.0

[a]From Häkkinen *et al.* (1973)

An 'oilman' (see p. 174) was exposed not only to biphenyl but also to tetrachloroethylene used for cleaning equipment. Such cleaning was done 5-10 times a year and took about 1 hour each time. Exposures are given in Table 9. The oilman was exposed annually to biphenyl for a total of 100-105 shifts of 8 hours each. The concentration was exceptionally high when biphenyl was added to the mixing container. In the oil room, biphenyl occurs both as a vapour and as dust; in the paper machine hall, it occurs predominantly in vapour form. Skin contact is likely to produce additional exposure (Häkkinen *et al.*, 1973).

Self-copying papers are another type that represents a health hazard. These papers have contained polychlorinated biphenyls, but in the Federal Republic of Germany, Japan, the Nordic countries, Switzerland, the UK and the US, this use has been prohibited. No substances are present in such papers which would vaporize in ambient temperatures. The coatings of these papers may, however, contain irritating agents, and skin symptoms have been observed (Central Board for Labour Protection, 1977).

Table 9. Measurements of tetrachloroethylene in a Finnish paper mill[a]

Sampling location	Average concentration (ppm)	
	June 1970	November 1970
paper machine hall		
in front of paper machine roll	9	30
near operator of paper machine	30	14
oil room		
near measuring container	75	34
near mixing container	40	
breathing zone of oilman during cleaning	32	35

[a]From Häkkinen *et al.* (1973)

2.4 Biological factors

(a) Pulp industry

Because wood contains various microbes, people employed in debarking, chipping and chip stocking may be exposed. For example, the fungus *Coniosporium certicola* has been shown to be the etiological agent in severe asthma attacks in workers in an Indian pulp mill involved in debarking (Gautam *et al.*, 1979). Many workers in a sulphite pulp mill in Finland that produces Torula yeast from 'black liquor' have been reported to have contracted a yeast allergy.

(b) Paper industry

Workers in paper mills that use wood as the raw material have been found to be exposed to *Aspergillus* and *Penicillium* spores. The results of a study made in a Polish paper mill of exposure to fungal spores are summarized in Table 10.

2.5 Current regulations and recommendations on exposures

See 'General Remarks on Wood, Leather and Some Associated Industries', p. 23.

2.6 Number of workers involved

See 'General Remarks on Wood, Leather and Some Associated Industries', p. 19.

Table 10. Exposure to spores in a Polish paper mill[a]

Sampling location	Number of spores per m^3
sorter	>334,000
conveyor belt	>334,000
dumping into boiler	>334,000
bark crumbler	<27,000
stockpiles	<27,000
cellulose filter	<27,000
paper winder	<27,000
paper cutter	<27,000

[a] From Halweg *et al*. (1978)

3. GENERAL TOXICITY DATA

3.1 Toxic, inflammatory and allergic effects in humans

In 31 workers involved in the preparation of biphenyl-impregnated fruit wrapping paper, the most common adverse health effects were headache, gastrointestinal symptoms, polyneuritis, general fatigue or giddiness. In one worker who died, autopsy showed liver necrosis. Needle biopsies from 3/8 workers showed hepatic cellular changes (Häkkinen *et al*., 1973).

Skalpe (1964) found significantly higher frequencies of symptoms of respiratory diseases (cough, expectoration, dyspnoea) in a group of 54 workers in 4 pulp mills exposed to sulphur dioxide at concentrations ranging from 2-36 ppm, than in a comparable control group. The expiratory flow rate was significantly lower in exposed workers, but vital capacity was not significantly different between the two groups.

Ferris *et al*. (1967), however, found no significant differences in the frequencies of these symptoms in similar observations in a pulp mill and in a paper mill. In a group of 271 men who worked in the same pulp and paper mills and who were followed up 10 years later (Ferris *et al*., 1979), analysis of retired categories suggested that a group of workers from a pulp mill, where they had been exposed to chlorine and sulphur dioxide, had slightly (though not statistically significantly) lower forced vital capacity and forced expiratory volume in one second than another, unexposed group of retired paper workers.

The occurrence of clinical symptoms, such as shortness of breath, cough, expectoration and frequent colds, in workers in a paper factory was related to the number of fungi in the air (Halweg *et al.*, 1978).

Lung hypersensitivity and granulomatous disease occur in workers in paper mills where maple logs are handled. Exposures are greatest in the winter months when the work is enclosed and are related to very high spore counts, which may comprise 85% of the dust counts. Pulmonary effects are believed to be due to a hypersensitivity reaction to the spores of the fungus *Cryptostroma (Coniosporum) corticale*, similar to 'farmer's lung', resulting in the formation of granulomas and fibrosis of the alveolar walls and eventually of the interstitium of the lung (Emanuel *et al.*, 1962, 1966).

Two men working in the recovery area of a sulphate pulp factory developed eczema of the hands and face. Routine patch testing gave positive reactions to both chromium and cobalt. In samples of water from the recovery process, chromium [III], chromium [VI] and cobalt were found (Fregert *et al.*, 1972). [See also p. 177 .]

3.2 Mutagenicity of effluents

Industrial effluents collected in Sweden from six mills where softwood kraft pulp was bleached were tested for mutagenicity in a streptomycin-dependent *Escherichia coli* strain and in histidine-requiring mutants of *Salmonella typhimurium* strains (Ander *et al.*, 1977). None of the effluents caused mutations in *E. coli*, but effluents from the chlorination stage induced mutations in *S. typhimurium* strains TA1535 and TA1537. After concentration, weak mutagenic activity was also shown by the effluent from the hypochlorite stage. Addition of a rat liver microsomal fraction to the assay reduced the mutagenicity of the effluent from the chlorination stage.

Industrial and laboratory-prepared effluents from the bleaching of softwood and hardwood kraft and sulphite pulps were tested for mutagenicity using *S. typhimurium* TA1535. Nearly all of the industrial effluents from the first chlorination stage were found to be mutagenic; the greatest effect was shown by the effluent from the softwood kraft pulp. Studies on laboratory-prepared effluents showed that first-stage bleaching with mixtures of chlorine and chlorine dioxide gave rise to mutagenic compounds. However, mutagenicity decreased linearly with an increasing chlorine dioxide/chlorine ratio (Eriksson *et al.*, 1979).

In another study (Lee & Mueller, 1979), various process streams and effluent types from one thermomechanical pulp mill, five kraft mills and one sulphite mill in Canada were assessed for the presence of DNA-damaging agents. Effluents *per se* and extracts were screened using the *Salmonella*/microsome test and the induction of chromosomal aberrations in Chinese hamster ovary cells. Both the *Salmonella* and the chromosome aberration tests were positive and demonstrated the presence of mutagenic agents - although of varying activity - in virtually all effluent types except those from thermomechanical pulping and from caustic extraction in kraft mills (Table 11). The mutagenic activity was highest and con-

Table 11. Pulp mill process streams and effluents with mutagenic activity, as monitored by the *Salmonella*/**microsome test and the chromosomal aberration test**[a]

Type of effluent	Mill	Mutagenic activity	
		Salmonella/ microsome test	Chromosomal aberration test
Woodroom effluent:			
softwood	A	+	+
hardwood	B	+	+
Thermomechanical pulping	C	-	-
Kraft mills:			
weak black liquor	D	++	+
1st chlorination stage (conventional chlorine bleaching)	D E F G	+++	+
1st chlorination stage (preceded by oxygen bleaching)	G	+++	+
1st chlorination stage (high levels of chlorine dioxide)	H	+++	+
alkaline extraction	D E F	-	-
untreated combined whole mill	D E F	+ - -	+ - +
aerated lagoon treated combined whole mill	D E F	- - -	+ - +
Sulphite mill:			
weak red liquor	A	-	+
1st chlorination stage	A	+++	+
alkaline extraction stage	A	+	+
untreated combined whole mill	A	-	+
aerated lagoon treated combined whole mill	A	-	+

[a]From Lee & Mueller (1979)

sistently present in first chlorination stage bleaching effluents from both the kraft and sulphite mills. Regardless of type of bleaching (conventional chlorine bleaching, oxygen pre-bleaching or bleaching with chlorine dioxide), the first chlorination stage effluents always caused high mutation rates in *S. typhimurium* and induced chromosomal aberrations in Chinese hamster ovary cells. When a rat liver microsomal fraction was added to the mutagenicity assay, mutagenicity was reduced by 50-70% in all experiments. The nature of the mutagenic compounds in chlorination stage effluents is not known; however, a large number of organic chemicals has been identified in effluents.

Ten resin acids that have been identified as constituents of pulp and paper mill effluents were assayed in the *Salmonella*/microsome assay. Only neoabietic acid was found to be mutagenic in TA1535, TA100, TA1538 and TA98 strains. Addition of liver postmitochondrial supernatant from Aroclor-induced rats reduced the mutagenic effect (Nestmann *et al.*, 1979).

4. CARCINOGENICITY DATA[1]

(a) Nasal cancer

No information was available to the Working Group.

(b) Laryngeal cancer

In reports by Decouflè *et al.* (1977) and Bross *et al.* (1978), men who had worked as 'operatives in paper industry' for 5 years or more showed a relative risk of 4.37 (P = 0.02) for laryngeal cancer (based on 5 cases). [See also monograph on carpentry and joinery, p. 152.]

(c) Lung cancer

A survey of lung cancer mortality in various US counties was carried out by Blot & Fraumeni (1976) for the period 1950-1969. The age-adjusted annual lung cancer mortality rates tended to be higher among white males (9%) (P < 0.05) in those counties of the eastern and southern (but not the western) part of the US where paper and pulp industries were located. The increased rates are not explicable by differences in demographic or socioeconomic factors or by the presence of other industries in the area. No similar correlation was found for white females, and there was only a small, non-significant increase for non-white males. No information on smoking histories was available.

---

[1] This section should be read in conjunction with Appendix 1, p. 295.

In a study of men who had died of lung cancers (Harrington *et al.*, 1978), a relative risk of 1.28 was found for lung cancer in workers in wood and paper industries in rural but not in urban areas. No information on smoking histories was available. [See also monograph on the lumber and sawmill industries, p. 88 .]

In a case-control study of lung cancer among males in coastal Georgia, occupational histories were obtained on 458 cases and 553 controls. Although the report of the study focused on the association between lung cancer and employment in shipyards during the Second World War, 1.7% of the 175 persons ever employed in shipbuilding and 7.8% of the 836 persons never so employed had worked in the paper industry. The relative risk for lung cancer associated with employment in paper mills (adjusted for cigarette smoking) was 1.0 (based on 68 cases and controls combined) (Blot *et al.*, 1978).

Ferris *et al.* (1979) followed a cohort of 271 US pulp and paper mill workers, identified in 1963. Thirty-three deaths had occurred by 1973, 16 in paper workers (to give an SMR of 162 for all causes of death), 9 in workers exposed to chlorine and 8 in people exposed to sulphur dioxide. No cause-specific SMRs were computed. Seven of the 33 deaths were due to cancer (1 of the kidney, 3 of the lung, 2 of the stomach/peritoneum and 1 lymphoma).

Menck & Henderson (1976) identified 2161 death certificates that had mention of lung cancer for white males who died between the ages of 20 and 64 in 1968-1970, as well as 1777 incident cases of lung cancer in white males of the same age group which had been reported to the Los Angeles County Cancer Surveillance Program in 1972 and 1973. They then classified subjects according to the last known industry in which they had been employed. Using 1970 census data, expected deaths and expected incident cases were calculated for each specific occupation, assuming that the age-specific rates of cancer in each occupation were the same as those for all occupations. A risk ratio of 1.71 ($P < 0.01$) (observed deaths plus incident cases divided by expected deaths plus incident cases) was calculated for 'paper manufacturing and sales', on the basis of 14 deaths and 14 incident cases and a census estimate of 11,900 men employed in this industry. No information on smoking histories was available.

A death certificate analysis was carried out by Gottlieb *et al.* (1979) on 3327 lung cancer deaths which occurred in the period 1960-1975 in Louisiana. Statements on occupation were compared with those of 3327 controls who had died of causes other than cancer, matched by sex, race, age and parish of residence. No excess risk was found among those employed in the paper industry. The RR was 1.05 (95% confidence limits, 0.79-1.40), on the basis of 103 cases and 98 controls. No information on smoking histories was available.

(d)   Haematopoietic and lymphoreticular cancer

In a study by Milham & Hesser (1967), 12 patients with Hodgkin's disease and 3 controls were paper mill workers, RR = 4 (P < 0.05). [See also monograph on the lumber and sawmill industries, p.   89   ].

In reports by Decouflè *et al.* (1977) and Bross *et al.* (1978), men who had worked as 'operatives in paper industry' for 5 years or more showed a relative risk of 2.45 for lymphomas (based on 4 cases). An excess was also found in labourers ever employed in the paper industry (based on 2 cases). [See also monograph on carpentry and joinery, p. 152 .]

(e)   Other cancers not previously specified

In reports by Decouflè *et al.* (1977) and Bross *et al.* (1978), men who had worked as 'operatives in paper industry' for 5 years or more showed a relative risk of 4.14 (P < 0.01) for oral and pharyngeal cancer (based on 14 cases). [See also monograph on carpentry and joinery, p. 152 .]

Blot & Fraumeni (1977) analysed US county mortality data in relation to oral and pharyngeal cancer between 1950 and 1969. A significantly increased mortality rate was observed among white males in eastern states (where many paper industries are located) but not in western states.

5. SUMMARY OF DATA AND EVALUATION

5.1 Summary of data

Information on the cancer experience of paper and pulp mill workers is limited. Most of the studies that assess risk are based on reviews of death certificate information on occupation; few studies had occupational histories or information on potentially influential variables such as cigarette smoking, and none followed the cancer mortality or morbidity of a large cohort of workers.

A case-control study in New York state of death certificates of Hodgkin's disease showed a four-fold excess of this cancer associated with employment in the paper industry. A similar study in Washington state subsequently showed a two-fold increase of Hodgkin's disease, as well as smaller, but significant increases for other lymphomas, but not for leukaemia. Elevated lymphoma risks were also reported for both operatives and labourers in the paper and allied products industry in a large multi-tumour-site case-control study in New York state.

Lung cancer mortality rates among males were elevated in eastern, but not western, US counties with paper or pulp mills. Death certificate surveys of occupation likewise show inconsistent results, with significant increases among paper workers in three studies: one in the south-east US where an excess was seen in rural, but not urban areas, although workers were employed in industries in both areas; the second in a cross-sectional study where occupational data were missing for one-third of the cases; and the third in which a small increase was seen in a national survey of deaths by occupation throughout the US. Increases were not seen in two other studies, nor in a detailed interview survey in which occupational histories and information on cigarette smoking were obtained.

A large, multi-tumour-site case-control study in New York state reported a four-fold excess of laryngeal cancer linked to five or more years' employment in the paper industry; and a 50% elevated ratio for this cancer was observed among paper workers in the Washington state mortality statistics. Both studies involved small numbers of cases among paper workers: five and six, respectively. A four-fold excess of oral and pharyngeal cancer was also seen in the New York study; and in US counties with paper or pulp manufacturing industries there tended to be slightly elevated rates of oral and pharyngeal cancer mortality among males.

The description of the industrial processes shows that some of the chemicals used are those for which there is evidence of carcinogenicity in humans and/or experimental animals (see Appendix 4). Although some of these chemicals are no longer used, others are still in use. The introduction of chlorination for treatment of effluents from pulping processes may cause transformation of molecular species to form carcinogenic and/or mutagenic chemicals.

5.2 Evaluation

The epidemiological data are not sufficient to make a definitive assessment of the carcinogenic risk of employment in the paper or pulp mill industries. Several studies suggest that an increased risk of lymphoproliferative neoplasms, particularly Hodgkin's disease and perhaps leukaemia, may be linked to employment in the paper and pulp industries.

Excesses of oral and pharyngeal and of laryngeal cancers were reported in two studies designed to generate hypotheses, and have not been evaluated in independent studies. There appears to be no moderate or large overall increased risk of lung cancer among paper workers. The excess risk of lung cancer observed in some subgroups of workers in two of the studies cannot be evaluated.

6. REFERENCES

Ahlberg, K. (1976) Slime-controlling agents: risk for cancer and foetal damage (Swed.). *Arbetsmiljö, 11,* 11-13

Ander, P., Eriksson, K.-E., Kolar, M.-C., Kringstad, K., Rannug, U. & Ramel, C. (1977) Studies on the mutagenic properties of bleaching effluents. *Sven. Papperstidn., 80,* 454-459

Anon. (1980) Pulp production: sprucing up old technology. *Chem. Eng. News,* 26 May, pp. 26-29

Ball, W.L. (1972) *Paper, paper pulp industry.* In: *Encyclopaedia of Occupational Health and Safety,* Vol. 2, Geneva, International Labour Office, pp. 997-1000

Blot, W.J. & Fraumeni, J.F., Jr (1976) Geographic patterns of lung cancer: industrial correlations. *Am. J. Epidemiol., 103,* 539-550

Blot, W.J. & Fraumeni, J.F., Jr (1977) Geographic patterns of oral cancer in the United States: etiologic implications. *J. chronic Dis., 30,* 745-757

Blot, W.J., Harrington, J.M., Toledo, A., Hoover, R., Heath, C.W., Jr & Fraumeni, J.F., Jr (1978) Lung cancer after employment in shipyards during World War II. *New Engl. J. Med., 299,* 620-624

Brecht, W. (1970) Paper manufacture in the last 100 years (Ger.). *Wochenbl. Papierfabr., 7,* 273-296

Bross, I.D.J., Viadana, E. & Houten, L. (1978) Occupational cancer in men exposed to dust and other environmental hazards. *Arch. environ. Health, 33,* 300-307

Carey, B.J.R. (1969) Paper and papermaking. Some notes on the history of the art. *Med. Sci. Law, 9,* 47-50

Central Board for Labour Protection (1977) *Kiertokirje 1/77 [Circular 1/77],* Tampere, Finland

Decouflé, P., Stanislawczyk, K., Houten, L., Bross, I.D.J. & Viadana, E. (1977) *A Retrospective Survey of Cancer in Relation to Occupation (DHEW Publ. No. (NIOSH) 77-178),* Washington DC, US Government Printing Office

Emanuel, D.A., Lawton, B.R. & Wenzel, F.J. (1962) Maple-bark disease. Pneumonitis due to *Coniosporium corticale. New Engl. J. Med., 266,* 333-337

Emanuel, D.A., Wenzel, F.J. & Lawton, B.R. (1966) Pneumonitis due to *Cryptostroma corticale* (maple-bark disease). *New Engl. J. Med., 274,* 1413-1418

Eriksson, K.-E., Kolan, M.-C. & Kringstad, K. (1979) Studies on the mutagenic properties of bleaching effluents. II. *Sven. Papperstidn., 82,* 95-104

Feiner, B. & Marlow, S. (1956a) Sulphur dioxide exposure and control. *Paper Ind., 38,* 37-40

Feiner, B. & Marlow, S. (1956b) Sulphur dioxide exposure and control. *Indian Pulp Paper, 11,* 112-116

Ferris, B.G., Jr, Burgess, W.A. & Worcester, J. (1967) Prevalence of chronic respiratory disease in a pulp mill and a paper mill in the United States. *Br. J. ind. Med., 24,* 26-37

Ferris, B.G., Jr, Puleo, S. & Chen, H.Y. (1979) Mortality and morbidity in a pulp and a paper mill in the United States: a ten-year follow-up. *Br. J. ind. Med., 36,* 127-134

Freeman, J.S. (1969) Chemicals: their critical role in the pulp and paper industry. *Pulp and Paper Magazine of Canada,* 6 June, pp. 37-41

Fregert, S., Gruvberger, B. & Heijer, A. (1972) Sensitization to chromium and cobalt in processing of sulphate pulp. *Acta dermatovenerol. (Stockh.), 52,* 221-224

Gautam, S.S., Venkatanarayanan, A.V. & Parthasarathy, B. (1979) Occupational environment of paper mill workers in south India. *Ann. occup. Hyg., 22,* 371-382

Gottlieb, M.S., Pickle, L.W., Blot, W.J. & Fraumeni, J.F., Jr (1979) Lung cancer in Louisiana: death certificate analysis. *J. natl Cancer Inst., 63,* 1131-1137

Häggblom, I. & Ranta, V. (1977) *Sellun Valmistus [Cellulose Production],* 3rd ed., Porvoo, Finland, Werner Söderström Osakeyhtiö

Häkkinen, I., Siltanen, E., Hernberg, S., Seppäläinen, A.M., Karli, P. & Vikkula, E. (1973) Diphenyl poisoning in fruit paper production. A new health hazard. *Arch. environ. Health, 26,* 70-74

Halpern, M.G. (1975) *Paper Manufacture,* Park Ridge, NJ, Noyes Data Corporation

Halweg, H., Krakówka, P., Podsiado, B., Owczarek, J., Ponahajba, A. & Pawlicka, L. (1978) Studies on air pollution by fungal spores at selected working posts in a paper factory (Pol.). *Pneumol. Pol., 46,* 577-585

Harrington, J.M., Blot, W.J., Hoover, R.N., Housworth, W.J., Heath, C.A. & Fraumeni, J.F., Jr (1978) Lung cancer in coastal Georgia: a death certificate analysis of occupation: brief communication. *J. natl Cancer Inst., 60,* 295-298

Jahn, E.C. & Strauss, R.W. (1974) *Industrial chemistry of wood.* In: Kent, J.A., ed., *Riegel's Handbook of Industrial Chemistry,* 7th ed., New York, Van Nostrand-Reinhold, pp. 435-487

Jensen, W. (1968) *Technical development and research in the pulp and paper industry* (Fin.). In: Laurila, J., Mäkinen, E. & Vuorimaa, H., eds, *Metsäteollisuus Itsenäisessä Suomessa [Forestry in Independent Finland],* Helsinki, Suomen Puunjalostusteollisuuden Keskusliitto, pp. 107-132

Kangas, J. (1980) *Foul-smelling compounds in pulp mills* (Fin.). In: *Työhygienian koulutuspäivät, Espoo, januari, 1980 [Course in Industrial Hygiene, Espoo (Finland), January 1980],* Helsinki, Suomen Työhygienian Seura r.y.

Kangas, J. & Turunen, E. (1978) *Various exposures to sulphur dioxide in a sulphite cellulose factory* (Dan.) (Abstract no. 28). In: *Nordiske Arbejdshygiejniske Møde i Danmark, nov. 1978, Resumèsamling [Nordic Conference of Industrial Hygiene, Denmark, November 1978, Abstracts],* Copenhagen, Arbejdsmiljøinstituttet, Arbejdstilsynet, p. 40

Kemppainen, T. (1978) *Puualan Perusoppi 1 [Fundamentals of Forestry 1]*, Helsinki, Otava

Kurkijärvi, E. (undated) *Selluloosateollisuudessa Esiintyvistä Kaasuista, Lähinnä Rikkidioksidista, Terveydelliseltä Kannalta [Studies on Gases Found in the Pulp Industry, with Special Reference to Sulphur Dioxide and Health Aspects]*, Helsinki, Teknillinen Korkeakoulu, Diplomityö n:o 246

Lee, E.G.-H. & Mueller, J.C. (1979) *Biological Characteristics of Pulp Mill Effluents, Part II, Final Report, CPAR Project Report 678-2,* Ottawa, Environmental Protection Service

Maksimov, V.F. (1957) Investigation of environmental air pollutants in the area of a sulphate cellulose industry and methods for reducing foul-smelling gases (Russ.). *Bum. Prom., 32,* 10-12

Menck, H.R. & Henderson, B.E. (1976) Occupational differences in rates of lung cancer. *J. occup. Med., 18,* 797-801

Milham, S., Jr & Hesser, J.E. (1967) Hodgkin's disease in woodworkers. *Lancet, ii,* 136-137

Nestmann, E.R., Lee, E. G.-H., Mueller, J.C. & Douglas, G.R. (1979) Mutagenicity of resin acids identified in pulp and paper mill effluents using the *Salmonella*/mammalian-microsome assay. *Environ. Mutagenesis, 1,* 361-369

Ryti, N. (1974) *Paperitekniikan Perusteet [Fundamentals of Paper Technology]*, Otaniemi, Finland, Teknillisen Korkeakoulun Ylioppilaskunta

Skalpe, I.O. (1964) Long-term effects of sulphur dioxide exposure in pulp mills. *Br. J. ind. Med., 21,* 69-73

Skyttä, E. (1978) *Tilasto Työhygieenisistä Mittauksista v. 1971-1976 [Statistics from Industrial Hygiene Measurements in 1971-1976]*, Katsauksia 17, Helsinki, Työtarveyslaitos

Wrist, P.E. (1970) 1920-1970: a technical perspective. *Paper Technol., 2,* 182-187

LEATHER

1. HISTORICAL OVERVIEW OF THE INDUSTRY

Tanning, the chemical process used to convert hides and skins to non-putrescible leather, is accomplished by the removal of the epidermis and the subcutaneous layer and the subsequent stabilization of the remaining middle portion.

Tanning has been practised since prehistoric times. Until the beginning of the industrial era the tanning industry developed slowly, using substances of animal and vegetable origin in the different processes necessary to obtain the finished goods. Since the end of the nineteenth century, much development has taken place in industrialized countries, taking advantage of chemical and mechanical innovations.

2. DESCRIPTION OF THE INDUSTRY

When the hide is removed from the animal, it is readily putrescible; it is converted to a non-putrescible, useful substance by the process of tanning. Leather production can be divided into three stages: preparation of the hide for tanning, which includes processes such as the removal of hair and adherent flesh; the tanning process; and finishing processes, which include colouring and producing surface effects. Figure 1 shows two typical processes for leather tanning: it must be emphasized that this is an illustration; in commercial practice, there is wide variation, for practical reasons and to meet changing market demands. In addition, in many parts of the world, leather tanning is carried out on a wide scale using primitive methods and largely manual operations.

2.1 Processes used previously and changes over time

From ancient times up to the nineteenth century, the only tanning method was the one in pits, i.e., the leathers were immersed in hollows, containing substances of natural origin necessary for the various process phases. At present, such methods are carried out only in countries with low levels of technology; however, a similar method is carried out in developed countries to obtain sole leathers of the best quality.

The method of tanning in rotating drums was introduced in the nineteenth century. Since then, this method has also been used for the operations preparatory to tanning (Bravo, 1964). Tanning in drums shortens the tanning time considerably, to only two to three days.

Some changes currently taking place which are important from the point of view of industrial hygiene, are:

Fig. 1. Typical process routes for leather tanning and finishing

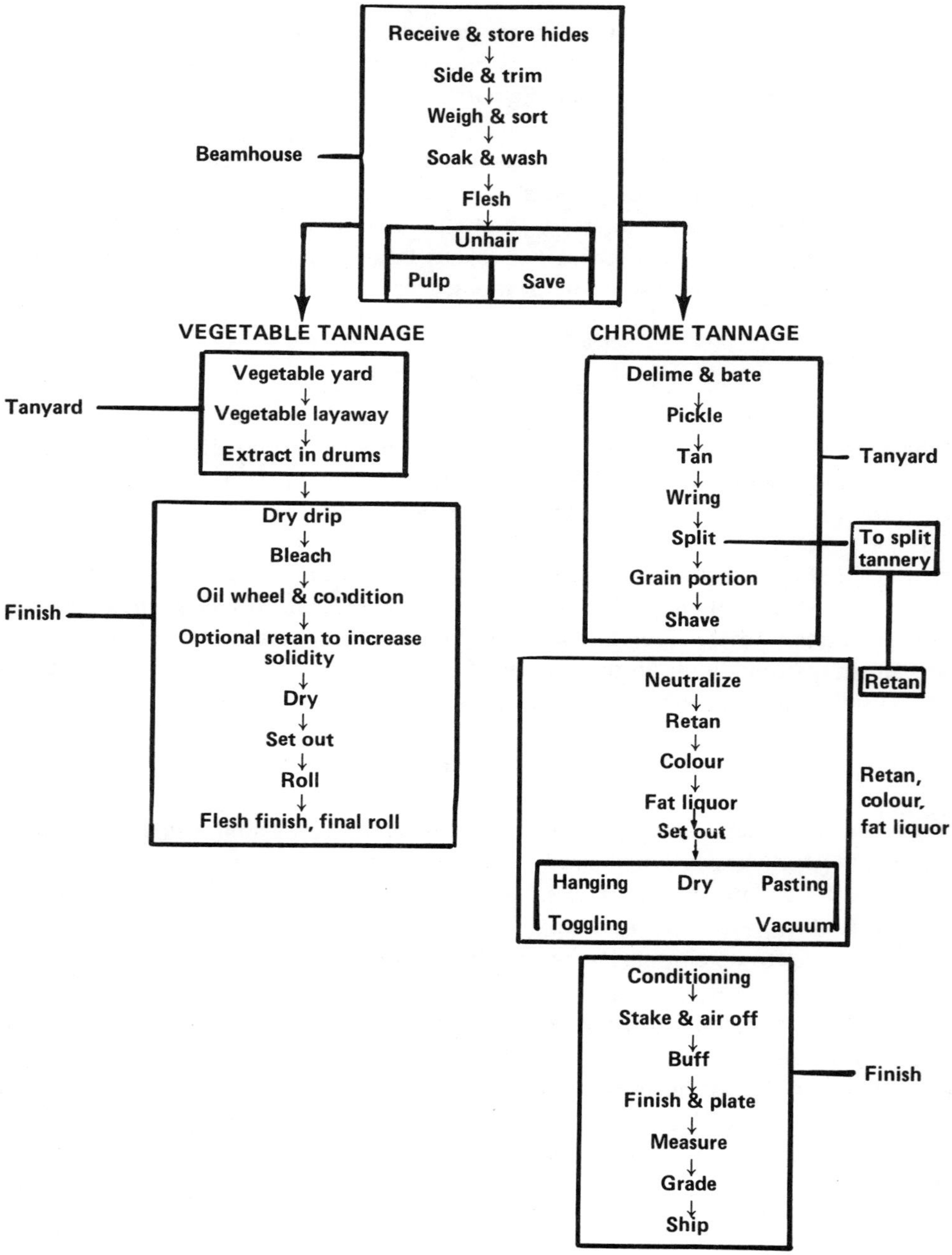

Beamhouse ——

Receive & store hides
↓
Side & trim
↓
Weigh & sort
↓
Soak & wash
↓
Flesh
↓
| **Unhair** | |
| Pulp | Save |

VEGETABLE TANNAGE   **CHROME TANNAGE**

Tanyard ——

Vegetable yard
↓
Vegetable layaway
↓
Extract in drums

Finish ——

Dry drip
↓
Bleach
↓
Oil wheel & condition
↓
Optional retan to increase solidity
↓
Dry
↓
Set out
↓
Roll
↓
Flesh finish, final roll

Delime & bate
↓
Pickle
↓
Tan
↓
Wring
↓
Split —— **To split tannery**
↓
Grain portion
↓
Shave

—— Tanyard

Retan

Neutralize
↓
Retan
↓
Colour
↓
Fat liquor
↓
Set out

| **Hanging** | **Dry** | **Pasting** |
| **Toggling** | | **Vacuum** |

Retan, colour, fat liquor

Conditioning
↓
Stake & air off
↓
Buff
↓
Finish & plate
↓
Measure
↓
Grade
↓
Ship

—— Finish

(1)   the practice of introducing the different chemical substances into drums through fixed pipes. This is both practical and labour-saving. The present method is to hand-load the various components from sacks, for the powdered substances, or pails, for the liquid ones. Generally, the newer systems thus reduce to a minimum, or fully eliminate, worker contact with these chemical substances.

(2)   the employment of 'closed' drums, which drain neither the rinse water nor the final bath onto the floor of the working place but canalize their waste directly into sewers. Such systems are already used for the dyeing phase and could be programmed for use in other working programmes. The method allows considerable savings of dyes and water and reduces both inside and outside pollution drastically.

(3)   the use of drainpipes, conveyed directly into a sewer system for traditional drums, too, so as to avoid flooding the floor during the rinsing phase. Furthermore, separate sewers are built for the water that comes from the various working phases (Zecchin, 1979), preventing the basic waters of the liming process from coming into contact with acid water and thus preventing the formation of hydrogen sulphide.

(a)   Manual operations

In the last 30-40 years, many operations that were previously carried out manually have been mechanized. The necessity of carrying out some manual operations has also been reduced by the introduction of chemical technology, e.g., manual unhairing has been replaced by a process whereby the hair is dissolved in a chemical bath.

Operations like fleshing, scudding, staking and finishing are now mechanized. Furthermore, chemical flow controls in modern tanneries are now computerized.

It must be emphasized, however, that in many parts of the world, most tanning operations are still carried out manually.

(b)   New operations in tanneries

The greatest modification in tanning has been brought about by the use of new chemical substances in all the working phases.

Preserving and disinfecting substances are widely used, in addition to the primitive system of dehydration which is still in use in some countries [see also section 2.2(a)].

At present, there is a growing propensity in developing countries to import hides and carry out tanning operations locally. It is estimated that in the next 10 years, 'wet-blue' leathers (i.e., leather already chrome-tanned) will account for 80% of all the raw leather imported into Europe. This trend is reinforced by the fact that all the operations preceding tannage create environmental pollution and are thus accepted with increasing difficulty in the developed countries, because of the specific laws against pollution.

One important aspect, introduced in the last 30-40 years, is the employment of anti-bacterial chemical substances, including chlorophenols, in disinfecting processes.

(c)   Tanning substances

Tanning is generally carried out by the use of either vegetable tanning materials or metal salts. The former are used largely, though not exclusively, for leather for shoe soles. Tanning of leather for shoe uppers is now carried out mostly by treatment with trivalent chromium salts.

Many other methods of tanning, e.g., the use of synthetic tanning materials, are available, but they are less used commercially than the two other methods.

The 'two-bath' tanning system used earlier is now nearly completely obsolete and is used only for special products, such as kid gloves. In this 'two-bath' method, the leather is immersed in a bath of hexavalent chromium salts (potassium or sodium dichromate), together with sodium chloride and sulphuric acid. When the leather has become impregnated, it is placed in a bath containing sodium thiosulphate and mineral acid that reduces the dichromate into tanning trivalent chromium salt.

At some tanneries, the chrome-tanning salt is prepared from the dichromates in the same factory. This operation is carried out in lead-sheathed vats, using sulphuric acid, dichromates and a reducing agent, in a highly exothermic developing reaction. The reducing agent is an organic substance, like glucose or starch dextrin or sulphur dioxide. This process exposes workers to hexavalent chromium compounds, and today, although it is sometimes carried out within the tannery, it is more often carried out in separate chemical factories. In Italy, some tanneries continued to prepare trivalent chrome in this way for 10-15 years after the Second World War.

Currently, in spite of the many new tanning agents introduced, single-bath chrome tannage is still the method most often used.

(d)   Leather finishing processes

Leather finishing has been highly modified both as to its execution and to the substances employed. For a long time, the substances employed were of animal and vegetable origin; however, over the last few years a wide range of synthetic compounds has been introduced.

Finishing agents used to be applied to the leather by hand spraying, but since the 1940s spray painting machines have been in use. Some such machines are completely ventilated, while others are only partly ventilated.

(e) Present trends

There have been many changes in the process of manufacturing leather, which have decreased the time of tanning and made the product more versatile. Some of the changes which have occurred are as follows:

(i) Curing - brine curing is replacing salt curing. 1,2- and 1,4-Dichlorobenzenes and phenols such as 2,4,5-tri- and pentachlorophenols, are being used as disinfectants.

(ii) Dimethylamine sulphate was introduced as an accelerating agent in the 1930s.

(iii) Sodium sulphydrate use has increased.

(iv) Hide-processing equipment changed from the paddle vat to the drum and now to the hide processor. The hide processor enables the operator to pump out the liquors, resulting in a cleaner, better controlled environment.

Tanning: Since chromium [III] is now usually supplied as such, it is handled as a bulk liquid. The shift from 'two-bath' to 'one-bath' chrome tannage should reduce worker exposure to chromium [VI].

Retanning: There is increased use of synthetic tannage, i.e., amino resin, phenol and naphthalene-based synthetics. Glutaraldehyde, introduced in the 1960s, is used to convey perspiration resistance to leather.

Colour: There is decreased use of benzidine-derived dyes, although they are still used in some tanneries.

Lubricants: There is a decreased dependence on natural marine oil (from sperm whales) and an increased use of synthetic oil, i.e., chlorinated paraffins, alkane sulphonates.

In most industrialized countries, the vegetable tanning industry has neither grown nor changed very much over the years. This is due to a decline of the leather industry in those countries and a greater emphasis on the more productive and rapid chrome-tanning process.

There is a growing trend to separate the wet process from the dry (finish) process. This is due, in part, to environmental pollution laws. The only advantage this change has to offer from a health perspective is that there is no cross-contamination of the workplace by the two processes: thus, employees in the finishing end are not exposed to chemicals used in the wet process.

2.2   Processes used currently

(a)   Preservation

Hides that arrive at a tannery may have been treated in one of the following ways:

Simple drying in the open air is carried out in countries where the climatic conditions are favourable.

Simple salting is carried out with sodium chloride (from the sea or from salt-mines) by scattering the fleshy side of the hide with a quantity of salt equivalent to 50% of the hide weight.

Brining involves immersion of the hide in a saturated solution of sodium chloride to which naphthalene may have been added.

Pickling comprises immersion of the hide in a bath of sodium chloride acidified with mineral acid.

In a process used in regions such as India, Pakistan and Africa, the skin is cured with a small quantity of vegetable tannins so that the hides can withstand transportation (Bayer, 1975).

(b)   Defestation and disinfection

Hides have been treated with DDT, zinc chloride (Gupta, 1972), mercuric chloride, sulphur dioxide, formaldehyde, formic acid, mineral oils, arsenious anhydride, anhydrous sodium sulphate, bisulphites, borax, boric acid, mercuric iodide, copper sulphate, arsenic, fluorides and phenols.

They may subsequently be refrigerated before being bought by tanneries.

(c)   Beamhouse process

(i)   *Sorting and trimming:* When received at the tannery, the hides are stored in warehouses until they are ready to be processed. The handling and processing of baled hides can result in exposure to dust, e.g., manure, hair, dirt. Foreign hides, if they have not been inspected at the country of origin, must be disinfected for such diseases as anthrax, bovine tuberculosis, brucellosis, Q fever and leptospirosis (Sommer *et al.*, 1971), usually by a 24-hour soaking in a 1:10,000 solution of sodium difluoride in water (O'Flaherty & Doherty, 1939). The hides are then trimmed and stamped with the pack number.

(ii) *Soaking:*   Soaking of salt-cured hides serves two purposes: first, washing removes any salt, dirt and blood remaining on the hide surfaces; second, it restores the moisture lost by the curing process.   The hides are soaked in water to which softening agents, such as sodium sulphide, sodium polysulphide or soda ash, have been added, in paddle vats or hide processors.   Disinfectants such as bleaching powder, chlorine or sodium fluoride may be added to inhibit putrefaction.   Soaking time ranges from 4-20 hours, depending on the thickness of the hide and the type of processing vessel being used.

(iii) *Fleshing:*   This is a mechanical operation designed to remove excess flesh and fatty substances, and may be carried out either before or after the liming operation.

(iv) *Unhairing:*   The hair is usually removed by a process called liming (New England Tanners' Club, 1965).   The hides are soaked in a solution of hydrated lime, which may contain sodium sulphide, sodium sulphite, cyanides or dimethylamine sulphate to accelerate the chemical reaction.   Sodium sulphide hydrolyses to produce sodium hydrogen sulphide.   If the sulphide solution is strong enough, the hair is partially or completely destroyed. It is removed mechanically by an unhairing machine.

Sheepskins are dewooled by painting a paste made of lime and sodium sulphide on the flesh side.   The paste penetrates the skin and loosens the wool, which is then pulled off.   Proteolytic enzymes and nonionic surfactants are also used in this process.

(v) *Scudding:*   The dirt and the remains of hairy bulbs are removed by machine.

(vi) *Deliming and bating:*   Bating is the first step in preparing the hide for the tanning process.   It is carried out in either vats, drums or hide processors.   The purpose of this process is four-fold:

(1)   delime hides,
(2)   reduce swelling,
(3)   peptize fibres, and
(4)   remove protein degradation products.

Buffering salts, such as ammonium sulphate or ammonium chloride, and the action of proteolytic enzymes neutralize the high alkalinity of limed hides.   The active ingredient of a bate is the proteolytic enzyme trypsin; before this enzyme became available, tanners used dog and pigeon manure as the bate material.   The enzymic action of the bate and the buffering salts reduces the swelling and softens the hide texture by removing residual unhairing chemicals and non-leather-making substances.

(vii) *Pickling:* In pickling, hides are placed in an acid environment consisting of a mixture of sodium chloride and sulphuric acid. The sodium chloride is added first to prevent swelling; the acid is necessary because chrome-tanning agents are not soluble under alkaline conditions. Vegetable-tanned hides do not need to be pickled. 2-Naphthol or *para*-nitro-phenol may be added to inhibit the formation of moulds.

(viii) *Degreasing:* This operation consists in removing fat and is normally applied only to sheep and pig skins. Emulsifying agents and solvents are used. In the 1930s hides were defatted by immersing them in benzene, kerosene or carbon tetrachloride (Schwartz, 1936).

(d) Tanning process

The tanning process consists in strengthening the collagen structure with a bond between the peptide chains. This effect is obtained because the tanning substance binds **at least** two reactive groups belonging to different peptide chains. The various tanning substances can be classified on the grounds of the kind of bond they acquire with the collagen-reactive groups:

• tanning substances that react with covalent bonds (e.g., formaldehyde, alkane sulphonic acid chlorides);

• salts of polyvalent metals that are made basic by the addition of alkalis. In this case the binding effect is very stable. The reactive sites in the collagen molecule are the carboxyl groups (COOH). Chrome, aluminium and zirconium tannins belong to this group.

• substances with several substituted aromatic rings which form dipolar bonds. Vegetable and synthetic tannins belong to this group.

(i) Mineral tannage:

• *Aluminium tannage* - This is one of the most ancient methods of mineral tannage, employed by the ancient Egyptians and since the 17th century in France. It is carried out with aluminium sulphate or potassium aluminium sulphate and is used for glove leathers.

• *Zirconium tannage* - Zirconium salts (generally sulphate and chloride) are used to tan very strong white leathers.

• *Chrome tannage* - The process most often used is the 'one-bath' method, in which basic chromium [III] sulphate is the tanning material. The hides are milled in a colloidal solution of basic chromium [III] sulphate until tanning is complete. The 'one-bath' method is more rapid than the 'two-bath' method, and it eliminates the handling of hides saturated with chromic oxide.

Chrome liquors (i.e., chromium salts dissoved in high concentration in water) are used in the most modern installations. They enter the drums directly from outer storage tanks, and worker contact with concentrated chrome liquors during the loading process is avoided.

With the 'two-bath' process, which is almost obsolete, the hides are placed in a solution of sodium dichromate and sulphuric acid and milled until the chromate penetrates the hides. The hides are then removed from solution, drained, and placed in a solution of sodium thiosulphate and hydrochloric acid for about 2 hours. The first bath saturates the hides with chromic oxide and the second bath reduces the chromium [VI] to basic chromium [III] sulphate. Remaining acid is neutralized by the addition of an alkali, such as sodium bicarbonate. It is during the manual handling of hides saturated with chromic oxide that formation of chrome sores or ulcers is most likely.

• *Iron tannage* - During the Second World War iron tannage was developed in Germany, but it has not been used since that time.

(ii) *Vegetable tannage:*   This is one of the oldest types of tannage, carried out since prehistory (Candura, 1974). It makes use of a group of substances (tannins) which can bind to dermal collagen, giving it the resistance and nondecaying properties characteristic of leather. The vegetable species most often used to supply tannins are the European chestnut, red quebracho, mimosa (Bayer, 1975), myrobalans and valonia (Candura, 1974).

Vegetable tannage may be carried out either in pits or in rotating drums. Rapid and ultrarapid tannages, in which high concentrations of tannins are used, are carried out in rotating drums. Slow tannage is carried out in pits: this ancient method is still used for the best sole leathers. Slow tannage takes about one month or more.

Vegetable tannins are characterized by the presence of molecules of considerable size with polyphenolic groups (carrying many OH groups in the benzene ring). The presence of these phenolic compounds allows a further subdivision into:

• Pyrocatechol tannins: containing pyrocatechol (1,2-dihydroxybenzene)
• Pyrogallic tannins: containing pyrogallol (1,2,3-trihydroxybenzene)

Another group of tannins is characterized by polyhydroxybenzenes bound to a sugar molecule, i.e., to a polyvalent alcohol through an ester bond.

• Ellagic tannins: the two carboxyl groups of ellagic acid (Costanza, 1977) are esterified with two hydroxyglucose groups.

(iii) *Tanning with synthetic tannins (syntans):* A group of organic synthetic tanning substances has an effect similar to that of vegetable tannins. They are products of condensing aromatic compounds with formaldehyde, the hydrophilic nature of which is increased by the introduction of sulphonic groups (Bayer, 1975). These can be divided into:

• *Auxiliary tannins* - endowed with less tanning power; products of sulphonation of naphthalene with sulphuric acid and then condensation with formaldehyde

• *Tannins of substitution* - endowed with remarkable tanning power; prepared from phenolic substances (mostly cresols) condensed with aldehydes.

• *Tannins of resinous substances* - products of reaction with substances that have amines as the active group; for example, the condensation of polyvalent phenols (e.g., resorcinol) with an aromatic base such as aniline. Solubility in water is increased by the introduction of a sulphonic acid group (Costanza, 1977).

Syntans are products of condensation of the formaldehyde with urea, dicyanodiamide (products of condensation of two molecules of cyanamide) or melamines (cyclic structures containing three molecules of cyanamide). They are used only in the retanning of leathers treated by chrome tannage. Copolymers of maleic anhydride with styrene are also used. This operation lasts 1-2 hours in a rotating drum.

(iv) *Oil tanning:* The tanning action is obtained by the oxidation of natural fish oils, usually from codfish.

(v) *Tanning with synthetic aliphatic compounds:* Leather may be tanned with formaldehyde or glutaraldehyde; however, these compounds are rarely used alone but usually in combination with other tanning agents.

(e) Wringing (sammying)

In this operation, excess water is removed from the leather so that it can be split.

(f) Splitting

Splitting is the longitudinal division of wet or dry leather that is too thick, for articles such as shoe uppers and leather goods. When the leather is split while dry, leather dust may be released (see Table 2).

(g)   Shaving

Roll machines with cutting blades are used to further reduce the leather to the thickness required. The workers uses both hands to introduce the leather between the rollers. During this operation a large amount of dust may be raised, depending on the degree of humidity of the leather.

(h)   Neutralizing

The chrome leather must be neutralized after being tanned. This normally forms the first part of the colour/retan/fat liquor operation and is carried out about 48 hours after the shaving. Salts with a weakly alkaline reaction, e.g., borax (hydrated sodium borate), sodium or ammonium bicarbonate, calcium or sodium formate are used to neutralize leathers.

(i)   Retanning

This is carried out on most chrome leathers to modify their physical properties. The leathers may be retanned with chromium or zirconium salts, but more often with vegetable and synthetic tannins or with resinous and synthetic aliphatic tanning compounds.

(j)   Bleaching

This is an optional operation, carried out only for some specialized leathers.

(k)   Colouring or dyeing

After tanning, most leathers, except sole leathers, undergo dyeing. The type of colouring used varies according to the tannage carried out on the leather. At present, the dyeing operation is usually carried out in drums at a temperature of about 50-60°C. During the rinsing process, the dyeing bath may be partially emptied from a small hatch in the drum, which is still rotating; so the floor of the workplace is often flooded and the working environment becomes polluted.

Generally, dyeing is performed in a batch mode; and retan, colouring and fat liquoring operations are all performed in sequence in the same drum without intermediate steps of washing and drying.

Hides at the blue stage are placed in drums, and retan formulations are added; at the appropriate time, a designated dye formulation is added, and mixing (by rotation) is continued. Fat liquoring chemicals are added at the prescribed time.

Three major types of dyes are used: acid, basic and direct. Acid dyes are usually azo, triarylmethane, or anthraquinone dyes with acid substituents such as nitro-, carboxy- or sulphonic acid. Basic dyes contain free amino groups. Direct dyes are principally water-soluble salts of sulphonic acids of azo dyes. All the dyes used in the tanning industry must be sufficiently water-soluble and have an affinity for leather, i.e., be protein-binding dyes. At the proper pH, both acid and basic dyes penetrate deeply into the hide; direct dyes do not penetrate when used on blue or vegetable-tanned leather. Acid dyes are fixed more readily at low pH but penetrate deeper as the pH increases. However, basic dyes must be used with a vegetable tanning material or an anionic syntan to dye chrome leather; thus, the uptake of dye by the leather is a function of the dye used, the pH, the syntans present and the float. Blends of dyes are used in order to obtain the exact shade desired, so the composition is not always known except by the supplier.

Providing a nitrosating agent is present, some of the basic dyes could give rise to *N*-nitroso compounds. For example, *N*-nitrosodimethylamine could result from nitrosation of the dye Basic Green 4.

A partial list of dyes known to be used in the leather industry is given in Appendix 6.

(l)   Fat liquoring

The purpose of fat liquoring is to lubricate leather to give it strength and flexibility. The process is carried out in the same processing equipment used for retan and colouring. Oils, natural fats, their transformation products, mineral oils and several synthetic fats are used. The latter include:

(1) chlorinated, unbranched paraffins, and
(2) high-molecular weight polyethers derived from vinyl alcohol.

Oils or fats are incorporated into the leather in an aqueous suspension which remains stable at the pH of the neutralized leather.

(m) Drying

The leathers now undergo a thermic treatment to eliminate excess water. Such drying operations may expose workers to contact with vapours emanating from the leather. The systems used at present are:

(i)   *Pasting:* The leathers are spread out with a starch paste onto glass sheets and introduced into an oven. It has been reported that 2,4,5-trichlorophenol or pentachlorophenol may be added to the paste as a biocide.

(ii) *Toggling (tacking):* The leathers are laid by hand on looms with fitting pliers and introduced into an oven in which the temperature and humidity are controlled.

(iii) The leathers are laid on plates heated from inside by hot water.

(iv) *Tunnel drying:* The leathers are hung on mobile chains which carry them through an oven.

(v) *Vacuum drying:* The leathers are pressed between a hot plate (about 85°C) and an absorbing surface.

(vi) *Drying with infra-red rays or with electromagnetic radiation (microwaves):* These are advanced technological processes, requiring the existence of a fully automatic cycle; not currently widely used.

(n) Finishing

(i) *Sole leather:* After drying, sole leather is subjected to simple mechanical operations (setting and rolling) and given a final polish.

(ii) *Chrome leather:* The finishing process comprises a sequence of operations that confer a specific feel and look to the tanned and dried leather. It includes a series of mechanical operations and, normally, the application of a covering layer to the leather surface. This layer may be produced with different substances, but it should be firmly bound and resistant to mechanical stress. The substances used are: sizes (usually colourless or coloured with aniline dyes) and substances containing pigments that can provide a deep covering action. The covering pigments are suspended in a 'binding' component of a colloidal nature which keeps them in suspension. Plasticizers are often added to improve the elasticity of the covering layer.

At various points during the finishing process, the leather may be pressed in a platen or rotary press, in which the press plate is usually heated.

• *Conditioning* - The moisture content of the leather is adjusted to the correct level. This is done, for example, by passing the hides under a spray of water and then stacking them overnight.

• *Staking* - This is a mechanical beating operation used to make the leather soft. It was once carried out by hand but is now largely carried out as follows:

(1) Staking with semi-automatic arms. The worker leans forward over the machine, holding the leather in both hands, while it is pressed by the mobile arm of the machine.

The working position enhances the inhalation of dust arising from the mechanical treatment.

(2) Automatic staking. This may be carried out by one or more workers. In most installations, automatic machines are rapidly replacing the semi-automatic method. The worker collects and introduces the leather into the machine on a conveyer belt. Dust is generated.

• *Buffing* - To improve the final appearance, the grain side of the leather is lightly buffed using a sanding drum. This process makes a tremendous amount of dust, made up of leather particles containing tanning chemicals. After the operation, the leather dust must be removed from the surface of the leather. Old methods included use of rotary brushes, jets of compressed air or a vacuum. Modern methods incorporate dust removal in one continuous operation.

• *Impregnating* - Sometimes, before application of the covering film, the leather is treated with aqueous acrylic resin emulsions or urethane solutions in organic solvents to increase the compactness of the fibre. This operation is carried out under the same conditions as the padding, spraying and flow-coating operations.

• *Dry drumming (fulling)* - This is an optional stage and is carried out to soften the leather. The leathers are put into the rotating drum with or without a small amount of water, or with wet sawdust. This operation can generate a mixture of leather dust and saw-dust.

• *Finishing with pads* - This consists of passing a pad impregnated with a covering dye over the surface of the leather. Once always done by hand, this is now usually carried out by automatic machines, such as seasoning machines. The finish is pumped through a trough and deposited on the leather which is moving on a conveyor by means of a rotating fluted roll. A rotary brush evens out the finish on the leather surface, and the leather is swabbed mechanically. Such installations have no aspiration systems. Some tanneries employ hand labour to impart the final finish by the use of hand pads.

• *Flow coating* - The finish is pumped into a reservoir above the conveyor carrying the leather and flows down onto it. In most cases, painted leathers are not dried in ovens but on trays on shelves; this provides a wide evaporating surface and contributes to air pollution.

• *Spraying* - Some leathers are sprayed by hand in booths with an external extraction system. Spraying may also be carried out in a tunnel through which the leathers are trans-ported on a conveyer belt where they are exposed to spray-guns. Such tunnels usually contain an aspiration system. In the US, leather for military use receives a final spray of *para*-nitrophenol as a preservative. The only system which is totally ventilated is the rotary spray system.

· *Doubling* - This special technique, which is not widely used, is employed only to cover a 'flesh split', i.e., the split from the flesh side of a hide, with an artificial film to feign the grain structure. The grain that is to appear on the finished product is recorded on matrices (often made of silicone), which are put on a conveyer belt and passed into an automatic spray box where they are covered with polyurethane compounds. They are then covered with leather and passed into an oven where polymerization takes place. When this is completed, the leathers are separated from the matrices, leaving the engraved polyurethane film (Bayer, 1975).

(o) Internal transport

Since the leathers are very heavy they are carried from one workplace to another by mechanical trolleys (within the factory), on pallets or in wooden or metallic containers called 'boxes'. Electric traction is uncommon, and the majority of the trolleys used have thermic traction with diesel motors or engines that run on liquefied gases (about 30% propane, 70% butane and traces of pentane and ethane). (See also section on *N*-nitrosamine formation, p. 235 .)

(p) Equipment used in chemical processes of tanning

(i) *Paddle vats:* The oldest method of hide processing employs a half-round, open, cylindrical vat into which a paddle wheel dips. The paddle wheel rotates into the soak liquor, which causes the hide to flex and absorb water. The introduction of the processing chemical into the vat and the removal of the hides from the vat are carried out manually.

(ii) *Rotating-drums:* These are wooden casks (with a diameter varying from 2-5 metres) which hold from 3700-63,000 litres and rotate about a central axle. Each drum is fitted with two hatches: a main one through which the leathers and the bath are loaded and unloaded, and a secondary one with a grille which allows liquid to drain out during the rotation but which holds back the leathers. These drums are usually situated above the floor level so that the leathers are unloaded into suitable containers by gravity. This operation often floods the floor below with the contents of the tanning bath and with the chemical substances it contains. Waste water is removed through drains in the floor. This method of unloading creates a microclimate in the work place that is characterized by a high relative humidity.

Almost all machines are supplied with water through fixed pipes, while the numerous chemical substances used are introduced manually by a worker who stands on an elevated platform. If there are no platforms, the worker climbs up a ladder to carry out the loading.

(iii) *Hide processors:* Such machines constitute the newest method of hide processing and consist of large cement-mixer-type, metal-reinforced plastic containers. With this method, all operations from soaking and washing to bate, pickle and tan can be carried out in the same machine. Use of the hide processor enables the operator to pump out the liquors, resulting in a more closely controlled environment. Modern methods incorporate computer controls to regulate the flow of the chemicals.

2.3 Qualitative and quantitative data on exposures

Table 1 is a list of chemicals that are or have been used in the tanning industry. (See also Appendix 5.)

(a) Dust exposure within tanneries

Dust is produced in a variety of tanning operations: chemical dust can be produced during the loading of hide-processing drums; and leather dust impregnated with chemicals is produced during some mechanical operations, including buffing.

Workers may be exposed to dusts other than leather dust; for example, in storerooms where initial sorting and trimming of hides is carried out, the airborne dust will contain fragments of hair, mould, excrement and general dirt brought in from outside the factory.

(i) *Leather dust:* Leather dust can comprise both fibres and grains. The fibres can vary from 30-1200 μm in length and from 10-30 μm in diameter; grains are usually below 10 μm in size. The wide variation results from the use of sanding papers of various coarsenesses on leathers of different types. Available data indicate that most dust from weighed samples is < 5 μm in diameter (Tables 2 & 3).

Buffing is the most readily identifiable source of dust in tanneries. The dust removal efficiency of buffing and brushing machines has greatly improved in recent years. The percentage of leather that is buffed on the grain has varied greatly over the last 40-50 years for commercial reasons.

The composition of dust varies widely. For example, the values reported for chromium (III) levels in dust from chrome-tanned leathers vary from 0.1-4.5% by weight.

Table 1. Chemicals used in leather tanning. Asterisks (*) indicate those that are or have been the most widely used. (See also Fig. 1, p.202 .)

BEAMHOUSE

Receive and store hides; side and trim; weigh and sort

Sodium chloride*	2,4,5-Trichlorobenzene
Sodium difluoride	2,4,6-Trichlorobenzene

Biocides/Fungicides (Use very variable so no classification possible)

Arsenious oxide	2-n-Octyl-4-isothiazolin-3-one
Cetyldimethylbenzylammonium chloride	Pentachlorophenol (free phenol and sodium and potassium salts)
Chlorine dioxide	Phenol
Copper sulphate	Phenylmercuric acetate
Mixed cresols and other phenols	Potassium N-hydroxymethyl-N-methyl-dithiocarbamate
DDT	
1,2- and 1,4-Dichlorobenzenes	Sodium fluoride
Diiodomethyl para-tolyl sulphone	Sodium difluoride
Ethylene oxide	Sodium ortho-phenoxyphenate
Formaldehyde (gaseous)	Sulphur dioxide
2-Hydroxypropylmethane thiosulphonate	2-(Thiocyanomethylthio)benzothiazole
Mercuric chloride	Tributyl tin chloride complex of ethylene oxide condensate of dihydroabietylamine
Mercuric iodide	
Methylene bis-thiocyanate	2,4,5-Trichlorophenol
Naphthalene	Zinc chloride
2-Naphthol	
para- Nitrophenol	

Table 1 (contd)

Soak and wash

Aliphatic amines and salts	Sodium carbonate (soda ash)
Aromatic amines and salts	Sodium citrate
Calcium chloride	Sodium fluoride
Chlorine	Sodium hydrogen sulphide
meta-Cresol	Sodium hydroxide
Formic acid	Sodium hypochlorite
Hydroxyethyl derivatives of alcohols	Sodium polysulphide*
2-Naphthol	Sodium sulphide*
Phenol	Sulphonated fatty alcohols
Potassium thiocyanate	Surfactants
Proteolytic enzymes	Urea
Sodium arsenates	Zinc chloride
Sodium bisulphite	

Unhair (liming)

Aliphatic amines, e.g., dimethylamine (and sulphate)	Sodium cyanide
Ammonia	Sodium hydrosulphide
Arsenic sulphide	Sodium hydroxide
Calcium chloride	Sodium nitrate (Centro **Tecnico** di Cuoio, Italy)
Calcium hydroxide*	Sodium nitrite (Centre Technique du Cuir, France)
Glucose	Sodium perborate
Hydroxyethyl derivatives of alcohols	Sodium sulphide*
Magnesium hydroxide	Sodium sulphite
Proteolytic enzymes	Urea
Salts and derivatives of thioglycolic acid	

Table 1 (contd)

TANYARD

Chrome tannage

(i)   Delime and bate

Aliphatic acids of low molecular weight*
  (e.g., acetic and formic acids)

Ammonium chloride

Ammonium sulphate*

Boric acid

Glycolic acid

Hydrochloric acid

Proteolytic enzymes (trypsin)*

Sodium bisulphite

Sulphonated aromatic acids

Sulphuric acid*

(ii)   Pickle

Butyric acid

Sodium chloride*

Sulphuric acid*

(iii)   Tan (and manufacture of trivalent chromium tanning salts)

Ammonium sulphate*

Borax

Chromium aluminium sulphate

Chromium (III) sulphate*

Chromium (III) sulphite

Formic acid*

Glucose

Hydrochloric acid

Lactic acid

Magnesium oxide

Potassium acetate

Sodium acetate

Sodium bicarbonate*

Sodium carbonate

Sodium chloride

Sodium dichromate (VI)* (in the past)

Sodium formate

Sodium hydroxide

Sodium sulphite

Sodium thiosulphate

Sulphur dioxide

Sulphuric acid*

Table 1

Vegetable tannage		
Anhydrous sodium sulphate		
Lactic acid		
Sodium polyphosphate*		
Sulphuric acid*		
Vegetable tannins*:		
Bark extracts	*Quercus robur*	(English oak)
	Q. cerris	(European Turkey oak)
	Q. ilex	(Holly oak)
	Q. suber	(Cork oak)
	Pinus halepensis	(Aleppo pine)
	Betula alba	(White birch)
	Rhizophora mangle	(Mangrove)
	Acacia	(Mimosa spp.)
	Salix	(Willow spp.)
	Eucalyptus occidentalis	(Mallet-bark)
Wood extracts	*Q. robur*	
	Q. cerris	
	Q. ilex	
	Q. suber	
	Castanea sativa	(European chestnut)
	Quebrachia lorentzii	(Red quebracho)
	Rhus pentaphilla	(Tizerah sumach)
Leaf extracts	*Rhus coriaria*	(Sumach spp.)
	Rhus cotinus	(Wig tree)
	Uncaria gambir	(Gambier)

Table 1 (contd)

Fruit extracts	*Q. aegilops*	(Valonia oak)
	Emblica officinalis	(Mirobalan)
	Libidibda coriaria	(Dividivi)
	Caesalpinia brevifolia	(Algarobilla)
Gall extracts	particularly oak-gall	
Root extracts	*Sabal palmetto*	(Palmetto)
	Rumex hymenosepalus	(Canaigre)

Synthetic tannins* (see text, p. 210)

Miscellaneous tannages

Aluminium chloride	Cod-liver oil
Aluminium sulphate	Formaldehyde*

RETAN, COLOUR AND FAT LIQUOR

Neutralizing

Ammonium bicarbonate	Sodium acetate
Borax*	Sodium bicarbonate*
Calcium formate*	Sodium formate

Retan

Glutaraldehyde*	Vegetable tannins
Synthetic tannins (see text, p. 210)	Zirconium (chloride and sulphate)

Bleaching

Hydrogen peroxide	Sodium thiosulphate
Oxalic acid	Sulphur dioxide
Sodium carbonate	Synthetic tannins (see text p. 210)
Sodium hypochlorite	

Dyeing

Auxiliary surfactants*	Sulphuric acid
Dyes* (see also Appendix 6)	Synthetic tannins* (see text, p. 210)
Formic acid*	

Table 1 (contd)

    Fat liquor (These substances may also be emulsified with cationic* or nonionic surfactants)

Animal oils (e.g., neatsfoot oil, sperm oil)*

Chlorinated paraffins

Fish oils (e.g., cod-liver oil)*

Greases

Mineral oil*

    Paste drying

Carboxymethylcellulose*

Fungicides (chlorophenols)

Starch*

Polyethers (high molecular weight from vinyl alcohol)

Sulphated oils*

Sulphited oils*

Vegetable oils (e.g., castor, colza and cottonseed oil)*

FINISH

    Solvents (widely variable use, so no classification possible)

Acetone

Amyl acetate

Amyl alcohol

Benzene

Butanol

Butyl acetate

Butyl Cellosolve

Cyclohexane

Dichloromethane

Diethyl ether

1,4-Dioxane

Ethanol

Glycols and glycol acetates

Isopropanol

Methanol

Methyl acetate

Methylcyclohexane

Methyl ethyl ketone

Methyl isobutyl ketone

Nitrobenzene

Petroleum distillates

Tetrachloroethane

Toluene

1,1,1-Trichloroethane

Trichloroethylene

Xylene

Table 1 (contd)

Plasticizers

Butyl stearate	Diethylphthalate
Camphor	Dimethylphthalate
Diamide phthalate	Tricresylphosphate
Dibutylphosphate	Triphenylphosphate
Dibutylphthalate	

Pigments (see also Appendix 6)

Aluminium oxide	Lead chromate
Barium sulphate	Lead hydrate
Cadmium selenide	Lead oxide
Cadmium sulphide	Lead sulphate
Carbon black	Phthalocyanine blue
Chrome green	Phthalocyanine green
Ferric ferrocyanide	Titanium dioxide
Iron blue	Zinc oxide
Iron oxide	Zinc sulphide
Lead carbonate	

Binders (in water solution, solvent solution or as emulsions)

Acrylonitrile-butadiene copolymer* (polybutadiene-acrylonitrile)	Nitrocellulose
Blood albumin	Polyacrylate resin emulsions (e.g., polybutyl methacrylate* polyethyl acrylate* polymethyl methacrylate* polyisobutyl methacrylate)
Carrageenan	
Casein	
Colophony	Polyurethane*
Egg albumin	Polyvinyl acetate
Linseed oil	Polyvinyl butyl ether
Melamine	Polyvinyl chloride

Table 1 (contd)

Binders (contd)

Polyvinylidene chloride*

Polyvinyl toluene

Shellac

Styrene copolymers

Impregnants (in organic solvents or surfactants)

Alkyl succinic compounds	Polyurethanes*
Chromium or aluminium salts of fatty acids	Silicone compounds
Polyacrylic resins*	

Miscellaneous finishing operations

Beeswax stearin	Surfactants
Formaldehyde*	Talc
Kaolin	Wood dust
Paraffin wax	

Pigmented polyols and isocyanates (for special leather
  finishes such as wet-look effects and patent leather)

DEGREASING (widely variable use, so no classification possible)

Alkanol ethoxylates	Pentachloroethane
Alkylbenzene sulphonates	Petrol (gasoline)
Alkylphenols	Polyoxyethylene
Alkyl phenyl ethoxylates	Quarternary ammonium salts
Alkyl sulphates	Soaps
Alkyl sulphites	Stoddard solvent (petroleum distillate)
Benzene	Surfactants
Carbon tetrachloride	Tetrachloroethane
Cetyl ammonium bromide	Tetrachloroethylene (perchlorethylene)
Dichloroethylene	Trichloroethylene
Kerosene	White spirit

The following dust levels (Table 2) were measured in various factories in three different countries. They are therefore not necessarily typical, although the wide range of figures may well accurately reflect widely different conditions. (Personal samples tend to reflect particular operator exposure, and static samples, the general background level.)

(ii) *Other dusts:* Workers may also be exposed to dusts other than those from leather. Total dust levels in a leather storehouse are shown in Table 3.

(iii) *Exposure to airborne chemical substances:* Chemicals used in the various tanning operations can become airborne by evaporation, by suspension in mists or by suspension around the area in which they are being used or produced and, to a lesser extent, in other stages of the tanning. The sources of workroom pollution are as follows:

· The operations of taking the substances out of the main containers and transferring them into containers of smaller capacity (casks or pails, often open) where they are weighed provide a possibility of exposure. If the containers are not airtight, there is a risk of vaporization during transport and when the substances are introduced into the rotating drums or into the tanks of painting machines.

· Another source of pollution is the scouring and emptying of the rotating-drum baths. The amount of pollution from this source increases when the bath temperature is increased because vaporization is facilitated.

· In addition to the chemical substances used, the worker may be exposed to other compounds formed by the reaction of the original compounds with other substances in the environment; hydrogen sulphide is an important example, since its production in drums may cause acute and even lethal poisonings (Strack, 1977). Hydrogen sulphide is also produced on the floor when the effluents from baths containing sulphide or sodium sulphydrate are acidified by those from pickling and tanning baths.

· The weighing and mixing of various compounds, when carried out without dust or vapour extraction is another source of exposure.

· One working procedure which causes a great deal of air pollution is leather painting. All methods of painting do so, but particularly that done with spraying equipment or flow-coating. Another source of pollution in these departments is drying of painted leathers not in a stove but on trays placed on shelves, providing a wide evaporating surface.

Table 2. Dust levels measured during various operation in factories in three countries

	Range (mg/m^3)	No. of samples
Buffing		
total dust, personal samples	0.1-16.0	56
total dust, static samples	0.1-4.1	20
dust ⟨ 5 μm, static samples	0.9 and 1.1	2
Staking - automatic (through feed)		
total dust, personal samples	0.2-2.9	11
total dust, static samples	3.8 and 4.8	2
dust ⟨ 5 μm, static sample	1.5	1
Staking - semi-automatic		
total dust, personal samples	0.5-21	12
total dust, static samples	2.0 and 14.6	2
Shaving		
total dust, static samples	1.4-4.2	3
dust ⟨ 5 μm, static samples	1.1-1.9	3
Splitting (of dry leather)		
total dust, personal samples	0.3-1.9	4
Dry fulling		
total dust, static sample (centre of workroom)	0.54	

Table 3. Dust levels in the storehouse of an Italian tannery

Sample position	total dust >5 μm (mg/m^3)	particles/ cm$^{2\,a}$	% dust <5 μm
Sorting table	3.4	-	-
Sorting table in workplace	-	50	50
Middle of the room	-	50	70
Opening of bales	-	250	80
Sorting table	4.3	-	-
Work place	-	60	70
Middle of the room	-	45	70
Opening of bales	-	300	70
Work place	-	100	50
Middle of the room	-	50	60

[a] As observed by light microscopy

• Another source of workroom pollution is the putrefaction of decaying flesh and other waste products. This produces, for example, ammonia.

• *Trivalent chromium salts* - Exposure may occur during the weighing and introduction of chromium salts into rotating drums; exposures occur more frequently in tanneries in which these operations are still carried out by hand. The exposure time is short. Workers may also be exposed by inhalation when the tanning baths are emptied.

• *Tannins* - Exposure to tannins occurs under the same conditions as for chromium when the operations are carried out in drums. When tanning is carried out in pits, the probabilities of contact with tannins are considerable because the pits are open and the leathers are often handled by the workers.

• *Sodium pentachlorophenate* - Since this substance may be used to prevent deterioration of leather during tanning and to protect from mould, worker exposure may occur. Treated hides may also be used in the production of gelatin, and low levels of pentachlorophenol (up to 8.3 μg/g) have been measured in some Mexican gelatin samples (Firestone, 1977).

While tannery workers may be exposed *via* inhalation to the various chemicals used and produced in the leather tanning process, few data are available. The following data on levels of airborne chemicals are based on measurements made in two areas: Europe and the US.

• *European data* - In 1950, surveys were carried out in 12 French factories to estimate the risk of benzene pollution due to hand spray-painting. The concentrations measured were reported to be lower or close to 100 mg/m^3; higher concentrations (300 mg/m^3) were measured in a continuous spray-painting installation. Concentrations of 200-350 mg/m^3 were measured during finishing with wads; and concentrations up to 600-750 mg/m^3 benzene were measured during a particular operation, which lasted only a short time, in which a very dilute pigment was applied to leathers treated with a synthetic resin (Vallaud & Durand, 1950).

The concentrations measured by personal samplers are higher than those measured by fixed sampling devices, and personal sampling permits a more exact evaluation of the real risk of inhalation of substances. Since some of the measurements of airborne dust and compounds listed in Table 4 and in the text were taken with static sampling devices, it must be remembered in evaluating them that they probably give values inferior to the concentrations actually inhaled by workers.

• *United States data* - In a study to assess the health risk of working in the US tanning industry, the industrial process was reviewed, and quantitative and qualitative levels of exposure were determined. Data from five industrial hygiene surveys in the US were collated: from the National Institute of Occupational Safety and Health, the Occupational Safety and Health Administration, and city and state health departments. The operations surveyed (both by area and personal sampling) in the tanneries and the chemicals sampled were the following:

Beamhouse
Hydrogen sulphide
Ammonia

Table 4. Air concentrations of various compounds in different
departments of two Italian tanneries

TANNERY NO. 1 (1977)

Tanning, retan, colour and fat liquoring departments (9 static samples)

Compound	Range (%)
Chromium [III]	0.0-0.005
Acetic acid	0.0-2.0
Formaldehyde	0.0-0.3
Ammonia	0.0-2.2
Hydrogen sulphide	0.0-14
Sulphur dioxide	0.0-0.7

Beamhouse (liming, during dispensing)

Compound	Concentration (%)
Sulphuric acid	0.9
Ammonia	12.5
Acetic acid	7.2

Solvent vapours in finishing department[a]
(13 static samples near spraying position, 2 in centre of room)[b]

Compound	Range (mg/m^3)	Average (mg/m^3)
Butyl acetate (in centre of room)	13-322 (8 and 14)	112.0
Methyl ethyl ketone (in centre of room)	25 - 105 (7 and 4)	50.4
Toluene (in centre of room)	49-429 (16 and 21)	150.2

Table 4 (contd)

Compound	Range (mg/m^3)	Average (mg/m^3)
Isobutanol (in centre of room)	7-203 (traces)	65.4
Trichloroethylene (in centre of room)	10-95 (47 and 68)	53.6

Total dust and chromium [III] concentrations during weighing in finishing department[a,c]

Sample position[d]	Total dust (mg/m^3)	Cr[III] (mg/m^3)
Weighing Blancorol RA	312.00	17.54
Centre of room	4.57	0.008
Weighing Baykanol SL	25.50	-
Centre of room	17.50	-
Weighing Tanigan PC	67.07	-
Weighing Salcromo 26	145.70	0.600
Weighing Derma/GB/BRN/GS/+KRLS	9.50	-
Centre of room	4.70	-
Weighing Derma Carbone GTS	5.10	-
Weighing Derma Van GB	40.75	-
Weighing Oropon	15.5	-

TANNERY No. 2 (1979)[a]

Compound	Type of sample	No. of samples	Concentration (mg/m^3)
Solvent vapours in finishing department (doubling)			
Acetone	static	1	2.7
	personal	1	18.5
Ethyl acetate	static	2	3.7, 9.0
	personal	1	19.4

Table 4 (contd)

Compound	Type of sample	No. of samples	Concentration (mg/m^3)
Finishing department (doubling) (contd)			
Methyl ethyl ketone	static	2	55.2, 265.6
	personal	1	547.9
Isobutyl acetate	static	2	2.3, 5.3
	personal	1	11.5
Toluene	static	2	8.4, 33.6
	personal	1	50.6
Butyl acetate	static	2	1.8, 2.9
	personal	1	9.9
Xylene	static	2	1.0, 1.9
	personal	1	2.4
Toluene-2,4-diisocyanate (TDI)	static	2	<0.005
4,4'-Methylenedianiline	static	3	<0.05
Solvent vapours in finishing department (flow-coating)[e]			
Acetone	static[f]	2	2, 14.9
	personal	6	7.6-44.1 (average: 28.1)
Ethyl acetate	static	2	8.6, 1200.2
	personal	6	426.8-3698.2 (average: 2137.1)
Methyl ethyl ketone	static	2	2.8, 120.8
	personal	6	42.2-313.5 (average: 187.9)
Isobutyl acetate	static	2	0.7, 62.3
	personal	6	108.1-368.1 (average: 190)
Toluene	static	2	15.6, 408.8
	personal	6	368.6-876.5 (average: 652.2)

Table 4 (contd)

Compound	Type of sample	No. of samples	Concentration (mg/m^3)
Butyl acetate	static	2	0.4, 7.2
	personal	6	14.9-54.1 (average: 36.1)
Xylene	static	1	11.3
	personal	6	2.0-23.4 (average: 12.8)

[a]From Coato et al. (1980)

[b]Benzene levels were not determined.

[c]Weighing is an intermittent operation.

[d]Only commercial names are given.

[e]The finishing workroom had no natural or mechanical ventilation. The painted leather was dried on trays placed on shelves in the same room. The paint used was a polyurethane compound.

[f]Static samples were collected 60 minutes before the flow-coating machine was started up, and 75 minutes after it had been stopped, as two samples.

Tanyard
Sulphuric acid
Chromium [VI]
Chromium [III]
Hydrogen sulphide
Sodium 2,4,5-trichlorophenate

Retan, colour, fat liquor
Formic acid
Chromium [III]
Copper
Cobalt
Ammonia
Benzidine
Benzidine-2,2'-disulphonic acid
1-Naphthalene sulphonic acid
3,3-Dimethoxybenzidine

Finishing
Petroleum distillates
Butyl Cellosolve
Tetrachloroethylene
Xylene
Methyl ethyl ketone
Butyl acetate
Toluene
Methyl isobutyl ketone
Acetone
Formaldehyde
Isopropyl alcohol
Benzene

The samples from the beamhouse were taken in one tannery, and they reflect exposure of workers operating paddle vats and defleshing machines. In 14 personal samples taken to determine the levels of hydrogen sulphide during the addition of sulphides and sulphydrates to the paddle vat or operation of the defleshing machines, which were next to the vats, levels ranged from 2-60 ppm. Levels in six area samples taken for ammonia during the addition of ammonium sulphate to the paddle vats ranged from 50-75 ppm. The beamhouse had no ventilation. The exposure of workers operating the defleshing machine is an example of 'cross pollution', whereby workers performing mechanical operations are exposed to chemicals in the air from another operation.

Two tanneries were surveyed in 1979 for five chemicals used in the tanyard. By far the most common chemical used in the tanning department of a chrome tannery is basic chromium sulphate. Six personal samples obtained for chromium [III] showed levels ranging from < 5.5 to 8.0 $\mu g/m^3$. Although chromium [VI] was not used in the tanneries, five personal samples were taken for analysis; none was found at a detection limit of 1.0 $\mu g/m^3$. Five personal samples were also taken to determine hydrogen sulphide levels during feeding of sodium sulphydrate: the levels ranged from 330-11,000 $\mu g/m^3$, with an average of 2800 $\mu g/m^3$. Determinations of sulphuric acid while it was being added to the chrome liquor showed levels of 20.5-130 $\mu g/m^3$, with an average of 66.8 $\mu g/m^3$. Finally, personal samples were obtained while workers were adding a 2,4,5-trichlorophenate formulation to the tanning liquors: no detectable levels were found.

The retanning, colouring and fat liquoring departments of two tanneries were surveyed for nine chemicals, using personal and wipe samples. (Although other chemicals were in use, the survey was limited by the air sampling and analytical techniques currently available.) Chromium [III] was detected at a level of 5.8 $\mu g/m^3$ in the only sample taken on a colour-drum operator but was not detected on a dye-room operator. Cobalt, copper, benzidine, 3,3'-dimethoxybenzidine and benzidine-2,2'-disulphonic acid were not detected in the dye room or on the colour-drum operator. Formic acid was detected in a range of 0.07-9.30 $\mu g/m^3$ in 14 personal samples, giving an average of 1.53 $\mu g/m^3$. One personal sample showed a level of 55,000 $\mu g/m^3$ ammonia.

The survey of finishing departments, in which 11 chemicals were analysed from charcoal-tube samples (Table 5), provided a great deal of information on exposures to a wide array of chemical solvents, pigments and waxes. In each of the five US tanneries surveyed, ventilation systems were fitted to the mechanized spray booths and drying ovens. The operating procedure was similar in all the tanneries: the hides were fed onto a motorized conveyor belt by one worker, treated with finishing compounds and dried by passing through a long drying oven, then removed by another worker. A third employee swabbed the hide after it had been colour-coated to ensure an even finish. It was considered that these workers probably had the greatest exposure. Samples were also taken in the room in which lacquers and solvents were stored; this was usually small and contained open drums of the chemicals.

Table 5. Concentrations of various compounds in the
finishing departments of five US tanneries

Compound	No. of samples	Range	Average
Butyl Cellosolve	30	0.24-5.85 mg/m^3	1.3 mg/m^3
Tetrachloroethylene	54	25-⟨300 ppm	57.9 ppm
Xylene	69	0-20.9 ppm	4.0 ppm
Dubois machine (area sample)	5	0-6.0 ppm	4.5 ppm
Methyl ethyl ketone	1[a]	100-500 ppm	
Butyl acetate (lacquer & solvent storage room, area samples)	4	0-34 ppm	20 ppm
Toluene	28	0.52-65.7 ppm	10.4 ppm
Methyl isobutyl ketone	16	0.21-20.9 ppm	4.62 ppm
Acetone	26	0.24-25.0 ppm	5.64 ppm
Formaldehyde	5	1.0-7.4 ppm	4.2 ppm
Isopropanol	5	4.0-69.0 ppm	22.5 ppm
Benzene (storage room)	5	0	0

[a]Using direct-reading instrument

(iv) *Motor exhaust emissions:* Another source of workroom pollution is motor exhaust emissions from fork-lift trucks with diesel, petrol or propane engines. The main gaseous emissions are oxides of nitrogen, carbon monoxide, sulphur oxides and hydrocarbons. The particulate fraction of exhaust from diesel engines contains polycyclic organic matter (e.g., benzo[a]pyrene) (Kotin *et al.*, 1955). Diesel engines may emit ten times as much benzo[a]pyrene as other engines that operate similarly (Schenker, 1980).

(v) *Occurrence of nitrosamines in leather tanneries:* If dimethylamine is used in the tanning process, *N*-nitrosodimethylamine may be produced.

The toxic and carcinogenic properties of *N*-nitroso compounds have been reviewed (IARC, 1978). Evidence that certain consumer and industrial products contain *N*-nitroso compounds (Fan *et al.*, 1977; Fine *et al.*, 1977; Ross *et al.*, 1977) led to speculation that workers in the industries which either use or manufacture nitrosamine precursors (amines and nitrogen oxides) may be exposed to these agents. One such industry is leather tanning. Dimethylamine sulphate (DMAS, a precursor of *N*-nitrosodimethylamine, NDMA) is used in some leather tanneries as a depilatory agent in the hide unhairing process (Walker *et al.*, 1976), although the extent to which it is used throughout the world is not known. *N*-Nitroso compounds have been found in five leather manufacturing facilities (Rounbehler *et al.*, 1981). The levels of NDMA found in the air in five US tanneries are given in Table 6.

Tannery A was the first tannery surveyed. It is located in New England and employs about 300 workers who process about 2000 hides per day into fully tanned and finished leather. During three visits to this factory, the entire tanning and finishing processes were sampled for the presence of *N*-nitroso compounds. Thirty-six area air samples, representing a cross-section of the air in the tannery, were collected; in addition, 27 bulk samples were taken, 11 of which were of chemicals or chemical mixes, two of hide and leather, two of waste-water, and 12 of process water from the wet operation.

NDMA was found in most of the air samples, at levels ranging from 0.1 μg/m^3 in the lunch-room area to 47 μg/m^3 in the retanning area. *N*-Nitrosomorpholine (NMOR) was also found, at a level of 2.0 μg/m^3 , in three air samples taken in the finishing area. Use of DMAS was then discontinued; on a subsequent visit, 50 days later, the NDMA level in the retanning area had dropped to 3.4 μg/m^3 .

Of the 27 bulk samples only four contained NDMA (Table 7). The highest level, 0.5 μg/g, was found in a sample of DMAS solution; 0.0014 μg/ml was found in process water from the re-lime pit (unhairing vat), and 0.004-0.006 μg/ml was found in the waste-water streams from the tannery. No NDMA was detected in salted cowhide (detection limit, 0.05 μg/g).

In order to produce the airborne concentrations of NDMA observed during the first two visits, there would have to be about 2 g NDMA in the air at any given time. Since the level of NDMA found as an impurity in the DMAS can account for only 60 mg/day and no alternative sources were evident, one explanation for the presence of the NDMA could be nitrosation of dimethylamine in the air or on surfaces. Crude measurements of the nitrosating capacity of the air suggest that exhaust from the propane-driven fork-lift trucks could serve as the nitrosating agent (Rounbehler *et al.*, 1979, 1981). The greatest amount of

Table 6. Levels of *N*-nitrosodimethylamine in the air of five US tanneries[a]

Tannery	Concentration ($\mu g/m^3$)	
	Maximum	Average
A[b]	33	13
A[c]	47	18
A[d]	3.4	2.4
B	8	1.5
C	2.0	1.6
D	trace	-
E	ND[e]	-

[a]From Rounbehler *et al*. (1981)

[b]Tannery A was the only one in which dimethylamine sulphate was used in the hide unhairing process.

[c]During visit to Tannery A two days after the first

[d]Third visit to Tannery A 50 days after the first visit, by which time dimethylamine sulphate was no longer used

[e]ND - None detected; detection limit, 0.05 $\mu g/m^3$

such nitrosating exhaust was found in the wet process area, where high levels of NDMA were found previously. It is in this area that propane-driven fork-life trucks are operated and where DMAS is used.

Tannery B employs 80 workers and processes 700 hides per day into fully tanned and coloured leathers, which are shipped to tannery E for surface and mechanical finishing. Dimethylamine sulphate was not used, although it had been in the recent past. Nineteen air samples and four bulk samples were collected; the latter consisted of two of waste-water, one of steam system condensate and one floor scraping from the dye room.

Again, NDMA was found in the atmosphere at all stages of production, with levels ranging from 0.03 $\mu g/m^3$ in the drying area to 8 $\mu g/m$ in an unused loft above the unhairing area. The further away from the unhairing process that the air samples were taken the lower the levels of NDMA. The high level found in the loft above the unhairing area may be the result of DMAS use in the past. A later study by the US Department of Agriculture found NDMA adsorbed on the structural wood of the loft. None of the bulk samples examined contained *N*-nitroso compounds. This tannery also used propane-driven fork-lift trucks.

Table 7. Levels of *N*-nitrosodimethylamine (NDMA) in liquid and solid bulk samples from a US tannery[a]

Sample	NDMA (μg/g)
Chemicals	
Azo rubine dye	ND[b]
Penetrator L-219	ND
Nigrosine blue L	ND
Polar Sol 5	ND
Betz Formula NA-6	ND
Boiler rush inhibitor mix	ND
Ammonia paste wash	ND
para-Nitrophenol	ND
KITO-40 (fungicide)	ND
Fresh brine	ND
Aqueous dimethylamine sulphate (36.5% solution)	0.5
Leather	
Chrome-tanned leather	ND
Raw-salted cowhide	ND
Waste-water	
Beamhouse waste-water	0.004
Tanning house waste-water	0.006
Process water	
Re-lime pit	0.0014
Bating solution (two samples)	ND
Pickling solution (two samples)	ND
Chrome-tanning solution (two samples	ND
Final rinse from chrome tanning (two samples)	ND
Wash out of colouring	ND
First rinse from fat liquoring	ND
Final rinse from fat liquoring	ND

[a] From Rounbehler *et al*. (1979)

[b] ND - None detected; detection limit, 0.5 ng/g

Tannery C, located in midwestern US, employs 135 workers who produce 3000 chrome-tanned hides per day, which are then shipped to tannery D for retanning, colouring and final finishing. No dimethylamine sulphate had been used in Tannery C, except in some pilot plant tests. Ten area air samples and five process air samples were collected, along with eight bulk samples; the latter consisted of six of process water, one of plant waste-water and one of steam system condensate. The process air samples were collected inside hide-processing drums.

NDMA was found in all of the air samples taken within this tannery, at levels ranging from 0.2 $\mu g/m^3$ in the chemical processing room (sulphide stripping) to over 3 $\mu g/m^3$ in the centre of the plant. Airborne levels of NDMA within the hide-processing drums were equal to or lower than those within the plant. No NDMA was detected in any of the bulk samples (detection limit, 0.05 $\mu g/ml$); however, experimental nitrosation of three of the bulk samples of process water resulted in the formation of 1.5-2.5 ng/ml NDMA. Similar nitrosation experiments with air samples indicated the presence of twice that level of NDMA; and, in a separate experiment, an airborne nitrosating agent was detected.

This plant uses propane-driven fork-lift trucks and direct, gas-fired air heaters, both of which contribute nitrogen oxides to the air.

Tannery D, located in New England, employs 560 workers who process 8000-10,000 hides per day and retan and finish chrome-tanned hides received from tannery C and other plants. Twenty-one air samples were collected at all stages of the operation. There was no reported use of dimethylamine sulphate or any other amines in this facility.

Two air samples were found to contain NMOR at levels of 0.1 and 0.25 $\mu g/m^3$; in addition, 0.05 $\mu g/m^3$ NDMA was found in the sample containing 0.1 $\mu g/m^3$ NMOR. These levels of *N*-nitroso compounds are considerably lower than those found in the plants performing wet-tanning operations.

Tannery E, also located in New England, employs 60 workers who apply surface finishes to leather that has been fully tanned and coloured at tannery B. Seventeen air samples were taken at all stages of production. Although many chemicals and dyes are used at this plant, there were no known sources of amines or nitrosating agents. No *N*-nitroso compounds were found in any of the air samples.

The authors (Rounbehler et al., 1981) concluded from their study that the presence of NDMA in tanneries may be the result of nitrosation of ambient dimethylamine by oxides of nitrogen, mainly in the wet-process areas.

2.4 Biological factors

The risk of contracting some zoonoses must be considered, especially during those operations preceding wet processing, i.e., during the phase in which undressed leathers are handled.

Colonies of fungi may develop on leathers and on the surface of the pit liquid. Two species, Aspergillus niger and Penicillum glaucum, have been noted particularly (Martignone, 1964). Several yeasts have been isolated from chrome-tanned leathers, wet-blue stock, reducing sugars and syrups, and scrapings from tannery drums. Yeasts of three genera, Rhodotorula, Cladosporium and Torulopsis, were found (Kallenberger, 1978).

To avoid the development of fungi, various chemicals are often used (Hollingsworth, 1976). Among these, chlorinated phenols, particularly pentachlorophenol and sodium pentachlorophenate, are used widely.

2.5 Current regulations and recommendations on exposures

See 'General Remarks on Wood, Leather and Some Associated Industries', p. 23.

2.6 Number of workers involved

See 'General Remarks on Wood, Leather and Some Associated Industries', p. 19.

3. TOXIC, INFLAMMATORY AND ALLERGIC EFFECTS IN HUMANS

In view of the large numbers of toxic chemicals used in the leather tanning and processing industry, it is surprising that no more reports on toxicological effects than those reported here were available to the Working Group.

Skin disorders as well as systemic poisoning may result from handling hides and skins which have been treated with arsenic or mercury as preservatives (McConnell et al., 1942).

Eczema and contact and allergic dermatitis have been diagnosed in tannery workers (Abrams & Warr, 1951; Sinitsyna, 1972) and in hide, leather and fur workers (Abrams & Warr, 1951).

According to the statistics of the US Bureau of Labor, the highest incidence of skin disease (mainly allergic eczematous dermatitis), contributing 21.2 per 1000 cases of occupational dermatoses, occurs in workers in the leather tanning and finishing industry (Anon., 1979).

Levels of chromium [III] ranging from 0-0.349 mg/l of urine have been found in workers employed in tanning departments in the leather industry (Tyras & Blochowicz, 1974).

Irritation of the mucous membranes of the throat and nose, and even perforation of the nasal septum, may occur after inhaling chromic acid fumes liberated during the chrome-tanning process or during direct contact with chromates (McConnell et al., 1942).

Anthrax was reported to be a serious health hazard resulting from the handling of hides, principally before the introduction of decontamination in a solution of lime or formaldehyde (Smyth & Bricker, 1922; Schwartz, 1936; McConnell et al., 1942).

Two cases of fatal inhalation anthrax (one of which was complicated by systemic sarcoidosis) associated with tannery work were reported (Brachman et al., 1961). Another case of fatal inhalation anthrax was observed in a man who had worked in a metal fabrication shop near a goat-hair processing plant. Exposure was via contaminated aerosols (LaForce et al., 1969). In the USA, industrial anthrax was reported in workers exposed to goat skins imported from countries where anthrax is prevalent (Brachman & Fekety, 1958).

During the phase in which the undressed leathers are handled, tetanus, leptospirosis, epizootic aphtha, Q fever and brucellosis may be contracted (Sommer et al., 1971; Sinitsyna, 1972; Valsecchi & Fiorio, 1978).

Several cases of 'farmer's lung', i.e., interstitial allergic alveolitis, due to colonies of fungi belonging to the Penicillium and Aspergillium genera have been found in tannery workers (Valsecchi & Fiorio, 1978).

Chronic bronchitis was reported in workers in leather industries in Kanpur, India (Gupta & Sidhu, 1970).

Morbidity due to catarrh of the upper respiratory tract, angina and bronchitis was higher among workers in the finishing department of a tannery than in those in other departments of the same factory (Makshanova, 1977).

Polyneuritis, myositis and arthritis of the hands have been observed in tannery workers (Sinitsyna, 1972).

4. CARCINOGENICITY DATA[1]

(a) Nasal cancer

Delemarre & Themans (1971) investigated the occupational histories of 16 patients admitted to a hospital in The Netherlands during the period 1944-1967 with a diagnosis of nasal adenocarcinoma. Thirty-three controls were chosen among patients with nasal cancers other than adenocarcinoma admitted to the same hospital in the period 1956-1968. Two patients had had exposures in leather industries (one tanner and one shoemaker) compared with none of the controls.

(b) Lung cancer

Kennaway & Kennaway (1947) carried out an analysis of occupational mortality data based on death certificates in England and Wales during two different time periods, 1921-1932 and 1933-1938. Between 1921 and 1932, there were 21 lung cancer deaths among men classified in the occupational category 'tanners, leather dressers, curriers', whereas 14.2 were expected; during 1933-1938, there were 30 observed deaths and 22 expected. For both time periods combined, the SMR for lung cancer is 141.

(c) Bladder cancer

Henry et al. (1931) undertook a death certificate analysis of all men who died of bladder cancer between 1921 and 1928 in England and Wales with regard to specific occupation. An increased risk was identified for persons employed in the category 'tanners, leather dressers, curriers'. Specifically, there were 17 observed deaths among men so employed in contrast to 10.1 expected on the basis of age-specific bladder cancer death rates for all men in England and Wales (SMR = 168).

A case-control study carried out in eastern Massachusetts (Cole et al., 1971, 1972) included 356 men and 105 women with cancer of the lower urinary tract (94% of the bladder), representing a sample of all cases newly diagnosed between January 1967 and June 1968 in the area. Each case was matched individually by age and sex to a general population control. Men who worked in preliminary processes and in tanning within the leather industry had a relative risk of 1.45 (not statistically significant), based on 8 cases.

---

[1] This section should be read in conjunction with Appendices 1 and 3, pp. 295 and 305.

5. SUMMARY OF DATA AND EVALUATION

5.1 Summary of data

There is only one case report of an adenocarcinoma of the nasal cavity occurring in a tanner. In a study in England and Wales covering the period 1961-1966, no leather tanners or processors were found among patients with adenocarcinomas or other types of nasal cancers. (See monograph on boot and shoe manufacture & repair, p. 268.)

No data specifically related to laryngeal cancer in leather tanners and processors were available. In a large, multi-tumour-site case-control survey in New York state, the relative risk for developing laryngeal cancer associated with employment for more than five years in the leather industry was 5.5 (based on 6 cases).

SMRs for lung cancer in male tanners, leather dressers and curriers estimated from mortality statistics in England and Wales during the period 1921-1938 were in the order of 150. No excess was found in the study in England and Wales in 1961. SMRs for 'leather workers' in England and Wales in 1971 and for 'leather operatives' in the US were not significantly different from 100. However, in a cross-sectional study in Los Angeles in 1972-1973, the risk ratio for men engaged in 'leather-manufacturing and sales' was 1.72 ($P < 0.05$).

The SMR for bladder cancer in male tanners, leather dressers and curriers estimated from mortality statistics in England and Wales in the 1920s was 170. More recent reports listing SMRs for comparable occupational groups were not available to the Working Group.

An association between work in the leather trades and bladder cancer is suggested by three of four case-control studies. The one study among these that subclassified leather occupations shows that eight patients were engaged in 'preliminary' processes and tanning within the leather industry (relative risk, 1.5; not statistically significant).

No studies specifically related to lymphoma in leather tanners or processors were available. The SMR for 'leather workers' in England and Wales in 1971 was 184 for non-Hodgkin's lymphomas and 77 for Hodgkin's disease. In a large, multi-tumour-site case-control study in New York state, the relative risk for all lymphomas among 'leather workers' was 3.4 in men (based on 7 cases, $P < 0.05$) and 2.6 in women (based on 8 cases, $P < 0.05$).

In a large, multi-tumour-site case-control study in New York state, the relative risk for cancer of the oral cavity and pharynx among male 'leather workers' was 3.2 ($P < 0.01$, based on 18 cases). A correlation study in the US showed mortality rates for oral and pharyngeal cancer to be slightly elevated in counties with leather manufacturing industries.

Vital statistics from England and Wales and from the US suggest that death rates from renal cancer among 'leather workers' and 'employees in the leather industry' are about 1.6 - 2.3 times greater than those in the general population.

The SMR for cancer of the stomach in tanners in England and Wales in 1961 was 135 (P < 0.05). No data on comparable occupational groups in England and Wales at other periods or in other countries were available to the Working Group.

Inhalation of both chemical vapours and dust (including leather and hide dust) and dermal contact with these agents could occur simultaneously. For most workers, the degree and types of exposure depend upon their specific occupation and work area within the tannery. For example, the unloading of a hide-processing drum may result in simultaneous contact with the chemical substances within the drum, by inhalation and dermal contact, and with the chemical dusts generated while recharging the drums. In the case of a tannery which incorporates all the processes of leather production, beamhouse workers may also be exposed to the organic vapours generated in the finishing department;   however, their exposure to these agents may be lower than that of those employed within the finishing area. Workers in the buffing area are exposed to leather dust and to its burden of tanning chemicals, while those working in the hide receiving and sorting area are exposed to hide dust. Buffing area workers may also be exposed to solvent vapours from the finishing area; due to the proximity of the hide-sorting area to the beamhouse, hide sorters may also be exposed to beamhouse contaminants. The chemical complexity of the tanning process and the wide variety of finishing agents used will almost certainly result in worker exposure *via* inhalation and dermal contact to multiple and changing chemical pollutants.

The industry is moving towards greater automation and mechanization. However, in many plants wet hides are still handled manually throughout the manufacturing process. Some workers may subject their hands and arms to tanning chemicals both by handling wet hides and by direct exposure to the chemicals.

It must be emphasized that often more than one of the operations are carried out in the same work room, and this results in cross pollution. Furthermore, in some operations, the work load and elevated temperature and relative humidity may change the environmental exposure. These features of the industry make evaluation of individual exposures difficult.

Employment in tanneries may entail exposure to a number of chemicals for which there is evidence of carcinogenicity in humans and/or laboratory animals (see Appendix 5).

5.2 Evaluation

Very few epidemiological studies or case reports deal specifically with workers engaged in leather tanning and processing. There is no evidence to suggest an association between leather tanning and nasal cancer. The suggested associations between employment in the leather industry (not further specified) and cancer of the lung, larynx, buccal cavity, pharynx, and kidney and lymphomas come from hypothesis-generating surveys. They do not refer specifically to workers in tanneries. A positive association between employment in the leather industry (not further specified) and bladder cancer is supported by a number of studies. The only study that dealt specifically with leather tanners, however, revealed a relative risk of 1.5, which is not statistically significant.

6. REFERENCES

Abrams, H.K. & Warr, P. (1951) Occupational diseases transmitted *via* contact with animals and animal products. *Ind. Med. Surg., 20,* 341-351

Anon. (1979) Assessing skin problems of occupational origin. *Occup. Health Saf., 48,* 18, 39-43

Bayer AG (1975) *Tanner - Teindre - Finir [Tanning-Dyeing-Finishing]*, Leverkusen, Federal Republic of Germany

Brachman, P.S. & Fekety, F.R. (1958) Industrial anthrax. *Ann. N.Y. Acad. Sci., 70,* 574-584

Brachman, P.S., Pagano, J.S. & Albrink, W.S. (1961) Two cases of fatal inhalation anthrax, one associated with sarcoidosis. *New Engl. J. Med., 265,* 203-208

Bravo, G.A. (1964) *Storia del Cuoio e dell' Arte Conciaria [History of Leather and of the Art of Tanning]*, Turin, Associazione Italiana dei Chimici del Cuoio, pp. 17-32, 169-199

Candura, F. (1974) *Elementi di Tecnologia Industriale a Uso dei Cultori di Medicina del Lavoro [Elements of Industrial Technology for Use in the Study of Industrial Medicine]*, Pavia, Aurora, pp. 659-671

Coato, F., Fiorio, A. & Lovato, L. (1980) Identification of some risk factors in the tanning industry (Ital.). *Quad. Ig. Lav.* (in press)

Cole, P., Monson, R.R., Haning, H. & Friedell, G.H. (1971) Smoking and cancer of the lower urinary tract. *New Engl. J. Med., 284,* 129-134

Cole, P., Hoover, R. & Friedell, G.H. (1972) Occupation and cancer of the lower urinary tract. *Cancer, 29,* 1250-1260

Costanza, G. (1977) *Il Tecnico Operaio Conciatore e Pelliciaio [Work Practices for Tannery and Hide Workers]*, Milan, U. Hoepli, pp. 1-611

Delemarre, J.F.M. & Themans, H.H. (1971) Adenocarcinoma of the nasal cavities (Dutch). *Ned. T. Geneeskd., 115,* 688-690

Fan, T.Y., Goff, U., Song, L., Fine, D.H., Arsenault, G.P. & Biemann, K. (1977) *N*-Nitrosodiethanolamine in cosmetics, lotions and shampoos. *Food Cosmet. Toxicol., 15,* 423-430

Fine, D.H., Rounbehler, D.P., Fan, T. & Ross, R. (1977) *Human exposure to N-nitroso compounds in the environment.* In: Hiatt, H.H., Watson, J.D. & Winsten, J.A., eds, *Origins of Human Cancer,* Book A, *Incidence of Cancer in Humans,* Cold Spring Harbor, NY, Cold Spring Harbor Laboratory, pp. 293-307

Firestone, D. (1977) Determination of polychlorodibenzo-*p*-dioxins and polychlorodibenzofurans in commercial gelatins by gas-liquid chromatography. *J. Agric. Food Chem., 25,* 1274-1280

Gupta, V.P. (1972) *Tanning, leather finishing.* In: *Encyclopaedia of Occupational Health and Safety,* Vol. II, Geneva, International Labour Office, pp. 1381-1383

Gupta, R.K. & Sidhu, C.M.S. (1970) Health hazards in leather industries of Kanpur. *Indian J. public Health, 14,* 136-148

Henry, S.A., Kennaway, N.M. & Kennaway, E.L. (1931) The incidence of cancer of the bladder and prostate in certain occupations. *J. Hyg., 31,* 125-137

Hollingsworth, B.S. (1976) Some methods for the evaluation of fungicides particularly in the leather industry (Fr.). *Rev. tech. Ind. Cuir, 68,* 310-317

IARC (1978) *IARC Monographs on the Evaluation of the Carcinogenic Risk of Chemicals to Humans,* Vol. 17, *Some* N-*Nitroso Compounds,* Lyon

Kallenberger, W.E. (1978) A study of yeasts in chrome tanning and processing. *J. Am. Leather Chem. Assoc., 73,* 6-21

Kennaway, E.L. & Kennaway, N.M. (1947) A further study of the incidence of cancer of the lung and larynx. *Br. J. Cancer, 1,* 260-298

Kotin, P., Falk, H.L. & Thomas, M. (1955) Aromatic hydrocarbons. III. Presence in the particulate phase of diesel-engine exhausts and the carcinogenicity of exhaust extracts. *Arch. ind. Health, 11,* 113-120

LaForce, F.M., Bumford, F.H., Feeley, J.C., Stokes, S.L. & Snow, D.B. (1969) Epidemiologic study of a fatal case of inhalation anthrax. *Arch. environ. Health, 18,* 798-805

Makshanova, E.I. (1977) Some morbidity indexes and non-specific responses of leather industry finishing department workers (Russ.). *Zdravookhr. Beloruss., 9,* 85-86

Martignone, G. (1964) *Corso di Conceria Pratica [Treatise on Practical Tanning],* Turin, Levrotto & Bella

McConnell, W.J., Fehnel, J.W. & Ferry, J.J. (1942) Potential health hazards of the leather industry. *J. ind. Hyg. Toxicol., 24,* 93-108

New England Tanners' Club (1965) *Leather Facts,* Peabody, MA

O'Flaherty, F. & Doherty, E.E. (1939) Foot-and-mouth disease. II. A method of sterilizing skins and hides against the virus of foot-and-mouth disease. *J. Am. Leather Chem. Assoc., 34,* 329-336

Ross, R.D., Morrison, J., Rounbehler, D.P., Fan, T. & Fine, D.H. (1977) *N*-Nitroso compound impurities in herbicide formulations. *J. Agric. Food Chem., 25,* 1416-1418

Rounbehler, D.P., Krull, I.S., Goff, E.U., Mills, K.M., Morrison, J., Edwards, G.S., Fine, D.H., Fajen, J.M., Carson, G.A. & Rheinhold, V. (1979) Exposure to *N*-nitrosodimethylamine in a leather tannery. *Food Cosmet. Toxicol., 17,* 487-491

Rounbehler, D.P., Reisch, J.W., Coombs, J.R. & Fine, D.H. (1981) *Occurrence of nitrosamines in industrial atmospheres.* In: *180th American Chemical Society National Meeting, Las Vegas, 1980* (in press)

Schenker, M.B. (1980) Diesel exhaust - an occupational carcinogen? *J. occup. Med., 22,* 41-46

Schwartz, L. (1936) Skin hazards in American industry. Part II. *Public Health Bull., 229,* 13-19

Sinitsyna, Y.L. (1972) Fundamental causes of occupational diseases in the tanning industry (Russ.). *Gig. Tr. Prof. Zabol., 16,* 25-27

Smyth, H.F. & Bricker, E. (1922) Analysis of 123 cases of anthrax in the Pennsylvania leather industry. *J. ind. Hyg., 4,* 53-62

Sommer, D., Hincker, E. & Mehl, J. (1971) Occupational pathology in tanneries (Fr.). *Arch. Mal. prof., Méd. Trav. Sécur. Soc. (Paris), 32,* 723-732

Strack, W. (1977) Hazards due to the toxicity of hydrogen sulphide used in modern technologies of leather production (Yugoslav.). *Koza Obuca, 26,* 283-285

Tyras, H. & Bochowicz, A. (1974) Appraisal of occupational exposure to chromium compounds in leather industry work-places (Pol.). *Bromat. chem. Toksykol., 7,* 143-149

Vallaud, A. & Durand, A. (1950) Contribution to the study of benzolic risk in tawing (Fr.) . *Arch. Mal. prof., 11,* 395-396

Valsecchi, M. & Fiorio, A. (1978) Operating cycle in the tanning industry and related risks (Ital.) *Securitas, 63,* 132-144

Walker, P., Gordon, J., Thomas, L. & Ouellette, R. (1976) *Environmental Assessment of Atmospheric Nitrosamines,* MITRE Corporation Report MTR-7152, EPA Contract 68-02-1495, McLean, VA

Zecchin, F. (1979) *Proposition for improving the legal risk factors in tanning processes* (Ital.). In: *L'Igiene Ambientale nell' Industria Conciaria [Environmental Hygiene in the Tanning Industry],* Montecchio Maggiore, Consorzio per il Servizio di Igiene e Medicina Preventiva del Lavoro

1. HISTORICAL OVERVIEW OF THE INDUSTRY

1.1 Boot and shoe manufacture

Climatic conditions and the nature of terrain have influenced the development of footwear, first used by man as protection against the heat of the ground and sharp stones, or to disguise his tracks. Wood, palm leaves and, particularly, skins were used. Sandals made of a single layer of leather with the 'flower', the outer surface, turned to the inside are the earliest known type of footwear, found in Egyptian tombs of the predynastic era (5000 BC) (Waterer, 1956). Later, more elaborate models were made, with soles comprising several layers.

Sandals, half-boots and buckskins were worn in ancient Greece and in countries of the Near East. The ancient Romans produced shoes - especially those for soldiers - on a large scale, in well organized 'factories'. The soles were made of two or three layers of leather, which were sewn and tacked, while the uppers were composed of strips. This design remained practically unchanged until the sixteenth century, although in northern countries the uppers were slightly modified to adapt them for wear in cold climates.

At the end of the sixteenth century, when footwear was strengthened to meet the needs of military campaigns, the main characteristics of the modern shoe were introduced; and heels and seaming largely as we known them today were developed at that time.

1.2 Boot and shoe repair

In the past, when shoes were made mainly of leather, it was usual for soles and heels to be repaired regularly. This was done by repairers or by the shoe manufacturers. As the durability of solings and the cost of repairs increased, the need for repairing declined and, with it, the numbers of shoe repairers. There are still many repairers, who specialize in the replacement of heels and soles and of uppers when necessary.

2. DESCRIPTION OF THE INDUSTRY

2.1 Processes used previously and changes over time

The parts for the upper were cut by hand with a shoemaker's knife to his own models. They were then sewn together, the edgings were made and any eyelets pierced. The inner linings, made of finer skins or thinner slices, were sewn and glued together with natural glues.

A piece of leather was then wetted and struck with a hammer, and a sole cut from it with a shoemaker's knife, either following a shape drawn on the leather, or by cutting around a template. The sole was applied to the upper with tacks, glued with natural fish, bone or flour glue, and subsequently sewn by hand.

Sewing was done with a needle and hemp thread that was reinforced at one end with pig hair embedded by hand. The thread was lubricated with natural wax and pitch. Small holes were made in the sole to facilitate sewing.

Afterwards, the edges were trimmed with a shoemaker's knife, polished with a file and glass paper and burnished with a warm metal plate. The surface of the sole was polished first with a file and then with the warm metal plate.

These traditional hand processes are still used in many countries.

In the twentieth century, what was once a handicraft industry has been industrialized by the introduction of machines and the splitting up of the production process into several separate operations. Different groups of workers have become responsible for designing and preparing the models, cutting the uppers and the soles, preparing the uppers, assembling the parts and packing.

From the beginning of the century machines were used for stitching the uppers, and the various stages of making up the shoes were organized on the principles of the assembly line, so that the finished product had passed through several hands.

Industrialization of shoemaking at first led to a concentration of the work force, although in some countries it was subsequently dispersed. In Italy, for example, more than 80% of the production units employ fewer than 20 people: the splitting up of the manufacturing process has made it possible to decentralize production. In other countries, however, shoemaking factories are fairly large (average: USA, 195.0 workers; UK, 116.5 workers; Federal Republic of Germany, 162.0 workers; France, 132.9 workers).

Prior to 1950, footwear was made mainly from leather uppers and soles usually stitched together. All cutting and preparation of leather was done in a shoe factory. The outer parts of uppers were made mainly of chrome-tanned leather and the linings of vegetable-tanned leather. Insoles and outsoles were made almost entirely of vegetable-tanned leather. Other materials used included cotton fabric linings; nitrocellulose toe puff and stiffener materials; some satin (silk) for evening wear; natural rubber; inorganic solvents and natural rubber latexes as adhesives. The current trend in many countries is the substitution of natural soles by synthetic materials.

The dustiest operations were the preparation of leather soles and insoles and the scouring and finishing of those components on the manufactured shoes. The latter operations produce the finest dusts. Cyclone extraction systems are available, but even so the workers were certainly subjected to dusty working conditions. The volume of adhesives used was small by comparison with that used in modern manufacturing methods, because most of the shoe bottoms were attached by stitching. Some exposure to solvents, such as petroleum hydrocarbons (naphthas), benzene, carbon disulphide, carbon tetrachloride, acetone and amyl acetate, occurred. Hydrocarbon mixtures, benzene and carbon tetra-chloride were used in rubber solutions for laminating linings to uppers and in attaching crepe and rubber soles. Acetone and amyl acetate were used for softening nitrocellulose products such as toe puffs. The adhesives used were natural rubber latex or solutions; water-based paste adhesives made of starch, dextrin or natural gums were used widely for laminating and for sock insertion.

In 1950, footwear was made largely from natural products such as leather and textile uppers, leather and crepe soles, and a proportion of vulcanized natural rubber soles. In the mid 1950s, in some countries, leather soles were slowly replaced by resin rubbers, which were sewn or stuck on, and by directly moulded-on rubber soles. These tough, durable rubbers were used particularly for work boots and childrens' shoes. During the mid 1960s, plasticized polyvinyl chloride (PVC) began to be used in place of moulded-on rubber, and stuck-on PVC units appeared on the market several years later. PVC-coated fabric upper materials were also being developed as a cheaper substitute for leather.

Later in the 1960s, polyurethane soling and better quality PVC-coated fabrics were developed. Research progressed on water-vapour-permeable upper materials (poromerics), which were designed to be as comfortable as upper leather. With improved polyurethane technology in the mid 1970s, the use of coated textiles as upper materials increased. Cellular polyurethane soles became popular at that time and continue to do so.

These developments in soling materials and constructions led to increased usage of solvent-based adhesives for attaching the soles to the uppers. Use of polychloroprene adhesives coincided with use of resin rubber and polyurethane adhesives with that of PVC; there were also considerable developments in use of hot-melt adhesives. The composition of many components, e.g., linings, toe puffs, stiffeners and insoles, was adapted to the newer processes or to use of cheaper alternatives.

2.2 Processes used currently

(a) Boot and shoe manufacture

The operations that may be used in the manufacture of the most usual types of shoes are shown in Figure 1, grouped in the order in which they are carried out. Some of the operations mentioned are optional. A short description of each step follows.

(i) *Typical operations:*

Clicking - cutting upper shoe components, by hand or machine. The most common machine in use is a swing-arm press; modern machines are hydraulically operated.

Splitting - producing a uniform thickness of leather with a band-knife splitting machine

Flow moulding - forming a surface pattern on PVC-coated upper fabric by high-frequency heating

Stitch marking - marking the position of subsequent stitching lines on the upper

Skiving - a machine process which reduces the thickness of the edges of materials to facilitate joining and folding

Cutting out - removing parts of the upper to produce an open-work effect on the shoe

Edge binding - binding the edges of the upper

Fitting - attaching linings to the upper

Attachment of toe puffs - attaching the stiffener which shapes the toe to the upper, usually by heat to activate the adhesive

Stitching - sewing together components and stitching decorative effects

Machine cutting - cutting sole materials, with machines such as a clicking press, a travelling head press or a revolution press

Bevelling - reducing thickness of the edge of the sole material

Evening and grading - sorting into consistent groups

Scouring - removing surface layer on heels and soles in preparation for staining and colouring

Rand attaching - attaching decorative edging materials to soles

Sole cementing - applying adhesive to soles

Fig. 1. Typical operations in shoe manufacture

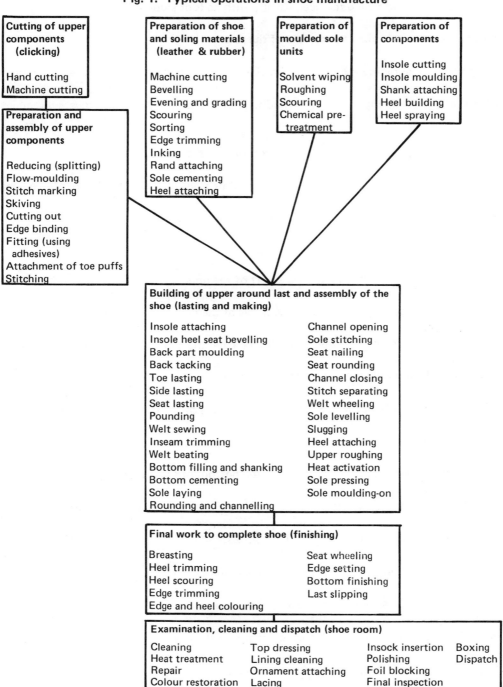

Cutting of upper components (clicking)

Hand cutting
Machine cutting

Preparation and assembly of upper components

Reducing (splitting)
Flow-moulding
Stitch marking
Skiving
Cutting out
Edge binding
Fitting (using adhesives)
Attachment of toe puffs
Stitching

Preparation of shoe and soling materials (leather & rubber)

Machine cutting
Bevelling
Evening and grading
Scouring
Sorting
Edge trimming
Inking
Rand attaching
Sole cementing
Heel attaching

Preparation of moulded sole units

Solvent wiping
Roughing
Scouring
Chemical pre-treatment

Preparation of components

Insole cutting
Insole moulding
Shank attaching
Heel building
Heel spraying

Building of upper around last and assembly of the shoe (lasting and making)

Insole attaching
Insole heel seat bevelling
Back part moulding
Back tacking
Toe lasting
Side lasting
Seat lasting
Pounding
Welt sewing
Inseam trimming
Welt beating
Bottom filling and shanking
Bottom cementing
Sole laying
Rounding and channelling

Channel opening
Sole stitching
Seat nailing
Seat rounding
Channel closing
Stitch separating
Welt wheeling
Sole levelling
Slugging
Heel attaching
Upper roughing
Heat activation
Sole pressing
Sole moulding-on

Final work to complete shoe (finishing)

Breasting
Heel trimming
Heel scouring
Edge trimming
Edge and heel colouring

Seat wheeling
Edge setting
Bottom finishing
Last slipping

Examination, cleaning and dispatch (shoe room)

Cleaning
Heat treatment
Repair
Colour restoration

Top dressing
Lining cleaning
Ornament attaching
Lacing

Insock insertion
Polishing
Foil blocking
Final inspection

Boxing
Dispatch

Heel attaching - attaching the heel, usually with nails or staples

Solvent wiping - cleaning the surface of the sole

Roughing - abrading surfaces to provide a rough surface for adhesive application

Chemical pretreatment - surface modification by chemicals to improve subsequent bonding

Insole moulding - shaping the insole to conform to the bottom shape of the last

Shank attaching - attaching a strip of wood or steel to the insole for reinforcement

Heel building - joining together layers of material comprising the heel

Heel spraying - surface coating of heel

Back part moulding - shaping the back part of the upper

Back tacking - tacking the upper to the insole at the back

Lasting (toe side seat) - pulling the upper over the last and fixing it to the insole

Pounding - beating the lasted margin of the upper

Bottom filling - filling the space between the edges of the lasted margin and the insole

Shanking - fixing the shank in the shoe

Bottom cementing - applying adhesive to the bottom of the upper

Sole laying - temporarily attaching the sole to the upper in the welted process

Rounding - cutting off surplus material from edge of sole

Channelling - making a groove to receive the welt seam

Seat nailing - tack-lasting the heel part of the shoe

Welt wheeling - pressing a pattern onto the top of the welt

Sole levelling - compressing the sole by levelling

Slugging - attaching the wearing surface of the heel

Heat activation - heating the adhesive-coated surface to facilitate bonding

Sole moulding-on - the moulding of a synthetic sole directly onto the lasted upper

Breasting - trimming the heel breast to shape

Edge setting - sealing the edge of the sole by applying heat and wax

Bottom finishing - finishing the sole after scouring

Last slipping - removing the completed shoe from the last

Heat treatment - application of heat to remove thread ends and wrinkles from the shoe upper

Top dressing - applying finishes to improve the appearance of the upper

Foil blocking - printing of gold or silver motifs on sole or sock

In modern factories, shoe components are transported on conveyors systems to machinery and work positions; in the past, shoe parts were moved to the various work stations on small trolleys pushed manually. Recently, conveyors have been fitted with a central extractor linked to the positions where cementing operations are carried out. The whole conveyor, or at least the parts nearest to the cementing positions, may be covered with transparent plastic sheets. Several completely automatic shoemaking systems, beginning with lasting and ending with sole attaching, have been designed, and these have worked successfully on long production runs of simple styles. Modular automatic systems are being developed for short runs of more intricate shoe designs.

(ii) *Significant processes used currently:*

Welting: A process by which the sole is attached to the upper by stitching to a presewn welt. Many operations are required in this process, and it is very labour intensive. The use of welted soles has declined over the years, and it will probably become a minor process. It is essentially used for men's footwear, especially for high-priced shoes.

Machine-sewing: Another process involving the stitching of soles onto uppers. It is widely used for the production of moccasins.

Veldts: A method of producing footwear by sewing the out-turned upper to a runner (an extended insole) and then sticking the outsole to the runner. It is widely used for childrens' sandals and for leisure footwear.

Moulded-on rubber: The uppers for outdoor footwear are made almost exclusively of full chrome leather, since it has sufficient heat resistance to withstand the pressure and temperatures involved. Basically, the upper is lasted, cemented (with a solvent-based adhesive) and placed in a heated mould containing an unvulcanized rubber blank. A cure time of about 10 minutes at 180°C is usually sufficient to cure the rubber adequately and to bond it to the shoe bottom.

At present, the process is used mainly for safety footwear. A similar process is still widely used for the production of slippers with sponge-moulded bottoms. Tennis and canvas uppered plimsolls are also made by the moulded-on process, although the techniques, e.g., autoclaving and preparation of the soles, are somewhat different.

Moulded-on plastics: The first plastic shoe bottoms of commercial value were made from injection moulded-on plasticized PVC. The main advantage of this process over rubber moulding is that the hot PVC melt is injected onto the cemented shoe bottom but the sole mould is not heated. Many other plastics, including thermoplastic rubber, solid polyurethane, nylon and polyesters, have been used successfully in this process; and thermoplastic rubber is likely to replace PVC, at least to some extent. Other plastics are used for special applications such as football boots.

The latest development, made in the early 1970s, is a moulded cellular polyurethane sole. The process involves a chemical reaction brought about by mixing and metering two reactive chemicals and pouring or injecting them into a mould to form the shoe sole. The final product is a tough, durable, cellular material. The process does not involve the use of adhesives.

Stuck-on process: This method of attaching a sole to a shoe upper is the most versatile of all sole attaching processes: it comprises applying adhesive to the shoe bottom and to the sole, allowing each adhesive to dry, reactivating the adhesive (usually by radiant heat) and then pressing the two coated surfaces together.

The stuck-on process makes particular use of prefabricated and premoulded units, which may be made or moulded in a shoe factory or be purchased. The units may be moulded from rubber, PVC, thermoplastic rubber, polyurethane, polyesters or nylon.

Since its development in the 1950s, the stuck-on process has been used widely and is likely to continue to be in the foreseeable future. Its versatility and simplicity are vital to the ability of the footwear industry to adapt to current fashions.

Finishing processes: Finishing processes involve many parts of the shoe. Some components (e.g., heels and units) may be prefinished before reaching the shoe factory. Depending on their properties, finishes may be applied by dip, sponge, brush or spray. When spray processes are used in shoe factories, extractor fans are normally available for removing the excess spray and hence the bulk of the chemicals.

(iii) *Materials used in footwear:*

Uppers: Currently, the uppers of footwear are made from leather (mainly full-chrome), textiles (natural and synthetic fibres), coated fabrics of various kinds (PVC- or poly-urethane-coated) and poromerics (porous polymeric material).

Linings: These may be of leather, nylon, textiles or coated fabrics.

Stiffeners: Premoulded stiffeners based on cellulose fibres and resin (polystyrene)-impregnated cloths, which are moulded by heating, are the most common types.

Toe-puffs: Nitrocellulose-impregnated cloths, softened with solvent before use, are used mainly for welted work. Impregnated fabrics and polymer films (extruded sheet or hot metal) that can be softened with heat are now more common. Some rubber-impregnated puffs are used when soft toes are required.

Insoles: Some vegetable-tanned leathers are used in men's high-grade footwear. More commonly, insoles are made of scrap leather (vegetable and/or chrome-tanned) bonded with natural rubber, or of cellulose fibres (fibreboard from chemical wood pulp) bonded with polychloroprene. Newer types of stitch-bonded textiles are becoming popular.

Insock: A cover for the insole of a shoe, made of coated fabrics or cork.

Heels: Low heels are usually moulded from polyethylene, while high heels are more often moulded from high-impact polystyrene, PVC or poly-acrylonitrile-butadiene-styrene (ABS). Leather and a special grade of polyethylene-impregnated fibreboard are also used in the manufacture of heels.

Soling materials: Leather for soling is usually vegetable-tanned but may be partially or fully chrome-tanned. Rubber is used widely, in the following forms: crepe (unvulcanized), vulcanized natural and synthetic, vulcanized butadiene-acrylonitrile copolymer and polychloroprene. Thermoplastic rubber (styrene-butadiene-styrene block copolymer) is the latest development in rubber injection moulding.

PVC is used widely in its plasticized form. Ethylene vinyl acetate (EVA) is used in two forms, depending on its end use: linear EVA for units and cellular cross-lined EVA for sheet soling.

Polystyrene, acrylonitrile-butadiene-styrene polycarbonate and rope have also been used. Polyurethane soling is made by mixing and metering two reactive chemicals (a polyol and an isocyanate) and pouring or injecting them into a mould to form the shoe sole. The process may be carried out in a shoe factory, or units may be purchased.

Cork: Cork is used in surgical footwear and unit soles. Shoe manufacturers can buy cork in precut, prefinished form, but they may shape the cork mechanically. Shaping of cork may also be done by specialized unit sole manufacturers. Cork for use in shoes comes in two forms: plank cork is the natural product and comes in sheet form; granulated cork is made up of cork particles bonded together into blocks ready for machining.

Wood: Wood, usually hardwood, is used for the manufacture of lasts, clogs, heels and shanks. Some rigid fibreboards used as footwear components are made from compressed wood pulp.

Lasts are made by last makers and purchased by shoe manufacturers.

Clogs may be made wholly of wood, or uppers may be attached. Clogs for industrial use may have grinding on the wearing surface; those for everyday use have rubber or plastic soles. The wood (solid or laminated) is usually shaped by unit manufacturers, but some shoe factories manufacture their own products. The wood is seamed and finally polished or coloured.

Wooden heels are usually produced in specialized factories and purchased by shoe manufacturers.

Shanks are slim pieces of roughly shaped wood placed between the sole and insole in the heel area.

Adhesives: Adhesives used in footwear manufacture fall into three main categories: latex, hot-melt and solvent solution adhesives.

Latex adhesives are made up of a dispersion of polymer (natural rubber, synthetic rubber or polyvinyl acetate) in water. They are widely used.

Hot-melt adhesives are solvent-free thermoplastic adhesives in rod, block or granule form. They are used essentially for lasting, folding and shank insertion (polyamide, EVA and polyester types); they are applied directly as a liquid hot melt and a bond is formed immediately. Hot-melt adhesives may be applied to components (such as toe puffs) and be reactivated by heat to form the bond.

Solvent solutions of rubber and polymers (natural, polychloroprene and polyurethane) are used widely. Natural rubber solutions are used for laminating, but the polychloroprenes and polyurethanes are used mainly for the bonding of soles to uppers. The adhesives may contain plasticizers, tackifiers and stabilizers. The solvents in rubber solutions are petroleum hydrocarbons or chlorinated hydrocarbons, and those in the synthetic rubber adhesives are mixtures of ketones, esters and hydrocarbons. Isocyanates may be incorporated into adhesives, but the use of two-component adhesives is not common in all countries.

(b) Boot and shoe repair

Many different types of repairs are carried out; the main ones are described below.

Welted leather soles: The worn out sole is removed and replaced with a half-sole using the same techniques as in shoe manufacture.

Cemented-on soles: The original sole is usually removed by ripping it off; the adhesive bond may be softened with heat or solvent to facilitate removal. The repair sole is stuck to the upper by the usual manufacturing procedure.

Stuck-on soles: These are premoulded or PVC soles which are stuck to the worn out, original sole without removing it from the shoe. The worn out sole may be levelled by scouring before the stuck-on sole is attached.

Heeling: This term applies to the replacement of the wearing surface of the heel of a shoe. The common materials for heeling are leather, rubber or plastics, and they are attached by adhesives after grinding. If the heel base requires levelling before being repaired, this is done by scouring.

Heel attaching: Heels, the base and the wearing surface, may need to be replaced completely. Sometimes they are removed from the plastic with heated pincers. New heel bases are attached after grinding.

Upper stitching: This repair is fairly uncommon. It may also be termed 'patching'. The patch is stitched.

Recolouring: This is occasionally done by repairers but is more often done by the owners of shoes who can buy recolour commercially.

Minor repairs: Loose buckles and trims are sewn on.

2.3 Qualitative and quantitative data on exposures

(a) Exposure to dust

Scouring and roughing operations produce the greatest volume of dust.

(i) *Scouring:* Scouring occurs most commonly during hand finishing (edges and bottoms), and the dust is fine. When plastic heel blocks and rubber top-pieces are used, the dust also contain particles of these materials. Dust extraction is widespread, and dust extractors are usually fitted to machinery used for scouring rubber soles.

(ii) *Roughing:* Upper materials are usually roughed by high-speed wire brushes using machines with dust extractors. Leather uppers are commonly prepared in this way, and the dust comprises leather and finish. Automatic roughing machines with built-in dust collectors are fairly common. Other materials may be roughed using similar techniques.

(iii) *Edge trimming and rounding:* These are cutting operations which produce small pieces of the soling material.

(iv) *Cutting:* When shoe components are cut to shape, various dusts can arise, consisting of leather (all tannages), rubber, textiles (cotton, nylon, wool, polyester, etc.). The handling both of the materials and the cut components can generate dust.

(v) *Moulded-on rubber sole process:* Unvulcanized rubber sheet used in this process is usually dusted with zinc stearate to prevent the sheets from sticking together. Over-dusting may contaminate the work place with zinc stearate dusts.

(vi) *Quantitative measurements:* The results of one survey carried out in the UK in the summer of 1976 are given in Table 1. The factory produced welted footwear with leather uppers and soles.

(b) Exposure to chemicals

The application of cleaners, adhesives and finishes is the main source of exposure to chemicals. These are listed in Table 2, although not all of them are used in all countries. (See also Appendix 5.).

(i) *Cleaner and adhesive application:* Cleaners and adhesives may be applied by hand or machine. The degree of exposure to evaporating solvents depends on the volume of cleaner or adhesive used, the conditions of drying and the use of extraction systems.

Table 1. Survey of dust levels in a footwear factory in the UK (summer, 1976)

| OPERATION | STATIC SAMPLES OF GENERAL WORKROOM AIR | | | | | PERSONAL SAMPLES | |
| | Concentration (mg/m³) | Particle size distribution (%) | | | | Concentration (mg/m³) | |
		< 1.53 µm	1.53-4.15 µm	4.15-13.65 µm	> 13.65 µm	Day 1	Day 2
Insole scouring	0.32	7	12	43	38	0.56	0.89
Upper cutting (hand)	0.17	14	17	41	28	0.48 / 0.34	0.41 / 0.26
Upper cutting (press)	0.30	31	12	32	25	0.30	0.27
Sole cutting (press)	0.12	73	13	14	0	0.49	1.10
Upper skiving (i)	0.37	34	9	38	19	0.46	0.28
Upper skiving (ii)	0.20	29	18	32	21	-	-
Sole stitching (i)	0.18	36	10	35	19	0.47	0.44
Sole stitching (ii)	0.23	31	23	26	20	-	-
Edge trimming	0.23	52	20	22	6	0.71	0.69
Heel scouring (i)	0.56	13	15	38	34	7.5	3.9
Heel scouring (ii)	0.27	42	11	28	19	0.88 / 0.20	0.91 / 0.05
Sole scouring	-	-	-	-	-	2.4 / 0.05	2.8 / 0.07
Upper roughing	-	-	-	-	-	0.50 / 0.68	0.58 / 0.49
Heel polishing	-	-	-	-	-	0.65	0.96
Edge polishing	0.15	26	17	33	24	0.29	0.30
Mean	0.26	32	15	32	21		

**Table 2. Chemicals that are or have been found in adhesives
and finishes used in boot and shoe manufacture**

Chemical	Use
Carbon disulphide	Rubber solvent and cleaner
Carbon tetrachloride	Rubber solvent and cleaner
Trichloroethylene	Rubber solvent and cleaner; adhesive solvent
Dichloromethane	Rubber solvent and cleaner
1,1,1-Trichloroethane	Rubber solvent and cleaner
Tetrachloroethylene	Cleaner
Benzene	Adhesive solvent
Toluene	Adhesive solvent
Xylene	Adhesive solvent
2-Methylpentane	Cleaner, diluent, adhesive solvent
3-Methylpentane	Cleaner, diluent, adhesive solvent
Hexane	Cleaner, diluent, adhesive solvent
Methylcyclopentane	Cleaner, diluent, adhesive solvent
Cyclohexane	Cleaner, diluent, adhesive solvent
Ethyl acetate	Adhesive solvent, lacquer solvent, cleaner
Butyl acetate	Adhesive solvent, lacquer solvent, cleaner
Amyl acetate	Adhesive solvent, lacquer solvent, cleaner
Acetone	Adhesive solvent, lacquer solvent, cleaner
Methyl ethyl ketone	Adhesive solvent, lacquer solvent, cleaner
Tetrahydrofuran	Cleaner
Methyl isobutyl ketone	Adhesive solvent, lacquer solvent, cleaner
Ethanol	Cleaner
Isopropanol	Cleaner

Table 2 (contd)

Chemical	Use
Dimethylformamide	Lacquer solvent
Surfactants	Cleaners
Ammonia	Cleaner
Waxes (natural)	Finishes
Shellac	Finish
Acrylic resins (various)	Upper and units finishes, emulsion or solvent-based
Nitrocellulose	Upper and units finishes, usually solvent-based
Cellulose acetate butyrate	Upper and units finishes, usually solvent-based
Polyurethanes (linear, one-part)	Upper and units finishes, usually solvent-based
Isocyanates (various)	Active primers and in two-part adhesives
Halogenation agents based on organic chlorine donors	Primers
Natural rubber	Adhesives
Polyvinyl acetate	Adhesives
Polychloroprene rubbers	Adhesives
Polyurethanes	Adhesives
Tackifying resins (unspecified)	Adhesive modifiers
Polyamides	Hot-melt adhesives
Polyesters	Hot-melt adhesives
Ethyl vinyl acetate	Hot-melt adhesive
Urea-formaldehyde resins	Toe puffs
Various plasticizers (e.g., tri-*ortho*-cresyl phosphate)	

(ii) *Finish application:* Both soles and uppers are cleaned before finishing. Finishes include coloured and transparent surface coatings for soles and uppers. Soles may be coloured by dipping, sponging or spraying. Uppers are sponged or sprayed. The degree of exposure depends on the volume of finish applied and the technique used. Extractors are commonly used to remove overspray, and, hence, chemicals in shoe upper finishing departments. A partial list of dyes known to be used in boot and shoe manufacture and repair is given in Appendix 6.

(iii) *Miscellaneous atmospheric contamination:* A number of shoe or component manufacturing processes involve special procedures, and atmospheric contamination may arise from:

· *release agents* (silicones and waxes) used to spray moulds

· *vinyl chloride monomer* (VCM): When two PVC compounds are welded together, hydrogen chloride and possibly VCM may be evolved; however, the operation is usually carried out by machines that are fitted with an efficient extractor system.

· *isocyanates* from the polyurethane unit and moulded-on processes. The processes may or may not be totally enclosed during the chemical reaction needed to produce the soling.

· *the heating of plastics* in general, especially when high temperatures are involved; e.g., the removal of grindery from acrylonitrile-butadiene-styrene components (heels and units) may lead to localized acrylonitrile pollution.

· *the fumes from hot vulcanized rubber* may result in exposure to petroleum distillates, curing agents, retarders, amines, sulphur and *N*-nitroso compounds. Although release of the latter has been suggested (Fajen *et al.*, 1979), no air measurements of these compounds in shoe factories have been reported in the published literature.

(iv) *Exposure to solvents:* It is unusual for an adhesive or finishing material to contain a single solvent; the solvent mixtures used in manufacture vary widely, not only between products but between different batches of the same product. A recognized technique for calculating the TLV of a mixture is given by the Health & Safety Executive (1978).

A survey of six shoe factories in the UK was carried out to determine the exposure of workers to solvent inhalation (Table 3). The atmospheric levels of solvent found, using personal samplers, are quoted as a fraction of the TLV calculated for the particular solvent mixture in the bulk product which was being used.

**Table 3. Solvent vapour levels found
in a survey of 6 UK shoe factories**

Operation	Efficiency of extraction	Level of solvent vapour
Sole cementing	satisfactory poor	½ x TLV 4 x TLV
Solvent cleaning	moderate poor	¾ x TLV 3 x TLV
Bottom cementing	none	¾ x TLV
Bottom filling	none	½ x TLV
Closing	none	¾ to 1¼ x TLV
Heel covering	none	3 x TLV

In a second survey of 28 factories, 17 were found to have areas in which the solvent vapour concentration was greater than the TLV. The areas with the highest concentrations were sole cleaning and cementing and bottom cementing, where racks were used to store the work during drying. When conveyor systems were used, the level of solvent vapour after cementing shoe bottoms was substantially lower.

Vigliani (1976) and Vigliani & Forni (1976) reported that benzene concentrations in the air in the working environments of shoe manufacturing industries in Pavia, Italy, ranged from 25 - 600 ppm, although in most analyses it was 200-500 ppm.

Levels of benzene in plants engaged in shoe, slipper and handbag manufacture in Istanbul, Turkey, reached a maximum of 210-650 ppm (Aksoy et al., 1974).

Carapella (1977), in a study in 19 shoe factories in the Marches (Italy), found concentrations of more than 500 ppm hexane in the air. De Rosa et al. (1977), in a study of solvent concentrations in the air in adhesive application areas in 20 shoe factories in Italy, found that in 45 of 71 working places examined the total concentration of solvents identified was higher than the mixture TLV, and that in 25 of 71 places hexane and its isomers occurred at levels of more than 500 ppm, the TLV of the American Conference of Governmental Industrial Hygienists (1979).

(c)   Boot and shoe repair

Shoe repairers may be exposed to all the chemicals contained in adhesives, paints and dust because one operator carries out all the operations. However, exposure to chemicals is usually limited to adhesives and paints for edges. Repairers are exposed to the dusts generated during scouring, which may be any of the materials used in shoe manufacture, but modern machines are usually fitted with extractors.

2.4 Biological factors

No data were available to the Working Group.

2.5 Current regulations and recommendations on exposures

See 'General Remarks on Wood, Leather and Some Associated Industries', p. 23 .

2.6 Number of workers involved

See 'General Remarks on Wood, Leather and Some Associated Industries', p. 19   .

3. TOXIC, INFLAMMATORY AND ALLERGIC EFFECTS IN HUMANS

The chronic toxic effects observed most frequently among shoemakers involve the haematopoietic system and the nervous system. Various peripheral blood abnormalities have been related to the use of benzene in the gluing process. Among these disorders, thrombocytopenia and depression of red blood cell, platelet and white cell counts have been described; pancytopenia, caused by chronic or acute bone-marrow atrophy, is the major such disorder (Robbins & Cotran, 1979). Although benzene appears to be the agent mainly responsible for this effect, some minor abnormalities of peripheral blood have also been attributed to the use in the gluing process of solvents other than benzene (Bartolucci *et al.*, 1978; Ceccarelli & Mastrangelo, 1978).

Peripheral neuropathy was found to be frequent among workers in leather goods and shoemaking factories in several countries. The preliminary symptoms of this disease usually occur bilaterally and include weakness and pain in the lower limbs, paraesthesia, sensitivity reduction and muscle spasms in the upper limbs and hands. At the same time, abnormally low maximal motor conduction velocity of the median nerve is observed; later, abnormally low nerve conduction velocity can occur, especially in the limbs (Buiatti *et al.*, 1978). This disease, which was first related to exposure to tri-*ortho*-tolylphosphate (Crepet *et al.*, 1968; Chauderon & Lévêque, 1969) is now mostly related on the basis of clinical and experimental data to exposure to low boiling-point solvents such as hexane (Inoue *et al.*, 1970; Foa *et al.*, 1976).

Electroencephalographic changes, possibly due to solvent exposure, have also been described in shoemakers (Guiliano *et al.*, 1974). Vestibular disorders were found to be more frequent in shoemakers exposed to solvents (D'Andrea *et al.*, 1979). Liver damage, as evidenced by increased γ-glutamyltranspeptidase (Bartolucci *et al.*, 1978), dermopathies (Fernandez, 1972) and behavioural changes (Murphy & Colligan, 1979) have also been reported in connection with exposure to solvents.

4. CARCINOGENICITY DATA[1]

(a)   Nasal cancer

During 1958-1968, 30 male patients with cancer of the nasal cavities were treated in a hospital in Belgium. Among 20 patients with adenocarcinoma, 2 were shoemakers (Debois, 1969). Among 16 patients with adenocarcinoma observed in The Netherlands during 1944-1967, one was reported to be a shoemaker (Delemarre & Themans, 1971). One further case of adenocarcinoma in a shoemaker was reported from the German Democratic Republic (Löbe & Erhardt, 1978).

One nasal cancer (histological type not given) in a shoe repairer was found in a general survey of relationships between occupation and cancer at the Roswell Park Memorial Institute in New York State (Decouflé, 1979).

Incident cases of nasal cancer diagnosed in Northamptonshire, UK, between 1953-1967 were identified by Acheson *et al.* (1970a). Of 46 cases collected, 29 were in males (10 adenocarcinomas, 15 squamous-cell carcinomas, 4 transitional-cell carcinomas) and 17 in females (3 adenocarcinomas, 7 squamous-cell carcinomas, 4 transitional-cell carcinomas and 3 unclassified tumours). Crude annual incidence rates per million were 5.1 in males and 2.3 in females for squamous-cell carcinomas and 3.4 and 1.0 for adenocarcinomas. For all but 9 cases the patient himself or a relative was questioned about occupational history. The proportion of men who had ever worked in the boot or shoe trade was 7/10 with adeno-carcinomas, 7/15 with squamous-cell carcinomas and 3/4 with transitional-cell carcinomas. Based on incidence rates for southern England, 0.2 cases of adenocarcinoma would have been expected in the population of shoe and boot workers in the area, compared with 7 observed [an observed/expected (O/E) ratio of 35]. The expected number for squamous-cell cancers was 1.6 (O/E ratio, 4) and that for transitional-cell cancers 0.4 (O/E ratio, 7.5). Two of the men with nasal adenocarcinoma had worked in the shoe and boot industry at a time prior to diagnosis. Of the women, 2 of the 17 had worked as boot and shoe operatives

[1] This section should be read in conjunction with Appendices 1 and 3, pp. 295 and 305.

and two others were the wives of a boot and shoe factory foreman and of a handbag manufacturer. Fifteen other cases of nasal cancer in Northamptonshire diagnosed before 1953 and after 1967 were collected: 5 of them were in workers in the shoe and boot industry. This brings to 61 the total number of cases observed in the population and to 26 those occurring among workers in the boot and shoe industry. Details on work in the boot and shoe industry have been obtained for 20 of the latter. Of these, 13 had been employed in the finishing room and 4 in areas where leather was sorted and cut for soles and heels.

In a subsequent report (Acheson et al., 1970b), crude annual incidence rates for male workers in different departments of shoe industries in Northamptonshire are given. The rates for workers in the press and finishing rooms were 7/100,000 for both adenocarcinomas and other nasal carcinomas. The incidence rate of all nasal cancers in other departments of the industry was 1/100,000. Less than 5% of women employed in the boot and shoe industry work in the press and finishing rooms, compared with 32% of men.

Acheson (1976) described 11 further cases of nasal cancer that occurred during 1970-1974 among boot and shoe workers in Northamptonshire. Two of the patients had worked in the shoe industry for only 6 months and 3 years. In a systematic search of the death register of the town of Northampton, no deaths from nasal cancer in workers in the boot and shoe industry were found before 1950.

Acheson et al. (1972) identified all cases of adenocarcinoma of the nasal cavity and sinuses recorded in cancer registries in England (except for the Oxford Regional Register) for the period 1961-1966. Each case was matched by age (within 5 years), sex and registry with a control patient with a nasal cancer other than adenocarcinoma. In response to a questionnaire requesting full occupational history, posted to both cases and controls, usable occupational data was obtained for 107 of the 149 cases (72%) and for 110 of 133 controls (83%). Among the men, 7/80 with adenocarcinomas (9%) reported employment as leather workers at some time; the corresponding proportion among controls was 1/85 (1%) (P < 0.001, according to the authors), and 0.5 cases of adenocarcinoma would have been expected in male leather workers on the basis of census data (O/E ratio, 14). In this series, a total of 12 cases and controls had at some time been leather workers, including 7 men and 1 woman with adenocarcinoma and 3 men and 1 woman with squamous-cell carcinoma. All had entered the leather industry before 1930; 4 had left it before 1945, 2 had left during the 1960s, and 4 were still working in the leather industry at the time of diagnosis. The occupations of the 8 patients with adenocarcinomas were reported as shoe repairer (3 cases), leather cutter in boot repair shop (1 case), supervisor in footwear retail and repair shop (1 case), worker in shoe factory (2 cases) and worker in glove trade and upholstery (1 case). The 4 patients with squamous-cell carcinomas reported employment as finisher and cleaner in a shoe factory, boot and shoe operative, shoemaker in a boot and shoe factory, handbag maker at home. It is stressed that the risk is limited to workers exposed to dusty work in the preparation and finishing departments; there is a suggestion of a risk among boot and shoe repairers.

Cecchi *et al.* (1980) collected 69 cases of nasal cancer diagnosed in the province of Florence during 1963-1977, i.e., 13 adenocarcinomas (12 in men), 38 epidermoid and anaplastic carcinomas (23 in men, 15 in women), 15 other primary cancers (11 in men, 4 in women) and 3 not histologically proven. Twenty-two hospital controls were matched to the 13 patients with adenocarcinoma (aged 44-73 years) by age (within 5 years), sex, place of residence, smoking habits and date of hospital admission (within 5 years). Occupational histories were collected from all patients or relatives and controls. Four patients (including 2 with adenocarcinoma) could not be located and were not included in the analysis. Seven of the 11 men with adenocarcinomas were shoemakers *versus* 0/22 controls. In an analysis of male patients aged 45-75, 6/9 adenocarcinomas, 2/19 epidermoid and anaplastic carcinomas and 0/5 other primary cancers occurred in shoemakers. Of the 7 shoemakers with adenocarcinomas, 5 were engaged in trimming, 1 was a shoemaker and repairer and 1 was a shoemaker also exposed to wood dust. In addition, one patient who had reported woodwork as his main occupation had repaired shoes at home for 10 years.

(b) Lung cancer

Menck & Henderson (1976) identified 2161 death certificates on which lung cancer was mentioned in white males between the ages of 20 and 64 for the years 1968-1970, as well as 1777 incident cases of lung cancer in white males of the same age group who had been reported to the Los Angeles County Cancer Surveillance Program for 1972 and 1973. They then classified subjects according to the last known industry of employment. Using 1970 census data, expected deaths and expected incident cases were calculated for each specific occupation, assuming that the age-specific rates of cancer in each occupation were the same as those for all occupations. The ratio of observed deaths plus incident cases to expected deaths plus incident cases was calculated as the risk ratio. Among 1350 shoe repairers, they found 3 deaths between 1968-1970 and 4 incident cases between 1972-1973, a risk ratio of 2.33 ($P < 0.05$). [No information was given on smoking habits.]

(c) Bladder cancer

Versluys (1949) compared the proportional mortality from cancer of different organs among shoemakers and shoehands to that of the general population in The Netherlands during 1931-1935. The comparison was restricted to persons over 30 years of age. A total of 317 male shoe workers died during 1931-1935. Occupations were identified from the death cards of each deceased person as either 'occupation' or 'former occupation'. Fourteen deaths from bladder cancer were observed *versus* 8.1 expected, a ratio of 1.7. No differences were observed among shoemakers' wives. [The expected numbers do not appear to have been age-standardized.]

Wynder et al. (1963) reported the results of a case-control study of bladder cancer (excluding papillomas) carried out in various hospitals in New York City during 1957-1961 inclusive. The study included 300 men and 70 women with transitional-cell or squamous-cell carcinoma and 15 men and 4 women with bladder adenocarcinoma. An equal number of age- and sex-matched controls were obtained from the same hospitals during the same period. Twelve cases and 3 controls reported long-term jobs involving shoe or leather repair or production. The 12 cases included 6 lifelong shoe repairers and one who had worked as a shoe repairer for 20 years. The remaining 5 cases reported pocket-book making (5 years), shoemaking (lifelong), shoe store owning (22 years), leather cutting (lifelong) and leather working (lifelong). Of the 3 controls without bladder cancer who had worked in the leather industry, 2 reported shoemaking for more than 5 years and one had been a shoe repairer for more than 5 years. Two of the 12 cases were nonsmokers, 2 smoked less than 20 cigarettes/day and 8 smoked more than 20 cigarettes/day. The smoking habits of the 3 controls were not given. None of the women with transitional-cell or squamous-cell carcinoma of the bladder nor their controls reported having worked in the leather/shoe industry; the same was true for all patients with adenocarcinoma and for their controls.

Veys (1974) analysed 144 death certificates in the period 1965-1970 on which a bladder tumour was mentioned in relation to a possible occupational exposure to carcinogens. Two shoe repairers were reported out of 36 male cases with suspected exposure. None of the female cases had an occupational history related to the leather industry.

(d) Haematopoietic and lymphoreticular cancer

Vigliani (1976) and Vigliani & Forni (1976) reported on benzene haemopathies seen at the Institutes of Occupational Health of Milan and Pavia (Italy). A total of 66 cases (37 men and 29 women) had been hospitalized in Milan since 1942, 11 of which were diagnosed as leukaemias; 18 patients (2 with leukaemia) had been engaged in shoe manufacture. During 1959-1974, 135 cases of benzene haemopathy associated with shoe manufacturing industries were seen in or reported to the Institute of Occupational Health in Pavia. Twelve of the patients died of acute myeloblastic leukaemia and one died of erythroleukaemia; the ages of 9 cases were reported: 3 were 40-49 and 6 were over 50 years old. The duration of exposure to glues and adhesives containing benzene was reported for 8 cases: less than 2 years in 2 cases, 8 years in 1 case and 30+ years in the remaining 5 cases. [See also section 2.3(*b*) (iv), p. 265 .]

Mazzella di Bosco (1964) described 3 cases of acute or subacute leukaemia diagnosed during 1961-1963 in 3 workers engaged in shoe production in the province of Florence (Italy), who were reported to have been exposed to benzene.

During 1967-1973, 26 workers engaged in the manufacture of shoes, slippers and handbags in Istanbul, Turkey, were admitted to one of the 4 major hospitals of that city and diagnosed with leukaemia. Fourteen were diagnosed as having acute myeloblastic leukaemia, 3 acute erythroleukaemia, 3 acute lymphoblastic leukaemia, 1 acute monocytic and 1 acute promyelocytic leukaemia. The remaining 4 cases were diagnosed as pre-leukaemia. Average age at diagnosis was 34.2 years (range, 16-58). All patients had been exposed to benzene, with an average exposure of 9.7 years (range, 1-15). [See also section 2.3 (b) (iv), p. 265 .] There were reported to be 28,500 workers in the shoe, slipper and handbag industries in the catchment area of the 4 hospitals, and a crude annual incidence rate of leukaemia of 13/100,000 was reported (19.7 during 1971-1973). This is compared with a crude rate of 6/100,000 in the general population (Aksoy et al., 1974).

A further 8 cases (3 acute erythroleukaemias, 3 other leukaemias and 2 preleukaemias), all of which involved exposure to benzene, were diagnosed in 1974. Five of the patients had worked in the shoe/leather industry and had been exposed to benzene for 1-20 years. On the basis of the 26 cases reported previously and the 5 cases reported in this study, a crude annual incidence rate of 13.5/100,000 was calculated for leukaemia in shoemakers (Aksoy et al., 1976).

It has been reported that since 1969, benzene has gradually been replaced by petrol in shoe manufacturing plants. The absolute number of newly diagnosed leukaemias among shoe workers in Istanbul decreased in 1974 and 1975, and none occurred in 1976 (Aksoy, 1978).

A total of 44 pancytopenic patients were observed in Istanbul in 1961-1977 who had previously been exposed to benzene. The adhesives for shoemaking that were prepared in benzene were both introduced and abandoned during this period. Thirty-four of the patients were shoeworkers. Average exposure to benzene was 6.7 years (range, 0.3-15). In 6 of the 21 patients who died, leukaemia developed after periods of 0.5-6 years (Aksoy & Erdem, 1978).

Cancer incidences in shoemakers were estimated in a historical cohort study in which rates were compared with those in the general population. A total of 579 diagnoses of cancer were identified, and a significant excess of leukaemia (ICD 204) was found (21 observed versus 13.5 expected; SMR = 156) (Englund, 1980).

(e)   Other cancers not previously specified

Versluys (1949) [see above, section (d)] also found 5 deaths from cancer of the mouth and pharynx in shoemakers/shoehands, compared with 1.9 expected, i.e., a ratio of 2.6.

In a general survey of the occupations of cancer patients undertaken between 1956-1965 at the Roswell Park Memorial Institute in New York State as a hypothesis-generating study, case-control analyses were performed for patients diagnosed with oral and pharyngeal cancer and for controls diagnosed with non-neoplastic diseases. Eight male patients had been employed as shoemakers or shoe repairers, resulting in a risk relative to that of clerical workers of 3.6 (P < 0.05). The relative risk was 3.0 among those employed 5 or more years (8 cases). The relative risk did not change substantially when smoking habits were taken into consideration (Decouflé et al., 1977; Decouflé, 1979).

5. SUMMARY OF DATA AND EVALUATION

5.1 Summary of data

The incidence rates of nasal cancers in workers engaged in boot and shoe manufacture in Northamptonshire, UK, in the 1960s were more than ten times greater than those of the general population. The relative risks were in the order of 35-fold for adenocarcinomas and 4 for squamous-cell carcinomas. A study in Florence has confirmed the association between shoemaking and nasal adenocarcinoma. This is also supported by a number of case reports from other countries.

A UK case-control study (in which the occupational histories of patients with nasal adenocarcinomas were compared with those of patients with other nasal cancers) indicated a relative risk of about 8 associated with work in the leather industry. A substantial proportion of the cases had been engaged in shoe production or repair. In the Northamptonshire study, the elevated risk was confined almost entirely to workers in the preparation and finishing departments: work in these areas entailed cutting, trimming and sanding, which were the dustiest operations.

A substantial proportion of the nasal cancer patients described in the study in Florence were engaged in trimming.

No observations on laryngeal cancer specifically related to boot and shoe manufacturers were available. In a large, multi-tumour-site case-control survey in New York State, the relative risk for development of laryngeal cancer associated with employment for more than five years in the 'leather industry' was 5.5 (based on six cases).

In England and Wales in 1951, SMRs for lung cancer in factory and non-factory-employed boot and shoemakers were 73 and 158, respectively (P < 0.05 for both); in 1961, the SMR for all shoemakers was 154 (P < 0.05). SMRs for lung cancer in footwear workers in the US and for shoemakers or repairers and leatherworkers in Washington State were slightly but not significantly elevated. In a cross-sectional study in Los Angeles in 1972-1973, the risk ratio for shoe repairers was 2.33 (P < 0.05, based on 7 cases).

None of these studies took smoking habits into consideration.

Increased risks of bladder cancer were found in death certificate surveys in The Netherlands in the 1930s (PMR = 170 for shoemakers) and in the US in 1950 (SMR = 288, based on 9 cases, for shoemakers and repairers). No increases were seen in the UK or in Washington State more recently.

An association between work in the leather industry and bladder cancer is supported by three (all in the US) of four case-control studies, with relative risks in the order of 2-6. In two of the studies, no distinction was made between shoemakers and other leather workers. In one of these, 8 of 16 cases among leather workers had worked in the same shoe-manufacturing company, which also included a leather tannery. In a third study, with equal numbers of cases and controls, there were seven shoe repairers and one shoemaker among the cases, and one shoe repairer and two shoemakers among the controls.

SMRs for leukaemia in England and Wales in 1951 and in 1961 and the PMR in Washington State ranged between 131 and 186, all based on 7 to 8 deaths.

Series of cases of benzene haemopathies[1] among shoemakers have been described in Italy and in Turkey. Erythroleukaemia was particularly frequent in these groups. Benzene was a constituent of the adhesives, and benzene levels were measured in some of the shoe factories in which leukaemia patients had worked. A study in Sweden showed 21 observed cases of leukaemia *versus* 13.5 expected. The association with benzene is further supported by a report suggesting that the occurrence of leukaemia in shoemakers has decreased following the replacement of benzene with petrol.

The PMR for lymphomas among shoemakers and repairers in Washington State was 40 (based on 2 deaths). In a large multi-tumour-site case control study in New York State, the relative risk for workers in the leather industry was 3.4 in men (based on 7 cases, P < 0.05) and 2.6 in women (based on 8 cases, P < 0.05).

The PMR for cancer of the oral cavity and pharynx among shoemakers/'shoehands' in The Netherlands in the 1930s was 260 (based on 5 deaths). In a large, multi-tumour-site case-control study in New York State, the relative risk for shoemakers/shoe repairers was 3.6 (P < 0.05, based on 8 cases).

---

[1] Benzene-associated haemopathies include pancytopenia, erythroleukaemia and leukaemia.

In England and Wales in 1951, SMRs for stomach cancer in factory- and non-factory-employed boot and shoemakers were 122 and 120, respectively; in 1961, the SMR for shoemakers was 106 and that for cutters in the footwear industry 135.

Handling of leather in boot and shoe manufacture may entail exposure to some of the chemicals used in the tanning and finishing processes and to other chemicals for which there is evidence of carcinogenicity in humans and/or experimental animals (see Appendix 5).

5.2 Evaluation

Employment in the boot and shoe industry is causally associated with the development of nasal adenocarcinomas; and relative risks well in excess of 10-fold have been reported in England and in Italy. It is most likely that exposure to leather dust plays a role in the association. There is also evidence that an increased risk may exist for other types of nasal cancers for employment in boot and shoe repairing shops.

There is evidence of an increased risk of bladder cancer associated with employment in the leather industry. Although boot and shoemakers were included in these studies, it is not possible to determine whether the risk relates to them in particular or to other occupational subgroups.

The occurrence of leukaemia and aplastic anaemia among shoemakers exposed to benzene is well documented (see also IARC, 1974).

Hypothesis-generating surveys have suggested associations between boot and shoe manufacture/repair and cancer of the lung, oral cavity and pharynx and stomach. The same surveys have suggested associations between work in the leather industry (occupation not further specified) and cancer of the larynx and lymphoma. Most of these associations were positive. In view of the design of the pertinent studies these findings cannot be evaluated.

6. REFERENCES

Acheson, E.D. (1976) Nasal cancer in the furniture and boot and shoe manufacturing industries. *Prev. Med.,* *5,* 295-315

Acheson, E.D., Cowdell, R.H. & Jolles, B. (1970a) Nasal cancer in the Northamptonshire boot and shoe industry. *Br. med. J., i,* 385-393

Acheson, E.D., Cowdell, R.H. & Jolles, B. (1970b) Nasal cancer in the shoe industry (letter). *Br. med. J., i,* 791

Acheson, E.D., Cowdell, R.H. & Rang, E. (1972) Adenocarcinoma of the nasal cavity and sinuses in England and Wales. *Br. J. ind. Med., 29,* 21-30

Aksoy, M. (1978) Benzene and leukaemia (letter). *Lancet, i,* 441

Aksoy, M. & Erdem, S. (1978) Followup study on the mortality and the development of leukemia in 44 pancytopenic patients with chronic exposure to benzene. *Blood, 52,* 285-292

Aksoy, M., Erdem, S. & Dinçol, G. (1974) Leukemia in shoe-workers exposed chronically to benzene. *Blood, 44,* 837-841

Aksoy, M., Erdem, S. & Dinçol, G. (1976) Types of leukemia in chronic benzene poisoning. A study in thirty-four patients. *Acta haematol., 55,* 65-72

American Conference of Governmental Industrial Hygienists (1979) *Threshold Limit Values for Chemical Substances and Physical Agents in the Workroom Environment with Intended Changes for 1979,* Cincinnati, OH, p. 36

Bartolucci, G.B., De Rosa, E., Cocheo, V., Manno, M., De Zanche, L., Negrin, P. & Fardin, P. (1978) Polyneuropathy in the shoe industry; an experimental, etiological and clinical contribution (Ital.). *Securitas, 63,* 187-206

Buiatti, E., Cecchini, S., Ronchi, O., Dolara, P. & Bulgarelli, G. (1978) Relationship between clinical and electromyographic findings and exposure to solvents, in shoe and leather workers. *Br. J. ind. Med.,35,* 168-173

Carapella, C. (1977) Toxic polyneuropathy in shoemakers: preventive aspects (Ital.). *Ann. Ist. Sup. Sanità, 13,* 353-366

Ceccarelli, S. & Mastrangelo, G. (1978) Polyneuritis in the footwear industry of the banks of the Brenta River (Ital.). *Securitas, 9-10,* 546-550

Cecchi, F., Buiatti, E., Kriebel, D., Nastasi, L. & Santucci, M. (1980) Adenocarcinoma of the nose and paranasal sinuses in shoemakers and woodworkers in the province of Florence, Italy (1963-77). *Br. J. ind. Med., 37,* 222-225

Chauderon, J. & Lêvêque, J. (1969) Thirteen cases of occupational poisoning by tri-cresyl-phosphate in handicraft making (Fr.). *Arch. Mal. prof., 30,* 716-719

Crepet, M., Gaffuri, E. & Picotti, G. (1968) The pathology of triarylphosphates in the shoemaking industry (Ital.). *Minerva med., 59,* 4073-4075

D'Andrea, F., Cavazzini, M., Perbellini, L., Apostoli, P. & Zampieri, P. (1979) Vestibular disorders in shoemakers (Ital.). *Med. Lav., 70,* 16-20

Debois, J.M. (1969) Tumours of the nasal cavities among woodworkers (Flem.). *Tijdschr. v. Geneeskd., 2,* 92-93

Decouflé, P. (1979) Cancer risks associated with employment in the leather and leather products industry. *Arch. environ. Health, 34,* 33-37

Decouflé, P., Stanislawczyk, K., Houten, L., Bross, I.D.J. & Viadana, E. (1977) *A Retrospective Survey of Cancer in Relation to Occupation (DHEW Publ. No. (NIOSH) 77-178),* Washington DC, US Government Printing Office

Delemarre, J.F.M. & Themans, H.H. (1971) Adenocarcinoma of the nasal cavities (Dutch). *Ned. T. Geneeskd., 115,* 688-690

De Rosa, E., Bartolucci, G.B., Cocheo, V. & Manno, M. (1977) The environment of shoemaking work: an investigation of solvents (Ital.). *Rev. Inf. Mal. prof., 64,* 215-222

Englund, A. (1980) Cancer incidence among painters and some allied trades. *J. Toxicol. environ. Health* (in press)

Fajen, J.M., Carson, G.A., Rounbehler, D.P., Fan, T.Y., Vita, R., Goff, U.E., Wolf, M.H., Edwards, G.S., Fine, D.H., Reinhold, V. & Biemann, K. (1979) *N*-Nitrosamines in the rubber and tire industry. *Science, 205,* 1262-1264

Fernandez, L. (1972) *Leather goods industry.* In: *Encyclopaedia of Occupational Health & Safety,* Vol. 2, Geneva, International Labour Office, pp. 772-773

Foa, V., Gilioli, R., Bulgheroni, C., Maroni, M. & Chiappino, G. (1976) The etiology of polyneuritis in glueworkers: experimental investigation into the neurotoxicity of *n*-hexane (Ital.). *Med. Lav., 67,* 136-144

Giuliano, G., Iannaccone, A. & Zappoli, R. (1974) Electroencephalographic study on workers in shoemaking exposed to the risk of poisoning by solvents (Ital.). *Lav. um., 26,* 33-42

Health & Safety Executive (1978) *Guidance Note EM 15/78,* London, Her Majesty's Stationery Office

IARC (1974)   *IARC Monographs on the Evaluation of Carcinogenic Risk of Chemicals to Man,* Vol. 7, *Some Anti-thyroid and Related Substances, Nitrofurans and Industrial Chemicals,* Lyon, pp. 203-221

Inoue, T., Takeuchi, Y., Takeuchi, S., Yamada, S., Suzuki, H., Matsushita, T., Miyagaki, H., Maeda, K. & Matsumoto, T. (1970) A health survey on vinyl sandal manufacturers with a high incidence of 'n-hexane' intoxication occurred (Jpn.). *Jpn. J. ind. Health, 12,* 73-85

Löbe, L.-P. & Ehrhardt, H.-P. (1978) Adenocarcinoma of the nose and paranasal sinuses - an occupational disease in workers in the wood industry (Ger.). *Dtsch. Gesundheitswes., 33,* 1037-1040

Mazzella di Bosco, M. (1964) Review of some cases of benzene leucoses in shoemaking workers (Ital.). *Lav. um., 16,* 105-121

Menck, H.R. & Henderson, B.E. (1976) Occupational differences in rates of lung cancer. *J. occup. Med., 18,* 797-801

Murphy, L.R. & Colligan, M.J. (1979) Mass psychogenic illness in a shoe factory. A case report. *Int. Arch. occup. environ. Health, 44,* 133-138

Robbins, S.L. & Cotran, R.S. (1979) *Pathologic Basis of Disease,* 2nd ed., Philadelphia, W.B. Saunders, pp. 712-739

Versluys, J.J. (1949) Cancer and occupation in The Netherlands. *Br. J. Cancer, 3,* 161-185

Veys, C.A. (1974) Bladder tumours and occupation: a coroner's notification scheme. *Br. J. ind. Med., 31,* 65-71

Vigliani, E.C. (1976) Leukemia associated with benzene exposure. *Ann. N.Y. Acad. Sci., 271,* 143-151

Vigliani, E.C. & Forni, A. (1976) Benzene and leukemia. *Environ. Res., 11,* 122-127

Waterer, J.W. (1956) *A History of Technology.,* Vol. 2, Oxford, Clarendon Press, pp. 150-189

Wynder, E.L., Onderdonk, J. & Mantel, N. (1963) An epidemiological investigation of cancer of the bladder. *Cancer, 16,* 1388-1407

1.   HISTORICAL OVERVIEW OF THE INDUSTRY

The use and manufacture of leather goods goes back to the paleolithic era. Technological improvements over the centuries were modest, and leather goods manufacture was one of the last industries to share the advantages of mechanization (Waterer, 1956). However, old-fashioned or primitive methods of leather manufacture are still in use in handicraft shops and in lesser developed countries.

A great many different goods were made out of leather in historical times, e.g., shoes, trousers, harnesses, water-bottles, sacks, sandals, bags, hats, gloves, book-bindings, curtains, parts of chairs and armchairs, stretchers, tubes, shields, mugs, parchments. For their manufacture, various animal skins were used, including those of camels, moufflons, deer, chamois, cattle, ovines, pigs, equines, reptiles, and fish such as skates and sharks (Bayer, 1975).

2. DESCRIPTION OF THE INDUSTRY

2.1 Processes used previously and changes over time

The main developments in the leather manufacturing process may be summarized as follows:

- The use of a large variety of animal skins was abandoned, and only a few species were selected, i.e., cattle, ovines, pigs, equines and reptiles.

- Tanning and leather manufacture became separate processes, often localized in different countries or in different regions of the same country.

- Tendons and leather thongs were replaced by hemp or linen sewing threads.

- Natural glues were introduced, and, later synthetic ones.

- Sewing machines came into use.

- Machines were invented for cutting, splitting, skiving and folding.

At the same time a noticeable transformation of the finished product occurred, with a reduction in the number of items made out of leather. At present, the most common leather goods are: bags, clothing, suitcases, gloves, artistic handicrafts, harnesses and shoes and leathers for industrial use.

2.2 Processes used currently

The processes involved in the production of leather goods that are described below take place after the tanning process, which is performed elsewhere.

(a) Outline of the production process

Several processes are common to the manufacture of a number of products, and these are described briefly (Fig. 1):

Fig. 1. Typical operations in leather goods manufacture

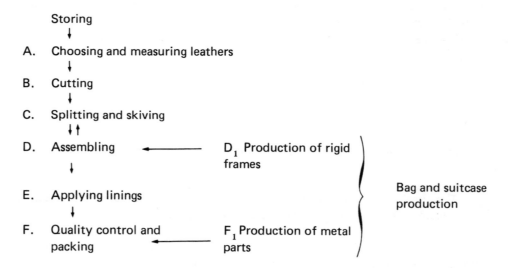

(A) *Choosing and measuring leathers:*   Leathers, which are stored in a special warehouse, are first chosen manually and then inspected for defects in the phases of pre-tanning, tanning, dyeing and finishing. Such inspection is particularly thorough for rare and valuable skins, such as reptile skins. Subsequently, the leather is measured; especially in large industries, this is done by machine.

(B) *Cutting:*   Even today, cutting is partly performed manually, with special knives or cutting blades, following the outline of previously prepared cardboard models.

In the 1950s, cutting machines were introduced which cut the leather by means of a sharp metal die to which intermittent pressure is applied. These machines were at first driven mechanically, and later equipped with hydraulic transmission. Nowadays they are usually operated automatically. Two types of cutting machine are commonly in use. In the first type, which is used for cutting large models, mainly in the manufacture of wearing apparel, a die is moved along a horizontal metal axis which is suspended over the cutting surface; in the second type, which is used for cutting small pieces, the die moves around a vertical axis which is perpendicular to the cutting surface. This surface, once made of wood, is now usually made of plastics and can be planed to repair wear damage.

(C) *Splitting and skiving:* Splitting is a process by which a piece of leather is reduced in thickness. Skiving is the reduction of leather thickness near the edges.

Splitting is carried out on thick leathers obtained from cattle; it was once done with a special knife or by scraping the surface with a piece of glass mounted on a wooden frame. About 50 years ago, the splitting machines that are now in use were introduced. With these machines, the leather is introduced into a slit and is cut by a bandsaw into two layers of the desired thickness. The blade of the saw is sharpened automatically. The latest models are equipped with an extractor to collect leather dust; and dust and leather cuttings are automatically collected in a closed container.

Skiving is necessary, for instance, for assembling parts in double layers. On small pieces or on reptile leather, it is still performed by hand (with a shoemakers' knife), but generally it is done with special machines. These machines, which were introduced at the same time as the splitting machines, have a cutting blade that trims the edges of the pieces of leather.

Although the processes of skiving and splitting are similar, the amount of dust produced during skiving is considerably higher. However, the latest skiving machines are also equipped with extractors and a closed container for collecting the leather cuttings and dust.

(D) *Assembling:* Assembling is the process of putting together the different pieces of leather. Some of the pieces must be strengthened prior to their final use. Reinforcing products (stiffeners) used are: cork mixed with glue (salpa), felt, hemp, polyurethanes (the latest were introduced only recently) and various natural and synthetic plastics. The stiffeners are glued or sewn to the leather at the points that are to be reinforced.

Stiffeners were once glued with natural glues derived from collagen, first described in 3000 BC; they were later supplemented with dextrins obtained from starchy materials. Glues in organic solvents were introduced about 60 years ago, and artificial latex glues about 20 years ago. Ten years ago, the thermoplastic process was introduced, whereby stiffeners are stuck onto leather by fusion at 170°C (Franco & Scarpa, 1978) with a thin layer of plastic that is applied to their surface. These plastics may include polyvinyl chloride (PVC).

After reinforcing, the different pieces of leather are glued and/or sewn together. Artificial glues and artificial latex are now mainly used in leather assembly. The glue or latex is usually spread with a brush, to which, during the last decade, a special container has been adapted to give a continuous supply of glue. Sometimes the brush is incorporated into the lid of the glue box, and the glue box must be closed by the worker each time the brush is not in use. Sometimes, however, in some countries, gluing is done using the fingers instead of brushes (Capellini et al., 1968; Franco & Scarpa, 1978), as was customary in the past. Some workers in the field claim that use of the fingers instead of a brush allows a more homogeneous spread over the whole surface and use of smaller amounts of glue; these factors, to their mind, justify this habit.

Sewing, once done by hand, is now performed with machines; these were introduced into the leather industry almost contemporaneously with the mechanization of the clothing industry, in the second half of the nineteenth century.

(E) *Application of linings:* Many leather goods are provided with linings, which are applied by the same methods described in the previous section. The linings are made of artificial or natural leather, or of fabric. Natural leather linings are usually made of thin, soft leather or with the thinner slice that is obtained during the splitting process. This layer, devoid of the natural brightness of the external part of the leather, is varnished with a spray finish and is glued onto a cloth base.

(F) *Quality control and packing:* Once finished, the product is inspected and packed for shipping.

(b) Specific processes

In addition to the general phases of leather manufacture described above, some specific processes may occur during the production of particular goods.

(i) *Production of bags, wallets and suitcases:* Trimming of the edges of bags and suitcases is performed by grinding, followed by polishing with felts and finally by painting with a brush. In the past, however, the edges were smoothed with a warm metal plate (burnishing).

Trimming can also be done by fitting the edges with a narrow band made of leather, reinforced with a cotton or plastic cord. This band is applied to the edges by sewing, gluing or by a thermoplastic process. These operations are performed by hand or by means of machines that were introduced about a decade ago.

Suitcases are almost all made either of cattle leather or of leather substitutes, which have replaced natural leather almost completely.

The factories that produce bags and suitcases often have sections for the production of rigid wooden, metal or PVC frames and of metal parts (such as locks, chains, rings), which are usually plated by a galvanizing process.

(ii) *Production of wearing apparel:* Ovine skins are used almost exclusively, since they are thinner and softer than other types, and splitting is therefore unnecessary. When skins are used with their fur, the skiving process may include shearing in addition to tapering the leather at the points to be superimposed. Shearing is done with scissors or with a shearing machine, introduced about 50-60 years ago. In this process, a considerable amount of hair may be spread throughout the working environment.

(iii) *Production of harnesses:* Only thick cattle or wild boar leathers are used, which are softened and polished with a large amount of wax.

(iv) *Artistic handicrafts:* This sophisticated technique is used to produce a series of objects that were once made almost exclusively of leather, such as boxes, book coverings, containers of different kinds, and to produce de luxe objects, such as beauty cases, wallets and bags.

Leather is bought from a market, perhaps dyed, and adjusted to size by splitting and skiving. Since thick leathers cannot easily be shaped to make boxes, a thin layer of leather imbued with water is wrapped several times around a wooden frame. The shrinking of the leather during drying induces layer adhesion; when gluing is necessary, natural glues are used. If the leather is not coloured, it may now be dyed, using a brush, and then waxed and burnished. Decoration may then be applied: a bas-relief effect is obtained by embossing the leather with warm metal dies; gilding is obtained by placing thin layers of gold on the leather and then pressing them with a warm die.

2.3 Qualitative and quantitative data on exposures (See also Appendices 5 and 6.)

(a) Table 1. Listing of substances, their occurrence in different phases of production, and routes of exposure

Substance	Occurrence in production[a]	Route of exposure
Dyes dissolved in ethanol	D (edge trimming)	skin contact
Artificial glues		
Polychloroprene, latex or solvent adhesives; butyl, phenol and formaldehyde resins (Calnan, 1973)	D-E	skin contact, inhalation (of ammonia)
Ethylene carboxylic glues: ethylene carboxylic resins in organic solvents (see polyurethane glues)	D-E	skin contact, inhalation (of solvents)
Phenolic glues: phenolic resins in organic solvents (see polyurethane glues)	D-E	skin contact, inhalation (of solvents)
Polyurethane glues: polyurethane resins dissolved in organic solvents (benzene, hexane, cyclohexane, methyl ethyl ketone (Carnevale & D'Andrea, 1977), acetone, methyl butyl ketone, ethyl acetate, propyl acetate, xylene, toluene, heptane, 2-methyl pentane, 3-methylpentane, trichloroethylene, dichloropropane, possibly with plastifiers such as tricresyl phosphate (TCP) (Carnevale & D'Andrea, 1977)	D-E	skin contact (with plastifiers), inhalation (of solvents)
Polyvinyl glues: polyvinyl acetate in water	D-E	skin contact
Leather substitutes: PVC elasticized with plasticizers (such as phthalates, sebacates, adipates, azelates, camphor, nitrobiphenyl and, in particular, TCP, at up to 35% of the weight of PVC (Capellini et al., 1968)	A-B-C-F and particularly D and E when TCP is solubilized with solvents; D (thermoplastic process)	skin contact (with TCP and other plasticizers) inhalation (of vinyl chloride monomer)

Table 1 (contd)

Substance	Occurrence in production[a]	Route of exposure
A mixture of ground cork with glue (salpa)	D	
Felt	D	
Foam rubber: polyurethanes	D	
Electroplated metals and plating solution	F_1	skin contact and inhalation (of various metals, metallic salts and solvents)
Natural and synthetic fabrics	D-E	
Natural glues		
Animal glues: collagen hydrolysed in hot water	D-E	
Gum arabic: exudate of *Acacia* in a water base	D-E	skin contact
Casein glue: alkaline extract of casein dissolved in water	D-E	skin contact
Colophony glue: rosin dissolved in organic solvents	D-E	skin contact, inhalation (of organic solvents)
Dextrins: rice and wheat starches hydrolysed in water	D-E	
Latex: natural rubber dispersed in ammonia	D-E	skin contact, inhalation (of ammonia)
Natural glue: resin from *Pistacia lentiscus* dissolved in water	D-E	skin contact
Soya glue: soya beans dissolved in alkaline water solution	D-E	

Table 1 (contd)

Substance	Occurrence in production[a]	Route of exposure
Nitrocellulose paint: nitrocellulose and synthetic resins dissolved in organic solvents (such as ethyl acetate, toluene); plasticizers, such as TCP, may be present at up to 5%	E	skin contact, inhalation (of solvents)
Adhesives for thermoplastics; TCP as plasticizer at up to 10%	D	skin contact (with plasticizers), inhalation (of vinyl chloride monomer)
Rigid polyvinyl chloride	D_1	inhalation (of vinyl chloride monomer) (?)
Tanned leathers and furs	A-B-C-D-E-F; C and edge trimming; shearing of fur	skin contact, inhalation (of dust), inhalation (of hair)
Wood dust	D_1	inhalation

[a] Letters refer to phases of production as listed on p. 280.

(b) Quantitative data on exposures to some substances present in the industrial process

No data were available concerning dust levels in the air of leather goods factories.

Solvent levels were measured in the air of three handbag factories in the area of Florence (Italy) by the Occupational Health Service of the District of Scandicci-Le Signe (Table 2). Vacuum pumps, localized near the workers and equipped with activated charcoal cartridges, sampled the air for periods ranging from 2 to 8 hours. Elution solvents on the cartridge were then identified and quantified using standard gas chromatographic techniques. The values obtained were compared with the 1979 TLVs for each solvent; TLVs for mixtures of solvents with similar toxicities were calculated using the following formula:

$$X_n = \frac{C_1}{TLV_1} + \frac{C_2}{TLV_2} + \cdots \frac{C_n}{TLV_n}$$

where, C = concentration of the solvent, and TLV = threshold limit value for the same solvent. Assuming an additive action of the components of the mixture, the sum X_n should not exceed 1. In the three plants studied, only one had a TLV for mixtures higher than 1.

Table 2. Solvent levels in the air of 3 handbag factories in the area of Florence, Italy

SOLVENT	CONCENTRATION (mg/m^3)		TLV (mg/m^3)[b]
PLANT 1 (17 employees)	at 4 gluing sites[a]	at 4 sites distant from gluing in the same room[a]	
2-Methylpentane	38.6 - 173.7	19.8 - 30.6	350
3-Methylpentane	69.5 - 189.9	ND[c] - 57.9	350
Hexane	136.2 - 365.5	122.3 - 191.2	(90)
Methylcyclopentane	31.3 - 222.4	18.4 - 25.4	360
Cyclohexane	103.7 - 173.7	18.8 - 87.0	1050
Ethyl acetate	15.7 - 30.8	2.7 - 16.0	1400
Trichloroethylene	15.8 - 24.3	3.0 - 12.7	(270)
Toluene	8.7 - 20.1	3.1 - 9.5	375
Methyl ethyl ketone	8.9 - 17.2	0.6 - 9.6	590
X_n for mixtures[d]	2.27 - 5.63	1.87 - 2.82	
PLANT 2 (13 employees)	at 6 gluing sites[a]	at 1 site distant from gluing in the same room[e]	
Pentane	ND	ND	360
Unspecified hexane isomers	10.68 - 46.49	10.62	(90)
Hexane	7.65 - 13.05	7.37	(90)
Cyclohexane	20.53 - 109.07	23.16	1050
Heptane	1.15 - 6.80	2.28	1600

Table 2 (contd)

SOLVENT	CONCENTRATION (mg/m^3)		TLV (mg/m^3)^b
PLANT 2 (13 employees) (contd)	at 6 gluing sites^a	at 1 site distant from gluing in the same room^e	
Ethyl acetate	2.55 - 16.80	3.60	1400
X_n for mixtures	0.25 - 0.67	0.22	
PLANT 3 (14 employees)	at 3 gluing sites^a	at 1 site distant from gluing in the same room^e	
Pentane	ND - 1.17	0.37	360
Unspecifed hexane isomers	ND - 24.5	0.31	(90)
Hexane	12.77 - 13.18	9.96	(90)
Cyclohexane	54.01 - 131.3	23.00	1050
Heptane	ND - 2.21	ND	1600
Ethyl acetate	ND - 5.91	ND	1400
Trichloroethylene	ND - 0.92	ND	(270)
Toluene	ND - 3.73	ND	375
X_n for mixtures	0.26 - 0.47	0.13	

^{a} Range of values, 1 determination at each site
^{b} Figures in parentheses are proposed values.
^{c} None detected
$^d X_n = \Sigma \dfrac{C}{TLV}$
^{e} 1 determination

2.4 Biological factors

No data were available to the Working Group.

2.5 Current regulations and recommendations on exposures

See 'General Remakrs on Wood, Leather and Associated Industries', p. 23.

2.6 Number of workers involved

See 'General Remarks on Wood, Leather and Some Associated Industries', p. 19.   .

3. TOXIC, INFLAMMATORY AND ALLERGIC EFFECTS IN HUMANS

No data specific to the leather goods manufacturing industry were available to the Working Group. See, however, the monograph on boot and shoe manufacture and repair, p. 266.

4. CARCINOGENICITY DATA[1]

(a) Nasal cancer

In a case-control study carried out in England and Wales by Acheson et al. (1970a, 1972), at least one adenocarcinoma was identified in the Yeovil glove and upholstery trades and a squamous-cell carcinoma in a handbag worker at home. In addition, the survey of nasal adenocarcinomas in operators in the boot and shoe industry in Northamptonshire since the 1950s by Acheson et al. (1970a,b) and Acheson (1976) included at least one case occurring in the wife of a handbag manufacturer. [See also monograph on boot and shoe manufacture and repair, p. 267 .]

(b) Bladder cancer

In a case-control study carried out in New York State in the late 1950s (Wynder et al., 1963), of the 12 cases and 3 controls who had worked in the leather industry, 1 (a case) had worked as a pocket-book maker. [See also monograph on boot and shoe manufacture and repair, p. 270.]

(c) Haematopoietic and lymphoreticular cancer

In a series observed in Istanbul by Aksoy et al. (1974, 1976), Aksoy (1978) and Aksoy & Erdem (1978), an unspecified number of 31 patients with leukaemia or 'preleukaemia' had worked in the slipper and handbag industry. In addition, among 44 pancytopenic patients 2 were manufacturers of leather objects and one a handbag worker. [See also monograph on boot and shoe manufacture and repair, p. 271.]

---

[1] This section should be read in conjunction with Appendices 1 and 3, pp. 295   and   305 .

Two cases of erythroleukaemia were observed in northern Italy, one in a beauty-case factory worker and one in a man who had glued artistic leatherware. Exposure had been for 7 and 3 years, respectively. Three further cases of leukaemia were observed in people working with imitation leather (Vigliani, 1976; Vigliani & Forni, 1976).

5. SUMMARY OF DATA AND EVALUATION

5.1 Summary of data

There have been a few case reports of nasal carcinomas among leather-goods manufacturers other than boot and shoemakers.

No observations on laryngeal cancer specifically related to leather-goods manufacturers other than boot and shoe manufacturers and tanners were available. In a large, multi-tumour-site study in New York State, the relative risk for laryngeal cancer associated with employment for more than five years in the leather industry (not further specified) was 5.5 (based on 6 cases).

No observations on lung cancer specifically related to 'other' leather goods manufacturers were available. The SMR for leather workers in England and Wales in 1971 was 104; SMRs for 'operatives, leather' and for 'leather except footwear' in the US were 103 (based on 37 cases) and 140 (based on 28 cases), respectively. In a cross-sectional study in Los Angeles in 1972-1973, the risk ratio for men engaged in 'leather manufacturing and sales' was 1.72 (P < 0.05). No information on smoking habits was given in these studies.

No observations on bladder cancer specifically related to leather-goods manufacturers other than boot and shoe manufacturers and tanners were available. In England and Wales, SMRs for 'leather workers' in 1961 and for 'leather' in 1971 were 122 (based on 8 cases) and 151, respectively. An association between work in the leather trades and bladder cancer is suggested by three of four case-control studies. In the one study among these in which occupations were reported by cases and controls, one of the 12 cases (a pocket-book maker) and three controls had been engaged in the production of 'other' leather goods.

No observations on lymphoma specifically related to leather goods manufacturers other than boot and shoe manufactures and tanners were available. The SMR for 'leather workers' in England and Wales in 1971 was 184 for non-Hodgkin's lymphomas and 77 for Hodgkin's disease. In a large, multi-tumour-site case-control study in New York State, the relative risk for all lymphomas for 'leather workers' was 3.4 in men (based on 7 cases; P < 0.05) and 2.6 in women (based on 8 cases; P < 0.05).

A number of cases of pancytopenia, erythroleukaemia and leukaemia have been observed among workers exposed to benzene during the manufacture of leather goods other than shoes and boots in Turkey and Italy.

The SMR for leukaemia for 'leather workers' in England and Wales in 1971 was 119, and that for 'operatives, leather' in the US was 73 (based on 6 cases).

No studies of other cancers specifically related to 'other' leather goods manufacturers are available. In a large, multi-tumour-site case-control study in New York State the relative risk for cancer of the oral cavity and pharynx for male 'leather workers' was 3.2 (based on 18 cases; $P < 0.01$). A correlation study in the US reported that mortality rates for cancer of the oral cavity and pharynx were slightly elevated in counties with leather manufacturing industries.

Vital statistics in England and Wales and the US suggest that death rates from renal cancers among 'leather workers' and 'employees in the leather industry' are greater than in the general population.

In addition to benzene, employment in the production and handling of leather goods (other than boots and shoes and tanning) may entail exposure to a number of chemicals for which there is evidence of carcinogenicity in humans and/or laboratory animals (see Appendix 5).

5.2 Evaluation

There are a few reports of cases of leukaemia following exposure to benzene (a known human carcinogen, see IARC, 1974) in the manufacture of leather goods other than boots and shoes or in tanning. The few cases of nasal cancers reported are insufficient to make an association with employment in the manufacture of leather goods (other than boots and shoes or tanning).

A positive association between employment in the leather industry (not further specified) with bladder cancer is supported by a number of studies; but the specific role of the production of leather goods (other than boots and shoes or tanning) cannot be evaluated. The suggested associations between employment in the leather industry (not further specified) and cancer of the lung, larynx, oral cavity and pharynx, kidney and lymphomas come from hypothesis-generating surveys. They do not refer specifically to workers engaged in the production of leather goods (other than boots and shoes or tanning).

6. REFERENCES

Acheson, E.D. (1976) Nasal cancer in the furniture and boot and shoe manufacturing industries. *Prev. Med.,* *5,* 295-315

Acheson, E.D., Cowdell, R.H. & Jolles, B. (1970a) Nasal cancer in the Northamptonshire boot and shoe industry. *Br. med. J., i,* 385-393

Acheson, E.D., Cowdell, R.H. & Jolles, B. (1970b) Nasal cancer in the shoe industry (letter). *Br. med. J., i,* 791

Acheson, E.D., Cowdell, R.H. & Rang, E. (1972) Adenocarcinoma of the nasal cavity and sinuses in England and Wales. *Br. J. ind. Med., 29,* 21-30

Aksoy, M. (1978) Benzene and leukaemia (letter). *Lancet, i,* 441

Aksoy, M. & Erdem, S. (1978) Follow-up study on the mortality and the development of leukemia in 44 pancytopenic patients with chronic exposure to benzene. *Blood, 52,* 285-292

Aksoy, M., Erdem, S. & Dinçol, G. (1974) Leukemia in shoe-workers exposed chronically to benzene. *Blood, 44,* 837-841

Aksoy, M., Erdem, S. & Dinçol, G. (1976) Types of leukemia in chronic benzene poisoning. A study in thirty-four patients. *Acta haematol., 55,* 65-72

Bayer AG (1975) *Tanner - Teindre - Finir [Tanning - Dyeing - Finishing]* , **Leverkusen,** Federal Republic of Germany

Calnan, C.D. (1973) Occupational leukoderma from alkyl phenols. *Proc. R. Soc. Med., 66,* 258-260

Capellini, A., Chiappino, G. & Zurlo, N. (1968) Clinical and experimental observations of the so-called polyneuritis of tricresylphosphates (Ital.). *Med. Lav., 59,* 721-759

Carnevale, F. & D'Andrea, F. (1977) Etiopathology of polyneuropathy in glue workers (Ital.). *Dif. Soc., 1,* 47-84

Franco, G. & Scarpa, G.L. (1978) Risks and prevention in the working of hides (Ital.). *Securitas, 63,* 43-51

IARC (1974) *IARC Monographs on the Evaluation of Carcinogenic Risk of Chemicals to Man,* Vol. 7, *Some Anti-thyroid and Related Substances, Nitrofurans and Industrial Chemicals,* Lyon, pp. 203-221

Vigliani E.C. (1976) Leukemia associated with benzene exposure. *Ann. N.Y. Acad. Sci., 271,* 143-151

Vigliani E.C. & Forni A. (1976) Benzene and leukemia. *Environ. Res., 11,* 122-127

Waterer, J.W. (1956) *A History of Technology,* Vol. 2, Oxford, Clarendon Press, pp. 150-189

Wynder, E.L., Onderdonk, J. & Mantel, N. (1963) An epidemiological investigation of cancer of the bladder. *Cancer, 16,* 1388-1407

APPENDICES

INDICES OF MORTALITY AMONG MALES FROM SELECTED CANCERS ACCORDING TO OCCUPATION AS RECORDED ON DEATH CERTIFICATES

The data given in this appendix were taken from extensive population-based mortality statistical studies which rely for cause of death and information about occupation on death certificates. The eight causes of death tabulated in Appendix 1 are the major ones referred to in the monographs. No statistics are given for some occupation/cause of death combinations, because these were not available in the original reports. In addition, the variety, length and detail of the decedents' employment were not determined, nor were the occupations verified. None of them allow the analyses to be controlled for various confounding variables.

The US (Guralnick) and UK (Registrar General) studies used death certificates and national census data on employed males aged 20-64 and 15-64 years, respectively, to estimate expected numbers of deaths for each occupation and/or industry. Standardized mortality ratios (SMRs) for each occupational category were calculated by dividing the observed number of deaths for each cause of death by the expected number of deaths and multiplying by 100. In the Washington State study (Milham), all deaths among males aged 20 or over were included, and proportionate mortality ratios (PMRs) were calculated on the basis of the ratio of the number of deaths from each cause of death to the total number of deaths. All studies used age-adjustment in calculating the expected number of deaths.

The occupational classifications used in the three studies differed. Within each of the UK series, there is some overlap of occupations: thus, some categories are sub-classifications of others, e.g., sawyers and woodworking machinists (Ib), cabinet-makers (IIa) and carpenters and joiners (IIIb) are subsets of woodworkers (IIIf).

These studies are useful in generating hypotheses that can be tested in cohort or case-control studies.

APPENDIX 1

Indices of mortality among males from selected cancers according to occupation as recorded on death certificates. Data are from three mortality series: (1) United States (US), 1950 (Guralnick, 1963a,b); (2) Washington State (WA), 1950-1971 (Milham, 1976); and (3) England & Wales (UK), 1970-1972 (Office of Population Censuses & Surveys, 1978), 1959-1963 (Anon., 1971), 1949-1953 (Anon., 1958a,b)

Occupation	SMR/PMR (observed no. of deaths) from							
	Stomach cancer ICD 151	Nasal cancer ICD 160	Laryngeal cancer ICD 161	Lung cancer[a]	Bladder cancer ICD 181	Lymphoma[b]	Hodgkin's disease ICD 201	Leukaemia ICD 204
I. SAWMILL, LUMBER WORKERS, LOGGERS								
a) Sawmills, planing mills, miscellaneous wood products, US				72 (23)				
b) Sawyers and woodworking machinists, UK 1971		886*(5)						
c) Sawyers, WA	120 (48)	170 (2)	153 (6)	92 (52)	89 (15)	73 (11)	113 (5)	106 (18)
d) Labourers-furniture, sawmills, miscellaneous wood, US	190 (38)			138 (44)				
e) Sawyers and woodworking machinists, UK 1951	111* (62)			91* (106)				67 (6)
f) Sawyers and woodworking machinists, UK 1961	98 (49)			99 (165)				155 (17)
g) Sawyers, planing mills, millwork, US	100 (70)			70 (75)				
h) Logging, US	157 (33)			91 (30)				

Appendix 1 (contd)

Occupation	SMR/PMR (observed no. of deaths) from							
	Stomach cancer ICD 151	Nasal cancer ICD 160	Laryngeal cancer ICD 161	Lung cancer[a]	Bladder cancer ICD 181	Lymphoma[b]	Hodgkin's disease ICD 201	Leukaemia ICD 204
i) Lumbermen, raftsmen, wood choppers, US	133 (28)			82 (28)				
j) Loggers, WA	120* (223)	87 (5)	84 (17)	93 (276)	62* (52)	73 (57)	65 (18)	84 (76)
k) Woodworkers, miscellaneous, WA	106 (139)	76 (3)	40* (6)		108 (66)	95 (54)	58 (10)	90 (57)
l) Plywood, WA	153 (32)		96 (3)	59 (50)	71 (7)	100 (12)	92 (4)	193* (23)
II. FURNITURE MAKERS								
a) Cabinet-makers, UK 1971		1318* (4)						
b) Cabinet-makers, UK 1961	87 (20)			130* (99)				100 (5)
c) Patternmakers, UK 1961	107 (15)			67 (32)				133 (4)
d) Furniture-fixtures, US	75 (27)			84 (47)				
III. CARPENTERS AND JOINERS								
a) Carpenters & cabinet-makers, WA	128* (271)	81 (5)	75 (17)	101 (325)	105 (102)	113 (93)	162* (38)	104 (99)
b) Carpenters & joiners, UK 1971				120* (572)	160* (54)			
c) Carpenters & joiners, UK 1961	93 (206)			109* (790)				81 (43)
d) Carpenters & joiners, UK 1951	96 (216)			104* (478)				108 (40)

Appendix 1 (contd)

Occupation	SMR/PMR (observed no. of deaths) from							
	Stomach cancer ICD 151	Nasal cancer ICD 160	Laryngeal cancer ICD 161	Lung cancer[a]	Bladder cancer ICD 181	Lymphoma[b]	Hodgkin's disease ICD 201	Leukaemia ICD 204
e) Carpenters, US	103 (187)			112* (316)	100 (47)	100 (82)		97 (58)
f) Woodworkers, UK 1971	108			113* (802)	145* (73)	99	58	91
g) Woodworkers, UK 1961	74 (29)			79 (101)				38 (3)
IV. PAPER - PULP WORKERS								
a) Paper, pulp, WA	115 (33)	91 (1)	146 (6)	89 (57)	45* (6)	165* (28)	192* (12)	140 (23)
b) Paper, allied products, US	89 (39)			114* (80)				
c) Paper-printing, UK 1971	101			86	120	113	105	104
V. LEATHER WORKERS								
a) Leather, UK 1971	102			104	151	184	77	119
b) Tanners, UK 1961	124 (21)			77 (44)				133 (4)
c) Shoemakers & repairers, UK 1961	106 (35)			154* (169)				133 (8)
d) Boot-shoemakers, not factory, UK 1951	120* (67)			158* (183)	120 (12)			186 (13)
e) Boot-shoemakers, factory, UK 1951	122* (73)			73* (90)				44 (9)
f) Cutters, footwear, UK 1961	135* (66)			91* (150)				70 (7)
g) Operatives, leather, US				103 (37)	97 (6)	54 (6)		73 (6)

Appendix 1 (contd)

Occupation	SMR/PMR (observed no. of deaths) from							
	Stomach cancer ICD 151	Nasal cancer ICD 160	Laryngeal cancer ICD 161	Lung cancer[a] ICD 162	Bladder cancer ICD 181	Lymphoma[b]	Hodgkin's disease ICD 201	Leukaemia ICD 204
h) Leather, except footwear, US				140 (28)				
i) Footwear, except rubber, US				115 (38)				
j) Shoemakers, repairers, leather-workers, WA	103 (13)		235 (3)	104 (17)	54 (3)	40 (2)	258 (3)	131 (7)
k) Leatherworkers, UK 1961					122 (28)			
l) Shoemakers & repairers, US				194 (33)	288* (9)			

[a] The ICD codes used for lung cancer were: WA: 162; US: 162, 163; UK 1971: 162; UK 1961: 162, 163; UK 1951: 162, 163

[b] The ICD codes used for lymphoma were: WA: 200, 202, 203, 205; UK 1971: 200; US: 200-203, 205

* Statistically significant according to the original reports, when tested

Note: For renal cancer, leather workers (UK 1961) have an SMR of 162 based on 21 deaths, and leather workers (US 1950) have an SMR of 234 based on 11 deaths.

REFERENCES

Anon. (1958a) *The Registrar General's Decennial Supplement, England & Wales, 1951, Occupational Mortality*, Part II, Vol. 1, *Commentary*, London, Her Majesty's Stationery Office

Anon. (1958b) *The Registrar General's Decennial Supplement, England & Wales, 1951, Occupational Mortality*, Part II, Vol. 2, *Tables,* London, Her Majesty's Stationery Office

Anon. (1971) *The Registrar General's Decennial Supplement, England & Wales, 1961, Occupational Mortality Tables*, London, Her Majesty's Stationery Office

Guralnick, L. (1963a) *Mortality by Occupation and Case of Death among Men 20 to 64 Years of Age: United States, 1950 (Vital Statistics - Special Reports, Vol. 53(3)),* Washington DC, US Department of Health, Education, & Welfare

Guralnick, L. (1963b) *Mortality by Industry and Cause of Death among Men 20 to 64 Years of Age: United States, 1950 (Vital Statistics - Special Reports, Vol. 53* (4)), Washington DC, US Department of Health, Education, & Welfare

Milham, S., Jr (1976) *Occupational Mortality in Washington State, 1950-1971 (DHEW Publ. No. (NIOSH) 76-175A, -BC),* Cincinnati, OH, National Institute for Occupational Safety & Health

Office of Population Censuses & Surveys (1978) *Occupational Mortality, The Registrar General's Decennial Supplement for England and Wales, 1970-72, Series DS No. 1*, London, Her Majesty's Stationery Office

OCCUPATIONAL RISKS ASSOCIATED WITH WOOD INDUSTRIES
NOT FURTHER SPECIFIED[1]

(a) Nasal cancer

Among 11 patients with adenocarcinomas of the nose and paranasal sinuses who were traced from Italian hospital records of 1963-1977, 3 were found to be woodworkers (Cecchi *et al.*, 1980).

(b) Nasopharyngeal cancer

In a review of 10 cases of nasopharyngeal cancer reported to the South Thames Cancer Registry between 1960 and 1974, 4 were found to have occurred in woodworkers (Mould & Bakowski, 1976).

(c) Laryngeal cancer

In a case-control study in the US, 258 men and 56 women with laryngeal cancer were matched by year of interview, hospital status and age at diagnosis (within 5 years) to 516 male and 168 female hospital controls. Of 18 male cases who were nonsmokers or long-term ex-smokers, 4 (22%) had been exposed to wood dust, whereas 0.2 (1.2%) would have been expected on the basis of the controls ($P<0.05$) (Wynder *et al.*, 1976).

(d) Lung cancer

Menck & Henderson (1976) found 20 deaths from lung cancer and 19 incident cases among men classified as 'lumber, wood and furniture workers', resulting in a standardized risk ratio of 114 (not statistically significant). No information on smoking histories was available. [See also monograph on the pulp and paper industry, p.

(e) Bladder cancer

In a case-control study of 300 male patients with bladder cancer in 7 US hospitals between 1957 and 1961 and of 300 controls matched for sex and age, 11 of the patients had been exposed to wood or sawdust for any duration, compared with 20 controls. Furthermore, 9 patients had been exposed for 5 years or more, compared with 16 controls (Wynder *et al.*, 1963).

---

[1] This appendix should be read in conjunction with sections 4 of the monographs on the lumber and sawmill industries (p. 87   ), the furniture and cabinet-making industry (p. 127   ), carpentry and joinery (p. 150), and the pulp and paper industry (p. 191   ), and with Appendix 1.

In Leeds, UK, and surrounding urban districts, 812 men and 218 women who were diagnosed with carcinoma or papilloma of the bladder between 1959 and 1967 were interviewed. Controls were patients with cancers at other sites, or surgical patients without cancer or with genito-urinary-tract disease, matched for sex, age (in decades), place of residence and smoking habits. Eighteen male cases (15 matched pairs) were found to have been woodworkers, whereas 23.7 (19 matched pairs) were expected on the basis of the controls (Anthony & Thomas, 1970).

In an area of eastern Massachusetts, including Boston, Cole *et al.* (1972) carried out a case-control study of 356 men and 105 women with cancer of the lower urinary tract (94% were of the bladder), representing a sample of all cases newly diagnosed between January 1967 and June 1968. Cases were matched individually by age and sex to an equal number of controls from the general population. Of the male patients, 22 had worked as carpenters and woodworkers, whereas 20.2 were expected (RR = 1.09).

Lockwood (1961) identified all cases of bladder cancer reported to the Danish Cancer Registry between 1942 and 1956 in persons still alive in March 1956: 519 cases were identified. Ten of the cancers were observed in 'workers in wood and furniture', while 6.3 cases were expected on the basis of incidence rates in the general population, resulting in an observed:expected ratio of 1.6.

(f) Haematopoietic and lymphoreticular cancer

In a study involving interviews with death-certificate informants, Petersen & Milham (1974) compared the occupations of 158 men who had died of Hodgkin's disease in Washington State between 1965 and 1970 with the occupations of men matched for age at death (within 5 years), year of death and county of residence, who had died of other causes. They found a 2.3-fold excess of Hodgkin's disease for men in wood-related occupations (carpenters, cabinet-makers, paper makers, sawyers combined) (P<0.05).

REFERENCES

Anthony, H.M. & Thomas, G.M. (1970) Tumors of the urinary bladder: an analysis of the occupations of 1,030 patients in Leeds, England. *J. natl Cancer Inst., 45*, 879-895

Cecchi, F., Buiatti, E., Kriebel, D., Nastasi, L. & Santucci, M. (1980) Adenocarcinoma of the nose and paranasal sinuses in shoemakers and woodworkers in the province of Florence, Italy (1963-77). *Br. J. ind. Med., 37*, 222-225

Cole, P., Hoover, R. & Friedell, G.H. (1972) Occupation and cancer of the lower urinary tract. *Cancer, 29*, 1250-1260

Lockwood, K. (1961) On the etiology of bladder tumours in København-Frederiksberg. An inquiry of 369 patients and 369 controls. *Acta pathol. microbiol. scand., 51 (Suppl. 145)*

Menck, H.R. & Henderson, B.E. (1976) Occupational differences in rates of lung cancer. *J. occup. Med., 18*, 797-801

Mould, R.F. & Bakowski, M.T. (1976) Adenocarcinoma of nasopharynx. *Lancet, ii*, 1134-1135

Petersen, G.R. & Milham, S., Jr (1974) Brief communication: Hodgkin's disease mortality and occupational exposure to wood. *J. natl Cancer Inst., 53*, 957-958

Wynder, E.L., Onderdonk, J. & Mantel, N. (1963) An epidemiological investigation of cancer of the bladder. *Cancer, 16*, 1388-1407

Wynder, E.L., Covey, L.S., Mabuchi, K. & Mushinski, M. (1976) Environmental factors in cancer of the larynx. A second look. *Cancer, 38*, 1591-1601

OCCUPATIONAL RISKS ASSOCIATED WITH LEATHER INDUSTRIES NOT FURTHER SPECIFIED[1]

(a) Nasal cancer

One man and one woman with nasal cancer, observed in a general survey of the occupations of cancer patients at Roswell Park Memorial Institute in New York State during 1956-1965, reported having been leather workers (Decouflé, 1979).

Of 179 patients with malignant tumours of the nose and sinuses observed in Jena, German Democratic Republic, between 1931-1977 and for whom a working history was available, a total of 5 had worked in the leather industries. Eighteen patients had adenocarcinoma, and one of these was among the 5 leather workers (Löbe & Ehrhardt, 1978).

Of 212 patients reported to the Swedish Cancer Registry with squamous-cell or poorly differentiated carcinoma of the nose and paranasal sinuses, 4 (1 male and 3 females) on whom information was available were leather workers. There were no leather workers among the 46 of these patients who had adenocarcinoma (Engzell et al., 1978).

(b) Laryngeal cancer

In the general survey of the occupations of cancer patients at the Roswell Park Memorial Institute (Decouflé, 1979), 7 male patients with laryngeal cancer had a history of employment in leather industries. The relative risk was 3.3 ($P < 0.05$). For 6 of these men, who had been employed for five or more years in the industry, the relative risk estimate was 5.48 ($P < 0.01$). Adjustment for smoking habits did not alter the risk estimates significantly. None of the female laryngeal cancer patients reported a history of employment in the leather industry. [See also monograph on boot and shoe manufacture and repair, p. 272 .]

---

[1] This section should be read in conjunction with sections 4 of the monographs on leather tanning and processing industries (p. 241), boot and shoe manufacture and repair (p. 267), and leather goods manufacturing industry (other than boot and shoe manufacture and tanning) (p. 289); and in conjunction with Appendix 1.

(c) Lung cancer

In a study by Menck & Henderson (1976), the ratio of observed deaths plus incident cases to expected deaths plus incident cases was calculated as the risk ratio among workers employed in 'leather manufacturing and sales'. Six deaths were found between 1968-1970 and 8 incident cases between 1972-1973, corresponding to a risk ratio of 1.72 (P<0.05). [See also monograph on boot and shoe manufacture and repair, p. 269 .]

(d) Bladder cancer

In a case-control study, 369 persons (282 men and 87 women) with a bladder tumour who were alive between 1956 and 1959 and were residents of the city of Copenhagen or the Borough of Frederiksberg were matched (one-to-one) by sex, age, marital status, residence and occupation to persons identified from local electoral rolls. Although occupational comparisons between cases and controls are not valid since occupation was a matching factor, the occupational distribution of male cases was compared with that of the general population of the area. Five of the male cases were classified as 'workers in skins, leather and rubber', whereas 1.6 would have been expected to be so employed. However, inclusion of the rubber industry, a known high-risk area for bladder cancer, makes interpretation of these results difficult (Lockwood, 1961).

Between 1957 and 1961, 300 males and 70 females with bladder cancer were identified from seven area hospitals in the US. They were matched by age and sex to an equal number of control subjects selected from patients at the same hospitals without cancer of the bladder, respiratory tract or upper alimentary tract and without myocardial infarction. No relative risk estimates were calculated; however, 12 male bladder cancer patients reported employment for five or more years in leather-related occupations, compared with 3 controls. The difference was accounted for almost entirely by shoe repairers (6 cases, 1 control); but 3 other male patients were described as 'leather workers', whereas no controls were so employed. No details were given concerning the specific duties of the latter group. None of the female patients reported employment in leather-related trades (Wynder *et al.,* 1963).

During 1959-1967, 1030 of 1422 patients hospitalized because of incident or prevalent bladder cancer in the main hospital in Leeds, UK, were questioned about all jobs undertaken throughout life. It is considered that this series included virtually all patients living in Leeds and a substantial proportion of those living in the surrounding urban and semirural districts. Smoking histories were known for 383 men and 57 women. Each of these was matched to two hospital controls, a 'surgical' control (excluding those with cancer and genitourinary diseases) and a 'cancer' control (mainly those with cancer of the lung). Matching was done on the basis of sex, decennial age class, smoking habits (5 categories) and residence (Leeds, urban suburbs, rural areas). Controls were interviewed during 1955-1958 and in 1968. The numbers of patients matched to a surgical control were 340 men and 50 women, and those matched only to a cancer control were 312 men and 39 women. Data on the 429 men and 161 women for whom no smoking history was taken were compared with data on all controls. None of the male patients with bladder cancer whose smoking history was known had had leather worker as their predominant occupation, whereas 7 among the surgical controls and 7 among the cancer controls had. In the series of 429 male bladder cancer patients with unknown smoking history, 9 had had leather worker as their predominant occupation; 9.2 were expected from controls. Among patients living in Leeds, 6 men and 2 women had leather worker as their predominant occupation, whereas 8.0 and 0.9 were expected from the 1951 census (Anthony & Thomas, 1970).

In a case-control study carried out in eastern Massachusetts (Cole *et al.*, 1972), 79 male cases were reported to have leather-related occupations whereas 42.4 were expected based on the distribution of occupations among the controls. This corresponds to a risk of 2 ($P<0.05$) relative to occupations not suspected of being associated with bladder cancer, when cigarette smoking habits have been controlled for. When subjects were further classified as to whether they had 'ever' worked in leather or leather products industries, 65 of the cases had so been employed compared with 32.7 expected when controlled for age, and 34.3 when controlled for age and for cigarette-smoking. Although leather-related occupations were reported for 8 female cases, the number differed very little from that expected (6.7) (7 observed *versus* 5.2 expected when cigarette-smoking was controlled for). The male cases with a history of leather-related employment were further grouped into subcategories, with the following results: finishing and associated processes (44 cases observed, 17.3 expected; relative risk: 2.65; $P<0.05$), contact with finished product or exposure type uncertain (13 cases observed, 8.1 expected; relative risk: 1.73; $P>0.05$). [See also monograph on the leather tanning and processing industries, p. 241.]

In the general survey of the occupations of cancer patients at the Roswell Park Memorial Institute during 1956-1965 (Decouflé *et al.*, 1977), 11 men with bladder cancer had been employed in the leather industry at some time during their working life, resulting in a relative risk estimate of 6.8 ($P<0.01$). The relative risk increased to 12.9 ($P<0.01$) among those employed five or more years (8 cases). When smoking habits were taken into consideration, a substantial excess persisted (relative risk: 4.0). Among female bladder cancer patients, 4 reported a history of employment in the leather industry, yielding a relative risk of 4.27 ($P<0.05$). [See also monograph on boot and shoe manufacture and repair, p. 272]

Of 16 male bladder cancer patients seen at Roswell Park Memorial Institute between 1956 and 1971 who reported employment in the leather industry, 8 had worked in a single large shoe manufacturing company which included a leather tannery (Decouflé, 1979).

(e) Haematopoietic and lymphoreticular cancer

In the general survey of the occupations of cancer patients at the Roswell Park Memorial Institute (Decouflè, 1979), 7 men with lymphoma or multiple myeloma had been employed in the leather industry for five or more years, yielding a relative risk of 3.42 (P<0.05). Among female lymphoma patients, 8 had a history of employment in the leather industry, resulting in a relative risk estimate of 2.63 (P<0.5). [See also monograph on boot and shoe manufacture and repair, p. 272.]

(f) Other cancers not previously specified

In the general survey of the occupations of cancer patients at the Roswell Park Memorial Institute (Decouflè, 1979), 18 male patients with oral and pharyngeal cancer had a history of employment in the leather industry, yielding a relative risk estimate of 3.22 (P<0.01). For 12 of these men who had been employed for at least 5 years in the industry, the relative risk estimate was 3.58 (P<0.01). Adjustment for smoking habits did not alter the risk estimates significantly. [See also monograph on boot and shoe manufacture and repair, p. 272.]

A survey of mortality from oral and pharyngeal cancer in US counties during the period 1950-1969 showed consistently elevated rates among white men in counties where there was a relatively high concentration (1% or more of total county population employed) of leather industries. The most striking differences were seen in counties in the central US, particulary in the State of Missouri. Mortality from oral and pharyngeal cancer among non-white males was increased in counties with leather industries but not significantly. Of 18 industries taken into consideration in this study, the highest risk for white males was found for the leather industry. However, the increase was only one-fifth as high as that associated with urbanization. The authors stated that the elevated mortality from oral and pharyngeal cancer associated with the leather industry cannot readily be explained by the tobacco or alcohol habits of the workers, although this possibility cannot be discounted completely (Blot & Fraumeni, 1977).

REFERENCES

Anthony, H.M. & Thomas, G.M. (1970) Tumors of the urinary bladder: an analysis of the occupations of 1,030 patients in Leeds, England. *J. natl Cancer Inst.*, *45*, 879-895

Blot, W.J. & Fraumeni, J.F., Jr (1977) Geographic patterns of oral cancer in the United States: etiologic implications. *J. chronic Dis.*, *30*, 745-757

Cole, P., Hoover, R. & Friedell, G.H. (1972) Occupation and cancer of the lower urinary tract. *Cancer*, *29*, 1250-1260

Decouflé, P. (1979) Cancer risks associated with employment in the leather and leather products industry. *Arch. environ. Health*, *34*, 33-37

Decouflé, P., Stanislawczyk, K., Houten, L., Bross, I.D.J. & Viadana, E. (1977) *A Retrospective Survey of Cancer in Relation to Occupation (DHEW Publ. No. (NIOSH) 77-178)*, Washington DC, US Government Printing Office

Engzell, U., Englund, A. & Westerholm, P. (1978) Nasal cancer associated with occupational exposure to organic dust. *Acta otolaryngol.*, *86*, 437-442

Löbe, L.-P. & Ehrhardt, H.-P. (1978) Adenocarcinoma of the nose and paranasal sinuses - an occupational disease in workers in the wood industry (Ger.). *Dtsch. Gesundheitswes.*, *33*, 1037-1040

Lockwood, K. (1961) On the etiology of bladder tumors in København-Frederiksberg. An inquiry of 369 patients and 369 controls. *Acta pathol. microbiol. scand.*, *51 (Suppl. 145)*

Menck, H.R. & Henderson, B.E. (1976) Occupational differences in rates of lung cancer. *J. occup. Med.*, *18*, 797-801

Wynder, E.L., Onderdonk, J. & Mantel, N. (1963) An epidemiological investigation of cancer of the bladder. *Cancer, 16*, 1388-1407

CHEMICALS USED OR PRODUCED IN WOOD AND ASSOCIATED INDUSTRIES (EXCEPTING DYES) AND CROSS REFERENCES TO *IARC MONOGRAPHS*

This list includes those chemicals used in or formed during the manufacture or treatment of wood or paper. No evaluation is made of the amounts of the chemicals that are actually used, of levels of exposure, or of temporal or geographical variations in their use during the various manufacturing processes. This list was compiled from information collected during the preparation of the present volume of *Monographs* and cannot pretend to be fully exhaustive for all situations in all countries. Evaluations of carcinogenicity are reported for those chemicals previously considered in the *IARC Monograph* series.

Appendix 4. Chemicals used or produced in wood and associated industries

Chemical	Industry	Use (or formation) in industry	Evaluation of carcinogenicity[a]
Abietic resins	Furniture	Water-repellent agents in wood preservatives	
Acaroid	Furniture	Varnish	
Acetic acid	Saw mills Pulp & paper Furniture	In wood preservatives Vapours from pulp production Hardener in melamine-formaldehyde glues	
Acetone	Furniture	Solvent in vinylic and neoprene glues, in cellulose varnishes, and in varnish removers; degreasing agent	
Acids	Furniture, plywood	Hardeners in formaldehyde-phenol and formaldehyde-cresol adhesives	
Organic acids	Furniture, plywood	Hardeners in melamine-formaldehyde glues	
Fatty acids	Furniture	In varnishes	
Acid copper chromate [VI] (Celcure)	Saw mills	Waterborne preservative	(See Chromates)
Acryl amide derivatives	Pulp & paper	Retention aids for inorganic fillers	
Acrylic resins	Furniture	Base component of polyurethane varnishes	Acrylic and polycrylic acid, ethyl and methyl acrylate: inadequate data in animals; no data in humans (Vol. 19, pp. 47-71) Acrylonitrile: probably carcinogenic in humans (Vol. 19, pp. 73-113; Supplement 1, p. 21) Acrylic fibres, acrylonitrile copolymers: inadequate data in animals; no data in humans (Vol. 19, pp. 86-113)

Appendix 4 (contd)

Chemical	Industry	Use (or formation) in industry	Evaluation of carcinogenicity [a]
Adipates	Furniture	Plasticizers in cellulose varnishes	
Adipic acid	Furniture, plywood	Condensed with a polyalcohol to make resins used in varnishes	
Albumin (from blood)	Furniture	Filler in glues	
Alcohols	Furniture	Solvents in glues and varnishes; higher alcohols, solvents in cellulose plasters and putties	
	Pulp & paper	By-product of pulping	
Aldonic acid	Pulp & paper	Vapours from pulp production	
Aldrin (in mixtures)	Furniture	Insecticide	Inadequate data in animals and in humans (Vol. 5, pp. 25-38)
Aliphatic hydrocarbons	Furniture	Diluting agent in wood preservatives	
Alkyds	Pulp & paper	Barrier coatings	
Alkyd resins	Furniture; carpentry	In cellulose plasters and putties; plasticizers in cellulose varnishes; base component of polyurethane varnishes; water-repellent agents in wood preservatives	
Alkyl phenols	Furniture	Emulsifiers in vinyl varnishes	
Alkyl resins	Furniture	Binders in glycerophthalic varnishes	
Allyl phthalate	Furniture; carpentry	Monomer in polyester varnishes	
Alum (sodium aluminate, aluminium sulphate)	Furniture / Pulp & paper	Adjuvant in gelatine glues / Sizing agent	
Alumina (hydrated)	Furniture	Water-based filler	
Aluminium salts	Pulp & paper	Additives to reduce viscosity of colour, to increase moisture resistance, or as humectants	
Aluminium oxide hydrate	Pulp & paper / Furniture	Coating pigment / Water-based filler	

Appendix 4 (contd)

Chemical	Industry	Use (or formation) in industry	Evaluation of carcinogenicity[a]
Aluminium silicate (kaolin)	Pulp & paper Furniture	Filler and coating pigment Filler in formaldehyde-melamine glues; in plasters and putties	
Aluminium sulphate	Pulp & paper Furniture	Used to precipitate sizing agent (rosin) Adjuvant in gelatin glues	
Amine products	Pulp & paper	Lubricants, plasticizers and flow modifiers used in coating	
Aminoplast	Furniture, plywood	Binder in urea-formaldehyde varnishes	
Ammonia and ammonium salts	Pulp & paper Furniture, plywood	By-product from paper machine Solubilizers in blood glues; hardeners in urea-formaldehyde and melamine-formaldehyde glues	
Ammoniacal copper arsenite (Chemonite)	Saw mills	Wood preservatives	*(See Arsenic and arsenical compounds)*
Ammonium bisulphite	Pulp & paper	Active chemical in sulphite pulping	
Ammonium carbonate	Furniture	Wood degreasing	
Ammonium hydroxide	Furniture	Solubilizer in blood glues	
Amyl acetate	Furniture	Solvent in cellulose and neoprene glues and in cellulose and polyurethane varnishes	
Amylased glues	Furniture	Glues	
Anhydrides	Furniture	Condensed with polyalcohol to make resins used in varnishes	
Anthracene oil	Furniture	Diluting agent in wood preservatives	
Aromatic hydrocarbons	Furniture	Diluting agents in wood preservatives	

Appendix 4 (contd)

Chemical	Industry	Use (or formation) in industry	Evaluation of carcinogenicity[a]
Arsenic and arsenical compounds	Saw mills Furniture	In wood preservatives Insecticides	Human carcinogens (Vol. 2, pp. 48-73; Vol. 23, pp. 39-141; Supplement 1, pp. 22-23)
Aryl alkyl sulphonate	Furniture	Emulsifier in vinyl varnishes	
Asbestos	Pulp & paper Furniture Carpentry	Tremolite asbestos may occur in talc used as coating pigment Filler in melamine-formaldehyde glues Insulating, flame-retardant and acoustic material	Carcinogenic in animals and in humans (Vol. 14; Supplement 1, p. 23)
Asphalt emulsions	Pulp & paper	Sizing agents	
Attapulgite	Pulp & paper	Coating pigment	
Barium sulphate	Pulp & paper Furniture	Coating pigment Filler in melamine-formaldehyde glues and in oil- and water-based plasters and putties; covering pigment	
Bases	Furniture, plywood	Hardeners in phenol-formaldehyde and cresol-formaldehyde glues	
Benomyl®	Saw mills	Antistaining agent	
Benzaldehyde	Furniture	In water-based plasters and putties	
Benzene	Furniture; carpentry	Varnish thinner and remover; diluting agent in wood preservatives	Human carcinogen (Vol. 7, pp. 203-221; Supplement 1, p. 23)
Benzoin	Furniture	Varnish	
Benzoyl peroxide	Furniture	Catalyst in polyester varnishes	
Biphenyl	Pulp & paper	In biphenyl papers	
Bis-1,4-bromoacetoxy-2-butene	Pulp & paper	Slime-controlling agent	
Bismuth salts	Furniture	Mordants in staining	
Bone powder	Furniture	Water-based filler	

Chemical	Industry	Use (or formation) in industry	Evaluation of carcinogenicity[a]
Borates, polyborates, boric acid	Furniture	Fungicides, insecticides, flame retardants	
2'-Bromo-4'-hydroxy-acetophenone	Pulp & paper	Slime-controlling agent	
2'-Bromo-2-nitropro-pane-1,3-diol	Pulp & paper	Slime-controlling agent	
Butadiene-styrene copolymers	Pulp & paper	Barrier coatings	Styrene: limited evidence in animals; inadequate data in humans (Vol. 19, pp. 252-274; Supplement 1, p. 17)
Butanol	Furniture; carpentry	Solvent and diluent in glues and varnishes; varnish remover	
Butyl acetate	Furniture; carpentry	Solvent in cellulose and poly-urethane varnishes and in glues; dilutent	
Butyl peroxide	Furniture	Catalyst in polyester varnishes	
Butyl phthalate	Furniture	Plasticizer in cellulose varnishes	
Calcium bisulphite	Pulp & paper	Active chemical in sulphite pulping	
Calcium carbonate (limestone)	Pulp & paper	Filler and coating pigment; formed during recovery process of sulphate pulping; used in acid sulphite pulping	
	Furniture	Adjuvant; solubilizer in glues; in fast colour plasters and putties	
Calcium hydroxide (slaked lime)	Pulp & paper / Furniture	Used in recovery of alkaline pulping / In varnish removers	
Calcium hypochlorite	Pulp & paper	Used in oxidative stages of pulp bieaching	
Calcium oxide (lime)	Pulp & paper	In recovery process of sulphate (kraft) pulping	
	Furniture	In varnish removers; adjuvant in vegetable glues; solubilizer in blood and casein glues; filler in urea-formaldehyde glues	

Appendix 4 (contd)

Chemical	Industry	Use (or formation) in industry	Evaluation of carcinogenicity[a]
Calcium phosphate	Furniture	Water-based filler	
Calcium sulphate	Pulp & paper	Coating pigment	
Calcium sulphate, crystalline hydrated (gypsum)	Furniture	Filler in melamine-formaldehyde glues	
Calcium sulphoaluminate (satin white)	Pulp & paper	Coating pigment	
Capryl alcohol (octan-2-ol)	Pulp & paper	Additive in pigment coating (foam-controlling agent)	
Carbon tetrachloride	Furniture	In varnish removers	Sufficient evidence in animals; probably carcinogenic in humans (Vol. 20, pp. 371-399; Supplement 1, p. 28)
Carborundum	Furniture	Abrasive in sanding	
Casein	Pulp & paper Furniture	Sizing agent Dry matter of casein glues; filler in urea-formaldehyde glues; in fast colour plasters and putties	
CCA salts (copper, chromium and arsenic oxides) (Cr-[VI] and As [V])	Saw mills; carpentry	Fungicides, insecticides	Arsenic, chromium: human carcinogens (Vol. 23, pp. 39-141, 205-323; Supplement 1, pp. 22-23, 29-30)
Cellulose (hydroxy-ethers)	Furniture	Solvent in varnishes, plasters, putties	
Cellulose acetate	Furniture	Dry matter of cellulose glues	
Cellulose derivatives	Pulp & paper	Barrier coatings	
Cellulose polymers	Furniture	Varnishes	
Nitrocellulose	Furniture	In cellulose plasters and putties	

Appendix 4 (contd)

Chemical	Industry	Use (or formation) in industry	Evaluation of carcinogenicity[a]
Nitrocellulose resins	Furniture; carpentry	Binders in cellulose varnishes	
Chlorine	Pulp & paper	Pulp bleaching (chlorination stage)	
Chlorine dioxide	Pulp & paper	Pulp bleaching (oxidative stages)	
Chlorinated resins	Furniture	Water-repellant agents in wood preservatives	
Chlorinated rubber	Furniture	In chlorinated rubber glues	
Chlorobenzenes (in mixtures)	Furniture	Insecticides	ortho & para-Dichlorobenzene: inadequate data in animals and humans (Vol. 7, pp. 231-244; Supplement 1, p. 45)
Chlorodibenzodioxins	Saw mills	Impurities in chlorophenols or formed by heating chlorophenols and chlorophenates	Inadequate data in animals and humans (Vol. 15, pp. 41-102) Produced liver tumours in Swiss mice (Toth et al., Nature, 1979, 278, 548-549)
Chlorodibenzofurans	Saw mills	Impurities in chlorophenols or formed by heating chlorophenols and chlorophenates	Not known if and to what extent polychlorinated dibenzofurans play a role in the observed carcinogenic effect of chlorinated biphenyls (Vol. 18, p. 84)
Chloronaphthalenes	Furniture	Softening agents in chlorinated rubber glues	

Appendix 4 (contd)

Chemical	Industry	Use (or formation) in industry	Evaluation of carcinogenicity[a]
Chlorophenols and chlorophenates	Pulp & paper Saw mills; carpentry Furniture	Slime-controlling agents Antistaining agents, wood preservatives Fungicides, insecticides, bactericides for wood, glues, textiles	Inadequate data in animals; no data in humans (Vol. 20, pp. 349-367). Subsequent to the meeting, a positive bioassay in mice and rats was published on 2,4,6-trichlorophenol (*NCI tech. Rep. Ser. No. 155,* 1979)
Chlorophenoxyphenols (pre-dioxins)	Saw mills	Impurities in chlorophenols or produced by heating chlorophenols and chlorophenates	
Chromium	Pulp & paper	Impurity in technical-grade chemicals used as make-up in recovery process of sulphate pulping	Chromium and certain chromium compounds: human carcinogens. Relatively insoluble Cr [VI]
Chromated zinc chloride	Saw mills	Wood preservative	salts: sufficient evidence in animals; Cr [III]: inadequate
Chromates and dichromates	Furniture Carpentry	Fungicides; insecticides; mordants; adjuvants in gelatine glues Wood preservatives	data in animals (Vol. 23, pp. 205-323; Supplement 1, pp. 29-30)
Potassium and sodium dichromates	Saw mills	In wood preservatives	
Chromium aluminium sulphate	Furniture	Mordants	
Chromium [VI] trioxide	Saw mills	In wood preservatives	

Appendix 4 (contd)

Chemical	Industry	Use (or formation) in industry	Evaluation of carcinogenicity[a]
Clay (hydrated silicates of aluminium mixed with various impurities)	Pulp & paper Furniture	Retention aid for inorganic fillers Filler in urea-formaldehyde glues	
Pipe-clay (loam or ball clay)	Furniture	Water-based filler; fast colouring plasters and putties	
Colloid clay	Furniture	Filler in urea-formaldehyde glues	
Coal-tar derivatives	Furniture	Colouring substances	Carcinogenic in humans (Vol. 3, pp. 25-29; Supplement 1, p. 43)
Coal-tar oil	Saw mills; furniture	Wood preservative	
Cobalt salts	Pulp & paper	Impurity in technical-grade chemicals used as make-up in recovery of sulphate pulping	
	Furniture	Dessicants in oil and glycerophthalic varnishes	
	Carpentry	Wood preservatives	
Cobalt hexonoate	Furniture	Catalyst in polyester varnishes	
Cobalt naphthenate	Furniture	Catalyst in polyester varnishes	
Cobalt octanoate	Furniture	Accelerator in polyester varnishes	
Cobalt sulphate	Furniture	Wood stain	
Colophony	Furniture	Found in wood	
Copal	Furniture	In cellulose plasters and putties; varnish	
Copper salts	Carpentry	Wood preservatives	
Copper acetate	Furniture	Mordant in staining	
Copper carbonate	Saw mills	In wood preservatives	

Appendix 4 (contd)

Chemical	Industry	Use (or formation) in industry	Evaluation of carcinogenicity[a]
Copper chloride	Furniture	Adjuvant in casein glues	
Copper hydroxide	Saw mills	In wood preservatives	
Copper 8-hydroxy-quinoline	Saw mills	Water-repellant preservatives	Inadequate data in animals; no data in humans (Vol. 15, pp. 103-110)
Copper naphthenate	Carpentry	In wood preservatives	
Copper oxide	Saw mills	In wood preservatives	
Copper sulphate	Saw mills; furniture, carpentry	Wood preservative	
Coumarin resins	Furniture	Water-repellent agents in wood preservatives	
Creosotes	Saw mills; furniture; carpentry	Wood preservatives	
Creosote oil	Saw mills	Fungicide, insecticide	
Cresols (chlorinated)	Furniture	Fungicides, insecticides; bactericides in amylased glues	
Cresol-formaldehyde resins	Furniture	In glues	
Cresol resins	Furniture	Dry matter in formol cresol glues	
Cyclohexane	Furniture; carpentry	Solvent in neoprene glues	
Cyclohexanol	Furniture	Solvent in cellulose varnishes; in varnish removers	
Cyclohexanone	Furniture	Solvent in vinylic and neoprene glues, cellulose and polyurethane varnishes; in varnish removers	

Appendix 4 (contd)

Chemical	Industry	Use (or formation) in industry	Evaluation of carcinogenicity[a]
Cyclohexanone peroxide	Furniture	Catalyst in polyester varnishes	
Cymene	Pulp & paper	Vapours from pulping	
Dammar	Furniture	Component of shellac; varnish	
Dazomet (3,5-dichloro-phenoxyacetic acid)	Pulp & paper	Slime-controlling agent	2,4-D and esters: inadequate data in animals and humans (Vol. 15, pp. 111-138)
DDT (in mixtures)	Furniture	Insecticide	Limited evidence in animals; inadequate data in humans (Vol. 5, pp. 83-124)
Dehydroabietylamine	Furniture	Fixative in wood preservatives	
Dextrin	Furniture	Fast colour in plasters and putties	
Diacetone alcohol	Furniture	Solvent in epoxide varnishes	
Diatomite	Furniture	Filler in formaldehyde-urea glues	
Dicarboxylic acids	Furniture	Condensed with polyalcohols to make resins used in varnishes	
Dichloromethane	Saw mills Furniture	Solvent for chlorophenols Solvent in vinylic glues, poly-urethane varnishes and varnish removers	Inadequate data in animals; no data in humans (Vol. 20, pp. 449-465)
Dichromates *(see Chromates)*			
Dicyanodiamide	Pulp & paper	Additive to reduce viscosity of colour, to increase moisture resistance, or as a humectant	

Appendix 4 (contd)

Chemical	Industry	Use (or formation) in industry	Evaluation of carcinogenicity[a]
Dieldrin (in mixtures)	Furniture	Insecticide	Limited evidence in animals; inadequate data in humans (Vol. 5, pp. 125-126; Supplement 1, p. 16)
Diethylene triamine	Furniture	Catalyst in epoxide varnishes	
Difluorides (sodium & potassium)	Saw mills	Antistaining agents	
Dimethyldisulphide	Pulp & paper	Produced during cooking stage of sulphate pulping	
N,N-Dimethyl dithio-carbamate	Pulp & paper	Slime-controlling agent	
Dimethylformamide	Pulp & paper	In solvent fraction of slime-controlling agents	
Dimethylsulphide	Pulp & paper	Produced during cooking stage of sulphate pulping	
Dinitrophenols	Saw mills Furniture	In wood preservatives In fungicides	
Dioctylphthalate	Furniture	Plasticizer in cellulose varnishes	
Elemi	Furniture	Varnish	
Emery	Furniture	Abrasive in sanding	
Epoxide resins	Furniture	Binders in epoxide varnishes; water-repellent agents in wood preservatives	Diglycidyl resorcinol ether: inadequate data in animals; no data in humans (Vol. 11, pp. 125-129; Supplement 1, p. 16)
Epichlorohydrin-based resins	Pulp & paper	Additives to improve wet strength of paper	Epichlorohydrin: limited evidence in animals; inadequate data in humans (Vol. 11, pp. 131-139)

Appendix 4 (contd)

Chemical	Industry	Use (or formation) in industry	Evaluation of carcinogenicity[a]
Epichlorohydrin reaction products	Pulp & paper	Retention aids in paper making	Styrene oxide: limited evidence in animals; inadequate data in humans (Vol. 11, pp. 201-208; Supplement 1, p. 17)
Epoxy resins	Furniture; carpentry	Water-repellent agents in wood preservatives; binders in epoxide varnishes	
Essential oils	Saw mills; furniture	Extractives in wood	
Esters	Furniture	Solvents in plasters and putties; used in degreasing	
Ester gum	Saw mills	'Bloom' preventative for chlorophenols	
	Furniture	In cellulose plasters and putties	
Ethanol	Pulp & paper Furniture; carpentry	Vapours from pulp production Solvent in vinylic and in cresol-formaldehyde glues; used in cellulose and urea-formaldehyde varnishes in degreasing	
Ethyl acetate	Furniture; carpentry	Solvent in cellulose and polyurethane varnishes and in cellulose and neoprene glues	
Ethyl benzene	Furniture; carpentry	Solvent in varnishes	
Ethylene-bis dithiocarbamate	Pulp & paper	Slime-controlling agent	Manganese ethylene-bis-dithiocarbamate, Maneb: inadequate data in animals; no data in humans (Vol. 12, pp. 137-149) Zinc ethylene-bis-dithiocarbamate, Zineb: inadequate data in animals; no data in humans (Vol. 12, pp. 245-257)

Appendix 4 (contd)

Chemical	Industry	Use (or formation) in industry	Evaluation of carcinogenicity[a]
Ethylenediamine	Pulp & paper	In solvent fraction of slime-controlling agents	
	Furniture	Catalyst in epoxide varnishes	
Ethylene glycol	Pulp & paper	In solvent fraction of slime-controlling agents	
	Carpentry	Solvent in varnishes	
Ethylene-vinyl acetate copolymer	Pulp & paper	Barrier coating	Ethylene and polymers: no data in animals or humans (Vol. 19, pp. 157-186) Vinyl acetate and polymers: inadequate data in animals; no data in humans (Vol. 19, pp. 341-366)
Ethyl glycol	Furniture	Solvent in epoxide varnishes	
Ethyl glycol acetate	Furniture	Solvent in epoxide and polyurethane varnishes	
Ethylglycol acetate copolymer	Pulp & paper	Additive in barrier coating	
Ethyl mercaptan *(see Mercaptans)*			
Ferrous sulphate	Furniture	Wood stain	
Fluor chrome arsenate phenol	Saw mills	Wood preservative	Arsenic, chromium: human carcinogens (Vol. 23, pp. 39-141; 205-323; Supplement 1, pp. 22-23, 29-30)
Fluorides (alkali), complex fluorides, fluorosilicates	Saw mills	Wood preservatives	
	Furniture	Fungicides; retarders in casein glues	
Sodium fluoride	Saw mills	In wood preservatives	
	Furniture	Adjuvant in casein glues	

Appendix 4 (contd)

Chemical	Industry	Use (or formation) in industry	Evaluation of carcinogenicity[a]
Formaldehyde (paraformaldehyde)	Pulp & paper Furniture, plywood; carpentry Carpentry	In sizing agents Bactericide in gelatine, casein and blood glues; hardener and catalyst in resorcinol-formaldehyde glues Released when handling chip-board	(See Resorcinol-formaldehyde resins)
Formaldehyde resins	Furniture, plywood; carpentry	Partially condensed with urea, melamine, resorcinol, phenol or cresol resins in formaldehyde-urea, melamine-formaldehyde, formal-dehyde-resorcinol, formaldehyde-phenol and formaldehyde-cresol glues; dry matter in formaldehyde and formal cresol glues	
Formic acid	Pulp & paper	Vapours from pulp production	
Fuel oil	Saw mills Pulp & paper Furniture	Solvent for chlorophenols Additive in pigment-coating (foam-controlling agent) Diluting agent in wood preser-vatives	
Furfural	Pulp & paper	Vapours from pulp production	
Gelatine	Furniture	Dry matter in glues	
Glass	Furniture	Abrasive in sanding	
Gluconic acid	Pulp & paper	Vapours from pulp production	
Glycerol	Furniture	Condensed with dicarboxylic acids to make resins used in var-nishes	
Glycerol derivatives	Pulp & paper	Additives to reduce viscosity of colour, to increase moisture resis-tance, or as humectants	
Glyceromaleic resins	Furniture	Insulating varnishes	
Glycerophthalic resins	Furniture	Water-repellent agents in wood preservatives; insulating varnishes; base components of polyurethane varnishes	

Appendix 4 (contd)

Chemical	Industry	Use (or formation) in industry	Evaluation of carcinogenicity[a]
Glycols	Saw mills	'Bloom' preventives in chloro-phenols	
	Furniture	Polycondensed to make polyurethane varnishes	
Glyoxal	Pulp & paper	Additive to reduce viscosity of colour, to increase moisture resis-tance, or as a humectant	
Guazatine [N,N-(iminodi-8,1-octanediyl)bis-guanidine]	Saw mills	Antistaining agent	
Gypsum	Furniture	Filler in melamine-formaldehyde glues	
	Carpentry	In plaster boards	
Halogenated hydro-carbons	Furniture	Diluting agents in wood preser-vatives	See Vol. 20
Hexachlorocyclohexane (in mixtures)	Furniture	Insecticide	Sufficient evidence in animals; inadequate data in humans (Vol. 20, pp. 195-239)
Hexamethylene diisocyanate (see Isocyanates)			
Hydrocarbon waxes	Pulp & paper	Sizing agents	
Hydrochloric acid	Furniture, plywood	Hardener in urea-formaldehyde glues; catalyst in urea-formal-dehyde varnishes	
Hydrogen peroxide	Pulp & paper	Vapours from pulp production; used in pulp bleaching (oxi-dative stages)	
	Furniture	Wood bleaching	
Hydrogen sulphide	Pulp & paper	Vapours produced during cooking stage of pulping (sulphate process)	

Appendix 4 (contd)

Chemical	Industry	Use (or formation) in industry	Evaluation of carcinogenicity[a]
Hydrosulphite (dithionite)	Pulp & paper	Pulp bleaching	
Hydroxy-ether (Cellosolve)	Furniture; carpentry	Solvent in varnishes	
Hydroxymethyl-furfural	Pulp & paper	Vapours produced during cooking stage of pulp production	
Hydroxysugiresinol	Furniture	Found in wood	
Hyposulphite (alkali)	Pulp & paper; furniture	Bleaching	
Iron sulphate	Carpentry	Wood preservative	
Isobutanol	Furniture	Solvent in varnishes	
Isobutyl acetate	Furniture	Solvent in varnishes	
Isocyanates	Pulp & paper Carpentry	Slime-controlling agents Released when spraying poly-urethane foam	Toluene diisocyanate: inadequate data in animals; no data in humans; highly toxic (Vol. 19, pp. 303-340)
Polyisocyanates	Furniture	Binders in polyurethane var-nishes	
Isopropanol	Pulp & paper Furniture	Solvent in slime-controlling agents Solvent in epoxide varnishes	Inadequate data in animals. Manufacture of isopropanol using the strong acid pro-cess is carcinogenic in humans (Vol. 15, pp. 223-243; Supplement 1, p. 36)
Isosequiric acid	Furniture	Found in wood	
Kerosene	Saw mills Furniture	Solvent for chlorophenols Varnish thinner and remover	

Appendix 4 (contd)

Chemical	Industry	Use (or formation) in industry	Evaluation of carcinogenicity[a]
Ketones	Furniture	Solvents in plasters and putties, in glues and varnishes; diluting agents in wood preservatives	
Lapachol	Furniture	Found in wood	
Latexes	Pulp & paper	Sizing agents	
Lead salts	Furniture	Dessicants in oil and glycero-phthalic varnishes; accelerators in polyester varnishes	*Sufficient evidence in animals; inadequate data in humans:* - lead acetate
Red lead (Pb_3O_4)	Furniture	Covering pigment in plasters and putties	- lead phosphate
White lead [$Pb(OH_{12})(CO_3)_2$]	Furniture	In putties; supporting pigment	- lead subacetate - lead chromate *Limited evidence in animals; inadequate data in humans:* - lead chromate oxide *Inadequate data in animals and humans:* - lead arsenate - lead carbonate - lead chloride - lead naphthenate - lead nitrate (Vol. 23, pp. 325-415)
Lime sulphate	Furniture	Filler in urea-formaldehyde glues	
Lindane (in mixtures)	Furniture	Insecticide	*Sufficient evidence in animals; inadequate data in humans (Vol. 20, pp. 195-239)*
Lithoprone (barium-zinc-sulphide-sulphate)	Pulp & paper Furniture	Filler pigment Covering pigment	
Magnesium bisulphite	Pulp & paper	Active chemical in sulphite pulping	
Magnesium carbonate	Pulp & paper Furniture	Preparation of bleaching solutions Water-based filler	

Appendix 4 (contd)

Chemical	Industry	Use (or formation) in industry	Evaluation of carcinogenicity[a]
Magnesium hydroxide	Pulp & paper	Preparation of magnesium bisul-phite; bleaching	
Magnesium silicate	Pulp & paper	Coating pigment	
Maleic resins	Furniture	Plasticizers in cellulose varnishes; in cellulose plasters and putties	
Manganese salts	Furniture	Mordants in staining	
Melamine resins	Furniture	Varnishes	
Melamine-aldehyde modified resins	Pulp & paper	Additives to improve wet strength of paper	
Melamine-formalde-hyde resins	Pulp & paper	Additives to reduce viscosity of colour, to increase moisture resis-tance, or as humectants	
	Furniture, plywood	Glues	
Mercaptans (ethyl, methyl)	Pulp & paper	Produced as vapours during cooking stage of alkaline (kraft) pulping	
Mercaptobenzothiazol	Pulp & paper	Slime-controlling agents	
Mercury compounds	Pulp & paper	Slime-controlling agents (almost obsolete)	
organic mercury compounds (acetate, oleate, ethylmercury, phenylmercury)	Saw mills	Antistaining agents	
Mercury dichloride	Furniture	Fungicide, insecticide	
Methanol	Pulp & paper	Vapours from pulp production	
	Furniture, plywood	Solvent in vinylic, phenol-formal-dehyde and cresol-formaldehyde glues; wood degreasing; French polishing	
Methyl acetate	Furniture	Solvent for varnishes	
N-Methyl dithio-carbamate	Pulp & paper	Slime-controlling agent	

Appendix 4 (contd)

Chemical	Industry	Use (or formation) in industry	Evaluation of carcinogenicity[a]
Methylene-bis-thio-cyanate	Pulp & paper	Slime-controlling agent	
Methyl ethyl ketone	Furniture	Solvent in vinylic and neoprene glues and in epoxide and poly-urethane varnishes	
Methyl ethyl ketone peroxide	Furniture	Catalyst in polyester varnishes	
Methyl isobutyl ketone	Furniture; carpentry	Solvent in varnishes	
Methyl mercaptan *(see Mercaptans)*			
Methyl methacrylate	Furniture	Monomer in polyester varnishes	Inadequate data in animals; no data in humans (Vol. 19, pp. 187-211)
Mineral oil	Saw mills	Solvent for chlorophenols	Carcinogenic in humans (Vol. 3, pp. 30-33; Supplement 1, p. 43)
Mineral wool	Carpentry	Insulating material	
Muscovite mica	Pulp & paper	Coating pigment	
Naphtha	Furniture	Varnish thinner	
Naphthol	Furniture	In water-based plasters and putties	
Neoprene (polychloro-prene)	Furniture	Neoprene glues	Inadequate data in animals and in humans (Vol. 19, pp. 141-156)
Nickel	Carpentry	Plating for screws	Nickel in some form(s) carcinogenic to humans (Vol. 11, pp. 75-112; Supplement 1, p. 38)

Appendix 4 (contd)

Chemical	Industry	Use (or formation) in industry	Evaluation of carcinogenicity[a]
Nitrocellulose *(see Cellulose)*			
N-[α-(1-Nitroethyl)-benzyl] ethylene-diamine	Pulp & paper	Slime-controlling agent	
1-Octanol (capryl alcohol)	Pulp & paper	Additive in pigment-coating (foam-controlling agent)	
Oils	Furniture	In plasters	
Oil of turpentine		Solvent in oil varnishes	
Dessicating oils		In insulating varnishes	
Semi-dessicating oils		In insulating varnishes	
Eucalyptus oil		In water-based plasters and putties	
Linseed oil		Binder in oil and glycerophthalic varnishes; fixative in wood preservatives; in putties	
	Carpentry	Wood preservative	
Pine oils	Pulp & paper	Additive in pigment coatings (foam-controlling agents)	
	Furniture	Varnish thinner and remover	
Stand oil	Furniture	Binder in oil varnishes	
Tall oil	Pulp & paper	By-product of sulphate pulping	
Organic sulphides	Pulp & paper	Vapours from pulp production	
Oxymethylfurfural	Pulp & paper	Vapours from pulp production	
Ozone	Pulp & paper	Released during paper laminating, printing and roller-cleaning	
Paraclox (N-4-dihydroxy-α-oxo-benzene ethanimidoyl chloride)	Pulp & paper	Slime-controlling agent	
Paraffins	Furniture	Water-repellent agents in wood preservatives	
Paraffin oil	Pulp & paper	Solvent for biphenyl	
	Furniture	Varnish thinner and remover	
Paraffin wax	Pulp & paper	Barrier-coating	

Appendix 4 (contd)

Chemical	Industry	Use (or formation) in industry	Evaluation of carcinogenicity[a]
Pentachlorophenol and pentachloro-phenates *(see Chlorophenols)*			
Pentadecylcatechol	Furniture	Found in wood	
Peroxides	Pulp & paper	Pulp bleaching	
Persulphates (alkali)	Furniture	Wood bleaching	
Petrol and petroleum products	Saw mills Furniture Carpentry	Solvents for chlorophenols in plasters In adhesives; on formworks; on screws	
Phenol	Pulp & paper; furniture; carpentry	Wood preservative	
Phenol-formaldehyde resins	Furniture, plywood	Glues	
Phenolic resins	Furniture	Fillers in resorcinol-formaldehyde glues; dry matter in formaldehyde glues	
N-(1-Phenyl-2-nitro-propyl)piperazine	Pulp & paper	Slime-controlling agent	
ortho-Phenylphenol	Furniture	Antiseptic in vegetable glues	
Phosphates (alkali)	Furniture	Fungicides, insecticides, flame retardants	
Phosphoric acid	Furniture, plywood	Hardener in urea-formaldehyde glues; catalyst in urea-formal-dehyde varnishes; hardener in varnishes	
Phthalates	Furniture	Plasticizers in cellulose varnishes	
Phthalic anhydride	Furniture	Condensed with polyalcohols to make resins used in varnishes	

Appendix 4 (contd)

Chemical	Industry	Use (or formation) in industry	Evaluation of carcinogenicity[a]
Plicatic acid	Furniture	Found in wood	
Polyacrylate acetate-based products	Pulp & paper Carpentry	Sizes used in conjunction with pigment coating In varnishes	Acrylic acid, poly-acrylic acid and acrylates: no data in animals or in humans (Vol. 19, pp. 62-71)
Polyalcohols	Furniture	Polymerized with dicarboxylic acids or anhydrides to make resins used in varnishes	
Polyamides	Pulp & paper	Barrier coatings	
Polyamide resins	Furniture	Base component of polyurethane varnishes	
Polychlorinated biphenyls	Pulp & paper	In self-copying papers	Sufficient evidence in animals for some PCBs; probably carcinogenic for humans (Vol. 18, pp. 43-103; Supplement 1, p. 41)

Polyesters
  containing free hydroxyls
  saturated polyesters
 	
  unsaturated poly-ester resins
	Pulp & paper
	Furniture; carpentry
	Furniture; carpentry
	Furniture; carpentry
		Barrier-coatings
		Binders in polyurethane varnishes
		
		Base components in polyurethane varnishes
		Binders in polyester varnishes	

Polyethylene	Pulp & paper	Barrier-coating	Inadequate data in animals and humans (Vol. 19, pp. 164-184)
Polyglycols	Furniture	Diluting agents in wood preservatives	
Polyisocyanates (see Isocyanates)			

Appendix 4 (contd)

Chemical	Industry	Use (or formation) in industry	Evaluation of carcinogenicity[a]
Polyphenolics	Saw mills	Extractives in wood	
Polyphosphate	Pulp & paper	Dispersive agent in pigment coating	
Polyurethane	Furniture; carpentry	In varnishes	
Polyurethane foam	Carpentry	Insulating material	Inadequate data in animals; no data in humans (Vol. 19, pp. 303-340)
Potassium carbonate (potash)	Furniture	In varnish removers	
Potassium fluoride	Saw mills	In wood preservatives	
Potassium hexacyano-ferrate	Furniture	Wood stain	
Potassium hydroxide	Furniture	In varnish removers	
Propanol	Furniture	Solvent in varnishes	
Pumice	Furniture	Water-based filler; abrasive in sanding	
Resins	Saw mills Pulp & paper Furniture	Extractives in wood Sizing agents In varnishes and glues	
Resorcinol-formal-dehyde resins	Furniture, plywood	Glues	Resorcinol: inadequate data in animals; no data in humans (Vol. 15, pp. 155-175)
Rosin	Pulp & paper Furniture	Sizing agent Modifier of maleic resins in cellulose plasters and putties; component of shellac; varnish	
Rubber derivatives	Pulp & paper	Barrier coatings	

Appendix 4 (contd)

Chemical	Industry	Use (or formation) in industry	Evaluation of carcinogenicity[a]
Shellac	Furniture	Hard putty; varnish; in French polish	
Silica	Saw mills	In wood and bark (cork)	
Silicones	Pulp & paper	Additives in pigment coating (foam-controlling agents); sizing agents	
Slate	Furniture	Filler	
Sodium aluminate	Pulp & paper	Size	
Sodium bicarbonate	Pulp & paper	Buffer in cooking liquor in neutral sulphite semi-chemical process	
Sodium bisulphite	Pulp & paper Furniture	Active chemical in sulphite pulping Wood bleaching	
Sodium carbonate (soda ash)	Pulp & paper Furniture	Preparation of sodium bisulphite; used in recovery process of alkaline (sulphate) pulping; buffer in cooking liquor in neutral sulphite semi-chemical process Wood degreasing	
Sodium chlorate	Pulp & paper	Used to generate chlorine dioxide for pulp bleaching	
Sodium hydroxide (caustic soda)	Pulp & paper Furniture	Treatment of chips in chemi-mechanical pulping process; active chemical in sulphate pulping; alkaline extraction in pulp bleaching; preparation of sodium bisulphite; buffer in cooking liquor in neutral sulphite semi-chemical process; in mist from pulp production In glues and varnish removers	
Sodium hypochlorite	Pulp & paper	Used in oxidative stages of pulp bleaching	
Sodium silicate	Pulp & paper Furniture	Sizing agent Adjuvant in vegetable and casein glues; dry matter of sodium silicate glues	

Appendix 4 (contd)

Chemical	Industry	Use (or formation) in industry	Evaluation of carcinogenicity[a]
Sodium sulphate	Pulp & paper	In recovery process; compensation chemical in sulphate (kraft) process	
Sodium sulphide	Pulp & paper	Active chemical in sulphate pulping; produced in recovery process of alkaline pulping	
Sodium sulphite	Pulp & paper	Cooking liquor in neutral sulphite semi-chemical pulping; used to treat chips in chemi-mechanical pulping process	
Sodium trichloro-phenate *(see Chlorophenols)*			
Soya oil	Furniture	Binder in varnishes	
Starch	Saw mills Pulp & paper Furniture	Extractive in wood Sizing agent Fast colour; filler in melamine-formaldehyde glues	
Starch derivatives	Pulp & paper	Retention aids	
Styrene	Furniture; carpentry	Solvent and monomer in polyester varnishes	Limited evidence in animals; inadequate data in humans (Vol. 19, pp. 231-274)
Dichlorostyrene	Furniture	Monomer in polyester varnishes	
Styrene-butadiene	Pulp & paper	Size used in conjunction with coating pigments	
Sugiresinol	Furniture	Found in wood	
Sulphur	Pulp & paper	Preparation of pulping liquors and bleaching solutions	
Sulphur dioxide	Pulp & paper	Produced in initial steps of sulphite pulping	
Sulphur trioxide	Pulp & paper	Accidental production during sulphite pulping	

Appendix 4 (contd)

Chemical	Industry	Use (or formation) in industry	Evaluation of carcinogenicity[a]
Sulphuric acid	Pulp & paper	Accidental production during sulphite pulping; addition to cooking liquor	
	Furniture	Wood bleaching	
Sulphurous acid	Pulp & paper	Used in acid sulphite pulping	
	Furniture	Wood bleaching	
Talc (magnesium silicate hydrate)	Pulp & paper	Coating pigment	
	Furniture	Water-based filler	
Tannins	Saw mills	Occur as extractives in wood and bark (cork)	Limited evidence in animals; no data in humans (Vol. 10, pp. 253-262)
	Furniture	Adjuvants in gelatine glues	
	Carpentry	Wood preservatives	
Tannin-based compounds	Furniture	Mordants	
Tetephthalic acid	Furniture	Condensed with polyalcohols to make resins used in varnishes	
Terpene compounds (α-pinene, β-pinene, δ-carene, plus other monoterpenes and some aromatic alkyl compounds)	Saw mills	Sawing vapours	
Tetrachloroethylene	Pulp & paper	Used to clean equipment in production of biphenyl papers	Limited evidence in animals; no data in humans (Vol. 20, pp. 491-514)
2,3,4,6-Tetrachloro-phenol (see Chlorophenols)			
Tetrahydro-3,5-dimethyl-2H-13,5-thiadiazine-2-thione (DMTT)	Pulp & paper	Slime-controlling agent	
Tetralin	Furniture	In varnish removers	

Appendix 4 (contd)

Chemical	Industry	Use (or formation) in industry	Evaluation of carcinogenicity[a]
2-(Thiocyanomethyl-thio)-benzathiazole	Pulp & paper	Slime-controlling agent	
Thiophenates	Saw mills	Antistaining agents	
Titanium salts	Furniture	Mordants in staining	
Titanium dioxide (amastase, rutile)	Pulp & paper	Filler pigment; coating pigment	
Toluene	Furniture; carpentry	Solvent in vinylic, neoprene and chlorinated rubber glues; solvent in glycerophthalic, urea-formaldehyde and poly-urethane varnishes; diluent in cellulose, epoxide and poly-urethane varnishes	
Toluene diisocyanate (see Isocyanates)			
para-Toluene sulphonic acid	Furniture	Hardener in varnishes	
Triallyl cyanurate	Furniture	Monomer in polyester varnishes	
Tributyl citrate	Pulp & paper	Additive to coating pigments (foam-controlling agent)	
Tributyl phosphate	Pulp & paper	Additive to pigment coating (foam-controlling agent)	
Tributyl tin compounds (bis(tributyl tin)-oxide, tributyl tin naphthenate, tris-(tributyl tin)phos-phate)	Saw mills; furniture; carpentry	Wood preservation	
111-Trichloroethane	Pulp & paper	In solvent fraction of slime-controlling agents	Inadequate data in animals; no data in humans (Vol. 20, pp. 515-531)

Appendix 4 (contd)

Chemical	Industry	Use (or formation) in industry	Evaluation of carcinogenicity[a]
2,4,5- and 2,4,6-Trichlorophenols (see Chlorophenols)			
Tricresyl phosphate	Furniture	Plasticizer in cellulose varnishes	
Tridecyl alcohol	Pulp & paper	Additive to pigment coating (foam-controlling agent)	
Triethylene tetramine	Furniture	Catalyst in epoxide varnishes	
Trihydroxymethyl-propane	Furniture	Condensed with resins to make varnishes	
Turpentine	Furniture	Solvent or thinner in varnishes; in plasters and putties; used for pumice sanding; found in wood	
	Pulp & paper	By-product of sulphate pulping	
Urea	Pulp & paper	Additive to reduce viscosity of colour, to increase moisture resistance, or as a humectant	
	Plywood	In urea-resin adhesives	
Urea-aldehyde modified resins	Pulp & paper	Additives to improve wet strength of paper	
Urea-formaldehyde resins	Pulp & paper	Additives to reduce the viscosity of colour, to increase moisture resistance, or as humectants	
	Furniture, plywood, carpentry	Glues, varnishes	
Usnic acid	Furniture	Found in wood	
Vanillin	Pulp & paper	By-product of sulphite pulping	
Vinyl resins	Furniture	Base components of polyurethane varnishes	

Appendix 4 (contd)

Chemical	Industry	Use (or formation) in industry	Evaluation of carcinogenicity[a]
Polyvinyl acetate (resin)	Furniture; carpentry	Dry matter of vinylic glues; binder in vinylic varnishes; in plasters and putties	
Polyvinyl acetate-based products	Pulp & paper	Sizes used in conjunction with coating pigments	Vinyl acetate, polyvinyl acetate and polyvinyl alcohol: inadequate data in animals; no data in humans (Vol. 19, pp. 341-366)
Polyvinyl acrylate	Carpentry	Glues	
Polyvinyl butyrate	Furniture	Dry matter of vinylic glues	
Polyvinylidene chloride	Pulp & paper	Barrier coating	
Polyvinyl resins	Furniture	Base components of polyurethane varnishes	Vinyl chloride: human carcinogen. Polyvinyl chloride and vinyl chloride-vinyl acetate copolymers: inadequate data in animals; no data in humans (Vol. 19, pp. 377-438)
Waxes	Saw mills Pulp & paper	Extractives in wood Sizing agents	
White spirit	Furniture	Solvent in oil and glycerophthalic varnishes	
Xylene	Furniture; carpentry	Solvent in vinylic, neoprene and chlorinated rubber glues; solvent in glycerophthalic, urea-formaldehyde and polyurethane varnishes; diluent in cellulose, epoxide and polyurethane varnishes	
Zinc salts	Pulp & paper	Additives to reduce viscosity of colour, to increase moisture resistance, or as humectants	
Zinc chloride	Saw mills Furniture	In wood preservatives Fungicide; insecticide	

Appendix 4 (contd)

Chemical	Industry	Use (or formation) in industry	Evaluation of carcinogenicity[a]
Zinc oxide	Saw mills Pulp & paper Furniture	In wood preservatives Coating pigment Water-based filler; in plasters and putties; supporting pigment	
Zinc stearate	Furniture	In alkyd resins used in cellulose plasters and putties	
Zinc sulphide	Pulp & paper	Filler pigment	
Ziram (zinc dimethyldithio-carbamate)	Saw mills	Antistaining agent	Inadequate data in animals; no data in humans (Vol. 12, pp. 259-270)

[a]For chemicals considered in *IARC Monographs*

CHEMICALS USED OR PRODUCED IN LEATHER AND ASSOCIATED INDUSTRIES (EXCEPTING DYES) AND CROSS REFERENCES TO
IARC MONOGRAPHS

This list includes those chemicals that are or were used in or formed during the manufacture or treatment of leather. No evaluation is made of the amounts of the chemicals that are actually used, of levels of exposure, or of temporal or geographical variations in their use during the various manufacturing processes. This list was compiled from information collected during the preparation of the present volume of *Monographs* and cannot pretend to be fully exhaustive for all situations in all countries. Evaluations of carcinogenicity are reported for those chemicals previously considered in the *IARC Monograph* series.

Appendix 5. Chemicals used or produced in leather and associated industries

Chemical	Industry	Use (or formation) in industry	Evaluation of carcinogenicity[a]
Acetic acid	Tanning & processing	Deliming and bating	
Acetone	Tanning & processing	Solvent in finishing	
	Leather goods	Solvent in ethylene carboxylic, phenolic and polyurethane glues	
	Boots & shoes	Adhesive and lacquer solvent; cleaner	
Acrolein	Tanning & processing	Tanning agent	Inadequate data in animals; no data in humans (Vol. 19, 479-494)
Acrylic resins (various)	Tanning & processing	Impregnants in finishing process	Inadequate data in animals; no data in humans (Vol. 19, pp. 47-71, 187-211)
	Boots & shoes	Upper and unit finishes, emulsion or solvent-based	
Polyacrylate resin emulsions (polybutyl methacrylate, poly-ethyl acrylate, poly-isobutyl methacry-late, polymethyl methacrylate)	Tanning & processing	Binders in finishing	
Polyacrylic resins	Tanning & processing	Impregnants in finishing	
Acrylonitrile	Boots & shoes	May be produced by heating of acrylonitrile-butadiene-styrene compounds	Limited evidence in animals; pro-bably carcinogenic in humans (Vol. 19, pp. 73-113; Supplement 1, p. 21)
Acrylonitrile-butadiene copolymer	Tanning & processing	Binder in finishing	
	Boots & shoes	Soling material	
Acrylonitrile-butadiene-styrene polycarbonate	Boots & shoes	Soles, heels	

Appendix 5 (contd)

Chemical	Industry	Use (or formation) in industry	Evaluation of carcinogenicity[a]
Adipates	Leather goods	Plasticizers in artificial leather	
Albumin (from eggs & blood)	Tanning & processing	Binders in finishing	
Aldehydes: unsaturated *(see Acrolein)*; **saturated** *(see Formaldehyde and Dialdehydes)*	Tanning & processing	Tanning agents	
Aliphatic acids of low molecular weight	Tanning & processing	Deliming and bating	
Aliphatic amines (including dimethyl-amine) and salts	Tanning & processing	Liming (unhairing); soaking and washing	
Alkane sulphonates	Tanning & processing	Lubricants	
Alkane sulphonic acid chlorides	Tanning & processing	Tanning agents	
Alkanol ethoxylates	Tanning & processing	Fat removal	
Alkylbenzene sul-phonates	Tanning & processing	Fat removal	
Alkylphenols	Tanning & processing	Fat removal	
Alkyl phenyl ethoxylates	Tanning & processing	Fat removal	
Alkyl succinic com-pounds	Tanning & processing	Impregnants in finishing	
Alkyl sulphates	Tanning & processing	Fat removal	
Alkyl sulphites	Tanning & processing	Fat removal	
Alum	Tanning & processing	Tanning agent	

Appendix 5 (contd)

Chemical	Industry	Use (or formation) in industry	Evaluation of carcinogenicity[a]
Aluminium [III] salts	Tanning & processing	Tanning agents	
Aluminium oxide	Tanning & processing	Pigment in finishing	
Aluminium salts of fatty acids	Tanning & processing	Impregnants in finishing	
Potassium aluminium sulphate	Tanning & processing	Tanning agent	
Amino resins	Tanning	Retanning agents	
Ammonia	Tanning & processing Leather goods Boots & shoes	Liming (unhairing); chrome tannage In neoprene adhesives and artificial latex Cleaner	
Ammonium bicarbonate	Tanning & processing	Neutralizer; used in dyeing	
Ammonium chloride	Tanning & processing	Deliming and bating	
Ammonium salts (quaternary)	Tanning & processing	Fat removal	
Ammonium sulphate	Tanning & processing	Deliming and bating; tanning	
Amyl acetate	Tanning & processing Boots & shoes	Solvent in finishing Adhesive and lacquer solvent; cleaner	
Amyl alcohol	Tanning & processing	Solvent in finishing	
Aniline	Tanning & processing Leather goods	Condensed with resorcinol to make synthetic tannins Oxidized with permanganate and dissolved in ethanol to make aniline black	Inadequate data in animals and humans (Vol. 4, pp. 27-38)
Aromatic amines and salts	Tanning & processing	Soaking and washing	

Appendix 5 (contd)

Chemical	Industry	Use (or formation) in industry	Evaluation of carcinogenicity[a]
Arsenic	Tanning & processing	Defestation, disinfection	Arsenic and arsenic compounds: carcinogenic in humans (Vol. 23, pp. 39-141; Supplement 1, p. 22)
Arsenic sulphide	Tanning & processing	Liming (unhairing)	
Arsenious anhydride	Tanning & processing	Defestation, disinfection	
Arsenious oxide	Tanning & processing	Defestation, disinfection	
Sodium arsenates	Tanning & processing	Soaking and washing	
Auxiliary surfactants	Tanning & processing	Dyeing	
Azelates	Leather goods	Plasticizers in artificial leather	
Barium sulphate	Tanning & processing	Pigment in finishing	
Beeswax stearin	Tanning & processing	Dressing in finishing	
Benzene	Tanning & processing	Fat removal (in the 1930s); solvent in finishing	Carcinogenic in humans (Vol. 7, pp. 203-221; Supplement 1, p. 24)
	Leather goods	Solvent in ethylene carboxylic, phenolic and polyurethane glues	
	Boots & shoes	Adhesive solvent	
Benzo[a]pyrene	Tanning & processing	Exhaust fumes	Carcinogenic in animals; no data in humans (Vol. 3, pp. 91-136)
Betanaphthol	Tanning & processing	Soaking	

Appendix 5 (contd)

Chemical	Industry	Use (or formation) in industry	Evaluation of carcinogenicity[a]
Bleaching powder (calcium hydroxide and chlorine)	Tanning & processing	Disinfection	
Borax (hydrated sodium borate)	Tanning & processing	Defestation, disinfection; tanning; dyeing; neutralizing	
Boric acid	Tanning & processing	Deliming and bating; defestation, disinfection	
Butane	Tanning & processing	In internal transport fuel	
Butanol	Tanning & processing	Solvent in finishing	
Butyl acetate	Tanning & processing	Solvent in finishing	
	Boots & shoes	Adhesive and lacquer solvent; cleaner	
Butyl Cellosolve	Tanning & processing	Solvent in finishing	
Butyl stearate	Tanning & processing	Plasticizer in finishing	
Butyric acid	Tanning & processing	Pickling	
Cadmium selenide	Tanning & processing	Pigment in finishing	Sufficient evidence in animals for cadmium sulphide; cadmium and certain cadmium compounds probably carcinogenic for humans (Vol. 11, pp. 39-74; Supplement 1, pp. 27-28)
Cadmium sulphide	Tanning & processing	Pigment in finishing	
Calcium chloride	Tanning & processing	Soaking and washing; liming	
Calcium formate	Tanning & processing	Dyeing; neutralizing	

Appendix 5 (contd)

Chemical	Industry	Use (or formation) in industry	Evaluation of carcinogenicity[a]
Calcium hydroxide (hydrated lime)	Tanning & processing	Liming (unhairing)	
Calcium oxide (lime)	Tanning & processing	Liming (unhairing)	
Camphor	Tanning & processing	Plasticizer in finishing	
	Leather goods	Plasticizer in artificial leather	
Caoutchouc	Boots & shoes	Soles, heels; adhesives	
	Leather goods	Adhesives	
Carbon black	Tanning & processing	Pigment in finishing	
Carbon disulphide	Boots & shoes	Rubber solvent and cleaner	
Carbon monoxide	Tanning & processing	Exhaust fumes	
Carbon tetrachloride	Tanning & processing	Fat removal (in the 1930s)	Sufficient evidence in animals; probably carcinogenic in humans (Vol. 20, pp. 371-399; Supplement 1, p. 28)
	Boots & shoes	Rubber solvent and cleaner	
Carboxymethyl-cellulose	Tanning & processing	Paste drying	
Carrageenan	Tanning & processing	Binder in finishing	Inadequate data in animals; no data in humans (Vol. 10, pp. 181-190)
Casein	Tanning & processing	Binder in finishing	
Casein (alkaline extract)	Leather goods	Glue	
Cellulose acetate butyrate	Boots & shoes	Upper and unit finishes, usually solvent-based	

Appendix 5 (contd)

Chemical	Industry	Use (or formation) in industry	Evaluation of carcinogenicity[a]
Cellulose fibres	Boots & shoes	Insoles	
Cetyl ammonium bromide	Tanning & processing	Fat removal	
Cetyldimethylbenzyl-ammonium chloride	Tanning & processing	Defestation, disinfection	
Chlorine	Tanning & processing	Preservation in beamhouse; soaking and washing	
Chlorinated hydro-carbons	Boots & shoes	Solvent in adhesives	(See Vol. 20)
Chlorinated paraffins	Tanning & processing	Fat liquoring	
Chlorine dioxide	Tanning & processing	Defestation, disinfectant	
Chlorophenols and chlorophenates	Tanning & processing	Defestation, disinfection; paste drying	Inadequate data in animals; no data in humans (Vol. 20, pp. 349-369). Subsequent to the meeting, a positive bioassay in mice and rats was published on 2,4,6-trichlorophenol (*NCI tech. Rep. Ser. No. 155,* 1979)
Chromium:	Tanning & processing	Chrome tannage	Chromium: human carcinogen. Relatively insoluble Cr[VI] salts: sufficient evidence in animals (Vol. 23, pp. 205-323; Supplement 1, pp. 29-30)
Chrome green	Tanning & processing	Pigment in finishing	
Chromium [VI] salts: potassium dichromate sodium dichromate	Tanning & processing	'Two-bath' chrome tannage 'Two-bath' chrome tannage; pickling	
chromic oxide		'Two-bath' chrome tannage	
Chromium [III] salts: chromium sulphate chromium sulphite chromium aluminium sulphate		Tanning agent	
Chromium salts of fatty acids		Impregnants in finishing, as water-oil repellents	

Appendix 5 (contd)

Chemical	Industry	Use (or formation) in industry	Evaluation of carcinogenicity[a]
Collagen	Leather goods	Glues	
Copper sulphate	Tanning & processing	Defestation, disinfection	
Cresols (mixed) and other phenols	Tanning & processing	Defestation, disinfection; in synthetic tannins	
meta-Cresol	Tanning & processing	Soaking and washing	
Cyanides	Tanning & processing	Liming, unhairing (sharpening agents)	
Cyclohexane	Tanning & processing	Solvent in finishing	
	Leather goods	Solvent in finishing and in ethylene carboxylic, phenolic and polyurethane glues	
	Boots & shoes	Cleaner; diluent; adhesive solvent	
DDT	Tanning & processing	Defestation, disinfection	Limited evidence in animals; inadequate data in humans (Vol. 5, pp. 83-104)
Dextrins	Leather goods	In natural glues	
Dialdehydes	Tanning & processing	Tanning agents	
Diamide phthalate	Tanning & processing	Plasticizer in finishing	
Dibutylphosphate	Tanning & processing	Plasticizer in finishing	
Dibutylphthalate	Tanning & processing	Plasticizer in finishing	
1,2- and 1,4-Dichloro-benzenes	Tanning & processing	Defestation, disinfectants	Inadequate data in animals and humans (Vol. 7, pp. 231-244)

Appendix 5 (contd)

Chemical	Industry	Use (or formation) in industry	Evaluation of carcinogenicity[a]
Dichloroethylene	Tanning & processing	Fat removal	
Dichloromethane	Tanning & processing	Solvent in finishing	Inadequate data in animals; no data in humans (Vol. 20, pp. 449-465)
	Boots & shoes	Rubber solvent and cleaner	
Dichloropropane	Leather goods	Solvent in ethylene carboxylic, phenolic and polyurethane glues	
Dicyanodiamide-formaldehyde condensation products	Tanning & processing	In retanning of leathers treated by chrome tannage	
Diethyl ether	Tanning & processing	Solvent in finishing	
Diethylphthalate	Tanning & processing	Plasticizer in finishing	
Diidomethyl *para*-tolyl sulphone (Amical 48)	Tanning & processing	Defestation	
Dimethylamine sulphate	Tanning & processing	Liming, unhairing (sharpening agent); accelerating agent	
Dimethylformamide	Boots & shoes	Lacquer solvent	
Dimethylphthalate	Tanning & processing	Plasticizer in finishing	
1,4-Dioxane	Tanning & processing	Solvent in finishing	Sufficient evidence in animals; no data in humans (Vol. 11, pp. 247-256)
Esters	Boots & shoes	Solvents in synthetic rubber adhesives	
Ethane	Tanning & processing	In internal transport fuel	
Ethanol	Tanning & processing	Solvent in finishing	

Appendix 5 (contd)

Chemical	Industry	Use (or formation) in industry	Evaluation of carcinogenicity[a]
Ethanol (contd)	Leather goods	Solvent	
	Boots & shoes	Cleaner	
Ethyl acetate	Tanning & processing	Solvent in finishing	
	Leather goods	Solvent in ethylene carboxylic, phenolic and polyurethane glues and in nitrocellulose paints	
	Boots & shoes	Adhesive and lacquer solvent; cleaner	
Ethyl acrylate	Tanning & processing	Binder in finishing	Inadequate data in animals and humans (Vol. 19, pp. 57-71)
Ethyl vinyl acetate	Boots & shoes	Hot-melt adhesive	
Ethylene carboxylic resins	Leather goods	In ethylene carboxylic glues	
Ethylene oxide	Tanning & processing	Defestation, disinfection	Probably carcinogenic in humans (Vol. 11, pp. 157-167; Supplement 1, p. 34)
Ethylene vinyl acetate	Boots & shoes	Soling material	Vinyl acetate: inadequate data in animals; no data in humans (Vol. 19, pp. 341-366)
Ferric ferrocyanide	Tanning & processing	Pigment in finishing	
Fluorides (sodium difluoride; sodium fluoride)	Tanning & processing	Defestation, disinfection; soaking, washing	
Formaldehyde	Tanning & processing	**Defestation, disinfection;** tanning agent; in synthetic tannins; dressing in finishing	
Formaldehyde resins	Leather goods	In adhesives	

Appendix 5 (contd)

Chemical	Industry	Use (or formation) in industry	Evaluation of carcinogenicity[a]
Formic acid	Tanning & processing	Soaking and washing; pickling; defestation; fixative in dyeing	
Glucose	Tanning & processing	Liming (unhairing); reducing agent in chrome tannage	
Glutaraldehyde	Tanning & processing	Tanning and retanning agent	
Glycols and glycol acetates	Tanning & processing	Solvents in finishing	
Glycolic acid	Tanning & processing	Deliming and bating	
Gold	Leather goods	Decoration	
Greases	Tanning & processing	Fat liquoring	
Gum arabic	Leather goods	Glues	
Halogenation agents based on organic chlorine donors	Boots & shoes	Primers	
Heptane	Leather goods; boots & shoes	Solvent in polyurethane, phenolic and ethylene carboxylic glues	
Hexane	Leather goods	Solvent in polyurethane, phenolic and ethylene carboxylic glues	
	Boots & shoes	Cleaner; diluent, adhesive solvent	
Hydrocarbons	Tanning & processing	Exhaust fumes	
	Boots & shoes	Solvents in synthetic rubber adhesives	
Hydrochloric acid	Tanning & processing	In 'two-bath' chrome tannage; deliming and bating; pickling	
Hydrogen chloride	Boots & shoes	Produced when two PVC compounds are welded together	

Appendix 5 (contd)

Chemical	Industry	Use (or formation) in industry	Evaluation of carcinogenicity[a]
Hydrogen peroxide	Tanning & processing	Bleaching; colouring in finishing processes	
Hydrogen sulphide	Tanning & processing	Produced by discharge of water from liming and pickling baths	
Hydroxyethyl derivatives of alcohols	Tanning & processing	Soaking and washing; liming (unhairing)	
2-Hydroxypropyl-methane thio-sulphonate	Tanning & processing	Defestation	
Iron salts	Tanning & processing	Tanning agents (in the 1940s)	
Iron blue	Tanning & processing	Pigment in finishing	
Iron oxide	Tanning & processing	Pigment in finishing	Not carcinogenic in animals; underground haematite mining is carcinogenic to humans (Vol. 1, pp. 29-39); Supplement 1, p. 34)
Isobutanol	Tanning & processing	Solvent in finishing	
Isobutyl acetate	Tanning & processing	Solvent in finishing	
Isocyanates (various)	Tanning & processing	Special leather finishes	2,4- and 2,6-Toluene diisocyanates: inadequate data in animals; no data in humans (Vol. 19, pp. 303-340)
	Boots & shoes	Reactive primers; in two-part adhesives	

Appendix 5 (contd)

Chemical	Industry	Use (or formation) in industry	Evaluation of carcinogenicity[a]
Isopropanol	Tanning & processing Boots & shoes	Solvent in finishing; imbuing to increase compactness of leather in finishing processes Cleaner	Inadequate data in animals; manufacture of isopropyl alcohol using the strong-acid process is carcinogenic in humans (Vol. 15, pp. 223-243; Supplement 1, p. 36)
Kaolin	Tanning & processing	Dressing in finishing	
Kerosene	Tanning & processing	Fat removal (in the 1930s)	
Ketones	Boots & shoes	Solvents in synthetic rubber adhesives	
Lactic acid	Tanning & processing	Chrome and vegetable tannage	
Lead carbonate	Tanning & processing	Pigment in finishing	Inadequate data in animals and humans (Vol. 23, pp. 325-415)
Lead chromate	Tanning & processing	Pigment in finishing	Sufficient evidence in animals; inadequate data in humans (Vol. 23, pp. 325-415)
Lead hydrate	Tanning & processing	Pigment in finishing	
Lead oxide	Tanning & processing	Pigment in finishing	Inadequate data in animals and humans (Vol. 23, pp. 325-415)
Lead sulphate	Tanning & processing	Pigment in finishing	
Magnesium hydroxide	Tanning & processing	Liming (unhairing)	

Appendix 5 (contd)

Chemical	Industry	Use (or formation) in industry	Evaluation of carcinogenicity[a]
Magnesium oxide	Tanning & processing	Basification (chrome tannage)	
Maleic anhydride-styrene copolymers	Tanning & processing	In retanning of leathers treated by chrome tannage	
Melamine	Tanning & processing	Binder in finishing	
Melamine-formal-dehyde condensation products	Tanning & processing	In retanning of leathers treated by chrome tannage	
Mercuric chloride	Tanning & processing	Defestation, disinfection	
Mercuric iodide	Tanning & processing	Defestation, disinfection	
Methanol	Tanning & processing	Solvent in finishing	
Methyl acetate	Tanning & processing	Solvent in finishing	
Methyl butyl ketone	Leather goods	Solvent in phenolic, polyurethane and ethylene carboxylic glues	
Methylcyclohexane	Tanning & processing	Solvent in finishing	
Methylcyclopentane	Leather goods Boots & shoes	Solvent in glues Cleaner; diluent; adhesive solvent	
Methylene-bis-thiocyanate	Tanning & processing	Defestation	
4,4'-Methylenedianiline	Tanning & processing	Solvent in finishing	Inadequate data in animals; no data in humans (Vol. 4, pp. 79-85
Methyl ethyl ketone	Tanning & processing	Solvent in finishing	
	Leather goods	Solvent in phenolic, polyurethane and ethylene carboxylic glues	
	Boots & shoes	Adhesive and lacquer solvent; cleaner	

Chemical	Industry	Use (or formation) in industry	Evaluation of carcinogenicity[a]
Methyl isobutyl ketone	Tanning & processing	Solvent in finishing	
	Boots & shoes	Cleaner; adhesive and lacquer solvent	
2-Methylpentane	Leather goods	Solvent in phenolic, poly-urethane and ethylene carboxylic glues	
	Boots & shoes	Cleaner; diluent; adhesive solvent	
3-Methylpentane	Leather goods	Solvent in phenolic and poly-urethane glues and in ethylene carboxylic glues	
	Boots & shoes	Cleaner; diluent; adhesive solvent	
Mineral acids	Tanning & processing	In 'two-bath' chrome tannage	
Mineral oil	Tanning & processing	Fat liquoring; defestation, disinfection	Carcinogenic in humans (Vol. 3, pp. 30-33; Supplement 1, p. 43)
Naphthalene	Tanning & processing	Defestation, disinfection; preservation; component of synthetic tannins	
Naphthalene-based compounds	Tanning & processing	Retanning agents	
1-Naphthalene sulphonic acid	Tanning & processing	Retanning, colouring and fat liquoring	
2-Naphthol	Tanning & processing	Pickling; soaking and washing; defestation, disinfection	
Natural rubber (see Caoutchouc)			
Nitrobenzene	Tanning & processing	Solvent in finishing	
Nitrobiphenyl	Leather goods	Plasticizer in artificial leather	4-Nitrobiphenyl: limited evidence in animals; no data in humans (Vol. 4, pp. 113-124)

Appendix 5 (contd)

Chemical	Industry	Use (or formation) in industry	Evaluation of carcinogenicity[a]
Nitrocellulose	Tanning & processing	Binder in finishing	
	Leather goods	In nitrocellulose paint	
	Boots & shoes	Upper and unit finishes, usually solvent-based	
Nitrogen oxides	Tanning & processing	Exhaust fumes	
para-Nitrophenol	Tanning & processing	Defestation, disinfection; spray finish for US military leather	
N-Nitrosodimethyl-amine	Tanning & processing	Produced from dimethylamine sulphate (unhairing)	Sufficient evidence in animals; no data in humans (Vol. 17, pp. 125-175)
N-Nitrosomorpholine	Tanning & processing	Produced from dimethylamine sulphate (unhairing)	Sufficient evidence in animals; no data in humans (Vol. 17, pp. 263-280)
Nylon	Boots & shoes	Sole units	
2-n-Octyl-4-isothiazo-lin-3-one	Tanning & processing	Defestation, disinfection	
Oils			
vegetable oils (castor, colza, cottonseed)	Tanning & processing	Fat liquoring	
animal oils (neatsfoot oil, sperm oil)	Tanning & processing	Fat liquoring	
fish oils	Tanning & processing	Fat liquoring; tanning	
linseed oil	Tanning & processing	Dressing in finishing	
Oxalic acid	Tanning & processing	Bleaching	
Paraffin wax	Tanning & processing	Dressing in finishing	
Pentachloroethane	Tanning & processing	Fat removal	

Appendix 5 (contd)

Chemical	Industry	Use (or formation) in industry	Evaluation of carcinogenicity[a]
Pentachlorophenol and pentachlorophenates (*See Chlorophenols*)			
Pentane	Tanning & processing	In internal transport fuel	
	Leather goods	Solvent in glues	
Petrol (gasoline)	Tanning & processing	Fat removal; solvent in finishing	
Petroleum distillates	Tanning & processing	Solvents in finishing	
Petroleum hydro-carbons (naphthas)	Boots & shoes	Solvents in adhesives	
Pitch (natural)	Boots & shoes	Thread lubrication	Carcinogenic in humans (Vol. 3, pp. 25-29; Supplement 1, p. 43)
Phenol	Tanning & processing	Defestation, disinfection; soaking and washing; retanning	
Phenolic resins	Leather goods	In artificial latex and phenolic glues	
Phenylmercuric acetate	Tanning & processing	Fat removal; defestation, disinfection	
Phthalates	Leather goods	Plasticizers in artificial leathers	
Phthalocyanine blue; phthalocyanine green	Tanning & processing	Pigments in finishing	
Polyacrylate resin emulsions *(see Acrylic resins)*			
Polyamides	Boots & shoes	Hot-melt adhesives	
Polychloroprene	Boots & shoes	Adhesive; soling material	Inadequate data in animals; no data in humans (Vol. 19, pp. 141-156)
	Leather goods	Adhesive	

Appendix 5 (contd)

Chemical	Industry	Use (or formation) in industry	Evaluation of carcinogenicity[a]
Polyesters	Boots & shoes	Hot-melt adhesives; sole units	
Polyethers of high molecular weight weight derived from vinyl alcohol	Tanning & processing	Fat liquoring	Polyvinyl alcohol: inadequate data in animals; no data in humans (Vol. 19, pp. 351-366)
Polyethylene	Boots & shoes	Heels; impregnant in fibreboard used for heels	Inadequate data in animals and humans (Vol. 19, pp. 164-184)
Polyols (pigmented)	Tanning & processing Boots & shoes	Special leather finishes Reactive chemical in polyurethane soles	
Polyoxyethylene	Tanning & processing Boots & shoes	Fat removal Heels	
Polystyrene *(see Styrene)*			
Polyurethanes	Tanning & processing Leather goods Boots & shoes	Binders and impregnants in finishing Adhesives; stiffeners; artificial leathers Adhesives; artificial leathers; sole units; coating on fabrics for uppers	Polyurethane foams (flexible and rigid): inadequate data in animals; no data in humans (Vol. 19, pp. 320-340)
Polyurethanes (linear, one-part)	Boots & shoes	Upper and unit finishes, usually **solvent-based**	
Polyurethane resins	Leather goods	Adhesives	
Polyvinyl acetate	Tanning & processing Leather goods Boots & shoes	Binder in finishing In polyvinyl glues In latex adhesives	Inadequate data in animals; no data in humans (Vol. 19, pp. 346-366)

Appendix 5 (contd)

Chemical	Industry	Use (or formation) in industry	Evaluation of carcinogenicity[a]
Polyvinyl butyl ether	Tanning & processing	Binder in finishing	
Polyvinyl chloride *(see Vinyl chloride monomer)*			
Polyvinylidene chloride	Tanning & processing	Binder in finishing	
Polyvinyl toluene	Tanning & processing	Binder in finishing	
Potassium acetate	Tanning & processing	Chrome tannage	
Potassium aluminium sulphate *(see Aluminium)*			
Potassium *N*-hydroxy-methyl-*N*-methyl-dithiocarbamate	Tanning & processing	Defestation, disinfection	
Potassium penta-chlorophenate *(see Chlorophenols)*			
Potassium thiocyanate	Tanning & processing	Soaking and washing	
Propane	Tanning & processing	In internal transport fuel	
Propyl acetate	Leather goods	Solvent in ethylene carboxylic, phenolic and polyurethane glues	
Proteolytic enzymes	Tanning & processing	Soaking and washing; liming (unhairing); deliming and bating	
Resin, natural	Leather goods	Natural glue	
Resins, synthetic: condensation products of: - formaldehyde with urea,	Tanning & processing	Retanning of leathers treated by chrome tannage	Styrene: limited evidence in animals; no data in humans (Vol. 19, pp. 231-274)

Appendix 5 (contd)

Chemical	Industry	Use (or formation) in industry	Evaluation of carcinogenicity[a]
Resins, synthetic: (contd)			
dicyanodiamide, melamines - styrene-maleic anhydride			
Resorcinol	Tanning & processing	Condensed with aromatic bases (such as aniline) to make synthetic tannins	Inadequate data in animals; no data in humans (Vol. 15, pp. 155-175)
Rosin (colophony)	Tanning & processing	Binder in finishing	
	Leather goods	In colophony glue	
Sebacates	Leather goods	Plasticizers in artificial leathers	
Shellac	Tanning & processing	Binder in finishing	
	Boots & shoes	Finish	
Silicone compounds	Tanning & processing	Impregnants in finishing; artificial grain matrices	
	Boots & shoes	Release agents in spray moulds	
Sodium acetate	Tanning & processing	Chrome tannage; dyeing	
Sodium arsenates (see Arsenic)			
Sodium bicarbonate	Tanning & processing	Chrome tannage; dyeing; neutralizing	
Sodium bisulphite	Tanning & processing	Soaking and washing; defestation, disinfection; deliming and bating	
Sodium carbonate (soda ash)	Tanning & processing	Chrome tannage; bleaching; soaking and washing	

Appendix 5 (contd)

Chemical	Industry	Use (or formation) in industry	Evaluation of carcinogenicity[a]
Sodium chloride	Tanning & processing	Salting, brining and pickling for preservation; in two-bath chrome tannage	
Sodium citrate	Tanning & processing	Soaking and washing	
Sodium cyanide	Tanning & processing	Liming (unhairing)	
Sodium dichromate (see Chromium)			
Sodium difluoride (see Fluorides)			
Sodium fluoride (see Fluorides)			
Sodium formate	Tanning & processing	Produced from formic acid used in deliming; chrome tannage; dyeing; neutralizing	
Sodium hydrogen sulphite	Tanning & processing	Soaking and washing; produced from sodium sulphide in liming process	
Sodium hydroxide	Tanning & processing	Chrome tannage; liming (unhairing); soaking and washing	
Sodium hypochlorite	Tanning & processing	Bleaching; soaking and washing	
Sodium nitrate	Tanning & processing	Liming (unhairing)	
Sodium nitrite	Tanning & processing	Liming (unhairing)	
Sodium-ortho-phenoxy-phenate	Tanning & processing	Defestation, disinfection	
Sodium pentachloro-phenate (see Chlorophenols)			
Sodium perborate	Tanning & processing	Liming (unhairing)	

Appendix 5 (contd)

Chemical	Industry	Use (or formation) in industry	Evaluation of carcinogenicity[a]
Sodium polysulphide	Tanning & processing	Soaking and washing	
Sodium polyphosphate	Tanning & processing	Vegetable tannage; soaking and washing	
Sodium sulphate (anhydrous)	Tanning & processing	Vegetable tannage; defestation, disinfection	
Sodium sulphide	Tanning & processing	Soaking and washing; liming, unhairing (sharpening agent)	
Sodium sulphite	Tanning & processing	Chrome tannage; liming, unhairing (sharpening agent)	
Sodium sulphydrate	Tanning & processing	Liming (unhairing)	
Sodium thiosulphate	Tanning & processing	In 'two-bath' chrome tannage; bleaching	
Sodium 2,4,5-tri-chlorophenate *(see Chlorophenols)*			
Starch	Tanning & processing	Paste-drying	
	Boots & shoes	Adhesive	
Starch dextrin	Tanning & processing	Reducing agent in chrome tannage	
Stearato-chromic chloride complex *(see Chromium)*			
Stoddard solvent (petroleum distillate)	Tanning & processing	Fat removal	
Styrene copolymers	Tanning & processing	Binders in finishing	Styrene: limited evidence in animals; inadequate data in humans (Vol. 19, pp. 231-274)
Styrene-butadiene-styrene block co-polymer	Boots & shoes	Soling material (rubber injection moulding)	

Appendix 5 (contd)

Chemical	Industry	Use (or formation) in industry	Evaluation of carcinogenicity[a]
Polystyrene	Boots & shoes	Soles, heels; stiffeners	Limited evidence in animals; inadequate data in humans (Vol. 19, pp. 245-274)
Sulphated oils	Tanning & processing	Fat liquoring	
Sulphited oils	Tanning & processing	Fat liquoring	
Sulphonated aromatic acids	Tanning & processing	Deliming and bating	
Sulphonated fatty alcohols	Tanning & processing	Soaking and washing	
Sulphonic acid	Tanning & processing	Soaking; in synthetic tannins	
Sulphur dioxide	Tanning & processing	Bleaching; defestation, disinfection; reducing agent in chrome tannage	
Sulphur oxides	Tanning & processing	Exhaust fumes	
Sulphuric acid	Tanning & processing	Deliming, pickling and bating; in 'two-bath' chrome and vegetable tannage; dyeing	
Surface-active compounds (cationic or nonionic)	Tanning & processing / Boots & shoes	Soaking and washing; unhairing; fat removal; impregnants and dressings in finishing / Cleaners	
Talc	Tanning & processing	Dressing in finishing	
Tannins *Vegetable tannins* - Pyrocatechol tannins containing 1,2-dihydroxybenzene	Tanning & processing	Tanning agents	Tannins and tannic acid: limited evidence in animals; no data in humans (Vol. 10, pp. 254-262)

Appendix 5 (contd)

Chemical	Industry	Use (or formation) in industry	Evaluation of carcinogenicity[a]
Vegetable tannins (contd)			
- Pyrogallic tannins containing 1,2,3-trihydroxy-benzene			
- Polyhydroxybenzenes bound to a sugar molecule			
- Ellagic tannins			
Synthetic tannins			
- Auxililary tannins: naphthalene sulphonated with sulphuric acid and condensed with formaldehyde			
- Tannins of substitution phenolic substances (mostly cresols) condensed with aldehydes			
Tannins of resinous substances: products of reaction of compounds with an amine group			Resorcinol: inadequate data in animals; no data in humans (Vol. 15, pp. 155-175) Aniline: inadequate data in animals and humans (Vol. 4, pp. 27-38)
Tetrachloroethane	Tanning & processing	Fat removal; solvent and oil repellent in finishing process	Limited evidence in animals; no data in humans (Vol. 20, pp. 477-489)
Tetrachloroethylene (perchloroethylene)	Tanning & processing Boots & shoes	Fat removal; solvent in finishing Cleaner	Limited evidence in animals; no data in humans (Vol. 20 pp. 491-514)
Tetrahydrofuran	Boots & shoes	Cleaner	

Appendix 5 (contd)

Chemical	Industry	Use (or formation) in industry	Evaluation of carcinogenicity[a]
2-(Thiocyanomethyl-thio)benzothiazole (Busan 30, Busan 72)	Tanning & processing	Defestation, disinfection	
Thioglycolic acid salts and derivatives	Tanning & processing	Liming (unhairing)	
Titanium dioxide	Tanning & processing	Pigment in finishing	
Toluene	Tanning & processing	Solvent in finishing	
	Boots & shoes	Adhesive solvent	
	Leather goods	Solvent in ethylene carboxylic, phenolic and polyurethane glues and in nitrocellulose paints	
Toluene-2,4-diisocyanate (TDI)	Tanning & processing	Solvent in finishing; tanning agent	No data in animals or humans (Vol. 19, pp. 303-340)
	Boots & shoes	Adhesive solvent	
Tributyl tin chloride complex of ethylene oxide condensate of dihydroabietylamine	Tanning & processing	Defestation, disinfection	
2,4,5- and 2,4,6-Tri-chlorobenzene	Tanning & processing	Defestation; conservation in beamhouse curing	
1,1,1-Trichloroethane	Tanning & processing	Rubber solvent and cleaner in finishing; toxic pollutant of raw wastewater	Inadequate data in animals; no data in humans (Vol. 20, pp. 515-531)
	Boots & shoes	Rubber solvent and cleaner	
Trichloroethylene	Tanning & processing	Fat removal; solvent and oil-repellent in finishing process	Limited evidence in animals; no data in humans (Vol. 20, pp. 545-572)
	Leather goods	Solvent in ethylene carboxylic, phenolic and polyurethane glues	
	Boots & shoes	Rubber solvent and cleaner; adhesive solvent	

Appendix 5 (contd)

Chemical	Industry	Use (or formation) in industry	Evaluation of carcinogenicity[a]
2,4,5-Trichlorophenol and trichloro- phenates (see Chlorophenol)			
Tricresylphosphate	Tanning & processing	Plasticizer in finishing	
	Leather goods; boots & shoes	Plasticizer in polyurethane glues, in artificial leathers and in nitrocellulose paints	
Triphenylphosphate	Tanning & processing	Plasticizer in finishing	
Trypsin (see Proteolytic enzymes)			
Urea	Tanning & processing	Soaking and washing; liming (unhairing)	
Urea-formaldehyde resins	Boots & shoes	Toe puffs	
Urea-formaldehyde condensation pro- ducts	Tanning & processing	In retanning of leathers treated by chrome tannage	
Vinyl chloride monomer	Leather goods	Vapours from PVC (?)	Carcinogenic in humans (Vol. 19, pp. 377-438; Supplement 1, p. 45)
	Boots & shoes	Possibly produced when two PVC compounds are welded together	
Polyvinyl chloride	Tanning & processing	Binder in finishing	Inadequate data in animals and in hu- mans (Vol. 19, pp. 402-438)
	Leather goods	In artificial leathers; rigid frames; stiffener	
	Boots & shoes	Heels, soles; coating on fabric for uppers	
Waxes (natural)	Boots & shoes	Thread lubrication; release agents in spray moulds; finishes	
	Leather goods	Softening, polishing	
White spirit	Tanning & processing	Fat removal	

Appendix 5 (contd)

Chemical	Industry	Use (or formation) in industry	Evaluation of carcinogenicity[a]
Wood dust	Tanning & processing	Dressing in finishing	
	Boots & shoes	Production of wooden soles, clogs	
	Leather goods	Production of rigid frames	
Xylene	Tanning & processing	Solvent in finishing	
	Leather goods	Solvent in ethylene carboxylic, phenolic and polyurethane glues	
	Boots & shoes	Adhesive solvent	
Zinc chloride	Tanning & processing	Soaking and washing; defestation, disinfection	
Zinc oxide	Tanning & processing	Pigment in finishing	
Zinc stearate	Boots & shoes	On unvulcanized rubber sheets	
Zinc sulphide	Tanning & processing	Pigment in finishing	
Zirconium salts	Tanning & processing	Tanning and retanning agents	
Zirconium chloride	Tanning & processing	Tanning and retanning agent	
Zirconium sulphate	Tanning & processing	Tanning and retanning agent	

[a]For chemicals considered in *IARC Monographs*

APPENDIX 6[a]

SOME DYES USED IN WOOD, LEATHER, AND SOME ASSOCIATED INDUSTRIES, WITH CROSS REFERENCES TO *IARC MONOGRAPHS*

[a]Evaluations of carcinogenicity are reported only for those chemicals evaluated in *IARC Monographs*.

Appendix 6. Some dyes used in wood, leather and some associated industries

C.I. Name	C.I. No.	CAS Reg. No.	Use	Evaluation of carcinogenicity[a]
Acid Black 1	20470	3121-74-2 (free) 1064-48-8 (Na$^+$ salt)	Leather dyeing	
Acid Black 2	50420	8005-03-6 12227-81-5	Leather dyeing	
Acid Black 52	15711	5610-64-0 (Na$^+$ salt) Cr[III] complex	Leather dyeing	
Acid Blue 1 (Blue VRS)	42045	129-17-9	Leather and paper dyeing	Limited evidence in animals; no data in humans (Vol. 16, pp. 163-170)
Acid Blue 9 (Brilliant Blue FCF)	42090	2650-18-2 (NH$_4$)$_2$ salt	Leather and paper dyeing; wood staining	Limited evidence in animals; no data in humans (Vol. 16, pp. 171-186)
Acid Blue 83	42660	25305-85-5 6104-59-2 (Na salt)	Leather dyeing	
Acid Brown 14	20195		Leather dyeing	
Acid Brown 354	20177		Leather dyeing	
Acid Fuchsine		3244-88-0	Wood staining	
Acid Green 3 (Guinea Green B)	42085	4680-78-8	Leather and paper dyeing; wood staining	Limited evidence in animals; no data in humans (Vol. 16, pp. 209-220)
Acid Green 5 (Light Green SF)	42095	5141-20-8	Leather and paper dyeing	Limited evidence in animals; no data in humans (Vol. 16, pp. 209-220)
Acid Green 35	13361		Leather dyeing	
Acid Orange 7	15510	573-89-7 (mono-Na salt, 633-96-5)	Leather dyeing	

Appendix 6 (contd)

C.I. Name	C.I. No.	CAS Reg. No.	Use	Evaluation of carcinogenicity[a]
Acid Orange 8	15575	18524-46-4 5850-86-2	Leather dyeing	
Acid Orange 10 (Orange G)	16230	1936-15-8	Leather and paper dyeing; wood staining	Inadequate data in animals; no data in humans (Vol. 8, pp. 181-187)
Acid Orange 20 (Orange I)	14600	523-44-4	Leather dyeing	Limited evidence in animals; no data in humans (Vol. 8, pp. 173-179)
Acid Orange 24	20170	1320-07-6	Leather dyeing	
Acid Orange 45 (Reddish Orange)	22195	2429-80-3	Leather dyeing	
Acid Orange 61	19320		Leather dyeing	
Acid Orange 63	22870		Leather dyeing	
Acid Orange 74	18745	10127-27-2	Leather dyeing	
Acid Red 1	18050	25317-20-8 3734-67-6	Leather dyeing	
Acid Red 14	14720	13613-55-3 3567-69-9	Leather dyeing; wood staining	Inadequate data in animals; no data in humans (Vol. 8, pp. 83-89)
Acid Red 73	27290	5413-75-2	Leather dyeing	
Acid Red 87	45380		Paper dyeing	
Acid Red 91	45400		Paper dyeing	
Acid Red 94	45440		Wood dyeing	
Acid Red 97	22890		Leather dyeing	
Acid Red 114	23635	6459-94-5	Leather dyeing	
Acid Red 151	26900		Leather dyeing	
Acid Violet 3	16580	1681-60-3	Leather dyeing	

Appendix 6

C.I. Name	C.I. No.	CAS Reg. No.	Use	Evaluation of carcinogenicity[a]
Acid Violet 49 (Benzyl Violet 4B)	42640	1694-09-3	Leather dyeing; wood staining	Sufficient evidence in animals; no data in humans (Vol. 16, pp. 153-162)
Acid Yellow 1	10316		Leather dyeing	
Acid Yellow 23	19140	118-26-3 1934-21-0 34175-08-1	Leather dyeing	
Acid Yellow 24	10315	605-69-6 887-79-6 10142-54-8	Leather dyeing	
Acid Yellow 36	13065	4005-68-9 587-98-4	Leather dyeing	
Acid Yellow 40	18950	6372-96-9	Leather dyeing	
Acid Yellow 42	22910	24382-22-7	Leather dyeing	
Acid Yellow 99	13900	10343-58-5	Leather dyeing	
Acid Yellow 151	13906	12715-61-6	Leather dyeing	
Basic Blue 6	51175	7057-57-0	Leather dyeing	
Basic Blue 9 (Methylene Blue)	52015	61-73-4	Leather dyeing	
Basic Brown 1	21000	1052-38-6	Leather dyeing	
Basic Brown 4	21010	4482-25-1	Leather dyeing	
Basic Green 1	42040		Leather dyeing	
Basic Green 4 (Malachite Green)	42000	569-64-2	Leather dyeing	
Basic Orange 1	11320	5042-54-6 4438-16-8	Leather dyeing	
Basic Orange 2 (Chrysoidine)	11270	495-54-5 532-82-1	Leather dyeing; wood and paper staining	Limited evidence in animals; no data in humans (Vol. 8, pp. 91-96)

Appendix 6 (contd)

C.I. Name	C.I. No.	CAS Reg. No.	Use	Evaluation of carcinogenicity[a]
Basic Red 1 (Rhodamine 6G)	45160	989-38-8	Leather dyeing; paper staining	Limited evidence in animals; no data in humans (Vol. 16, pp. 233-239)
Basic Violet 1 (Methyl Violet)	42535	8004-87-3	Leather dyeing	
Basic Violet 3 (Crystal Violet)	42555	548-62-9	Leather dyeing	
Basic Violet 10 (Rhodamine B)	45170	81-88-9	Leather dyeing; wood and paper staining	Limited evidence in animals; no data in humans (Vol. 16, pp. 221-231)
Basic Violet 11	45175	2390-63-8	Leather dyeing	
Basic Yellow 2	41000	2465-27-2	Leather dyeing	
Basic Yellow 37	41001	6358-36-7	Leather dyeing	
Carbon black	77266	1333-86-4	Paper dyeing	
Croceine			Wood staining	
Developer 4 (Resorcinol)	76505	108-46-3	Wood staining	Inadequate data in animals; no data in humans Vol. 15, pp. 155-175)
Developer 13 (para-Phenyl-enediamine)	76060	106-50-3	Wood staining	Inadequate data in animals; no data in humans (Vol. 16, pp. 125-142)
Direct Black 4	30245	2429-83-6	Leather and paper dyeing	
Direct Black 38	30235	1937-37-7	Leather and paper dyeing; wood staining	Contains, as impurities, 4-aminobiphenyl: carcinogenic in humans (Vol. 1, pp. 74-79; Supplement 1, p. 22); para-dimethyl-

Appendix 6 (contd)

C.I. Name	C.I. No.	CAS Reg. No.	Use	Evaluation of carcinogenicity[a]
Direct Black 38 (contd)				aminobenzene: sufficient evidence in animals, no data in humans (Vol. 8, pp. 125-146)
Direct Blue 1	24410	2610-05-1	Leather dyeing	
Direct Blue 2	22590	2429-73-4	Leather and paper dyeing	
Direct Blue 6	22610	2602-46-2	Leather and paper dyeing	
Direct Blue 14 (Trypan Blue)	23850	72-57-1	Leather and paper dyeing	Sufficient evidence in animals; no data in humans (Vol. 8, pp. 267-278)
Direct Blue 53 (Evans Blue)	23860	314-13-6	Leather and paper dyeing	Limited evidence in animals; no data in humans (Vol. 8, pp. 151-156)
Direct Brown 1	30045	2586-58-5	Leather and paper dying	
Direct Brown 2	22311	2429-82-5	Leather and paper dying	
Direct Brown 6	30140		Leather and paper dyeing	
Direct Brown 31	35660	2429-81-4	Leather and paper dyeing	
Direct Brown 59	22345		Leather dyeing	
Direct Brown 74	36300		Leather dyeing	
Direct Brown 95	30145	16071-86-6	Leather and paper dyeing	
Direct Brown 111			Leather dyeing	
Direct Brown 154	30120	6360-54-9	Leather and paper dyeing	
Direct Green 1	30280	3626-28-6	Leather and paper dyeing	
Direct Green 6	30295	4335-09-5	Leather and paper dyeing	
Direct Green 8	30315	5422-17-3	Leather and paper dyeing	

Appendix 6 (contd)

C.I. Name	C.I. No.	CAS Reg. No.	Use	Evaluation of carcinogenicity[a]
Direct Orange 1	22370	6459-87-6	Leather and paper dyeing	
Direct Orange 8	22130	2429-79-0	Paper dyeing	
Direct Red 1	22310	2429-84-7	Leather and paper dyeing	
Direct Red 10	22145	2429-70-1	Leather dyeing	
Direct Red 13	22155	1937-35-5	Leather and paper dyeing	
Direct Red 23	29160	3441-14-3	Leather dyeing	
Direct Red 28	22120	5730-58-0	Paper dyeing	
Direct Red 37	22240	3530-19-6	Leather and paper dyeing	
Direct Red 81	28160	2610-11-9	Leather dyeing	
Direct Violet 1	22570	2586-60-9	Leather and paper dyeing	
Direct Violet 22	22480	6426-67-1	Leather dyeing	
Direct Yellow 12	24895	2870-32-8	Leather dyeing	
Direct Yellow 20	22410	6426-62-6	Leather dyeing	
Disperse Yellow 3	11855	2832-40-8	Sheepskin and fur dyeing	Inadequate data in animals; no data in humans (Vol. 8, pp. 97-100)
Fluorescent Brightening Agent 30	40600		Paper dyeing	
Food Red 3 (Carmoisine)	14720	3567-69-9	Leather dyeing; wood staining	Inadequate data in animals; no data in humans (Vol. 8, pp. 83-89)
Food Red 5 (Ponceau MX)	16150	3761-53-3	Leather dyeing; wood staining	Sufficient evidence in animals; no data in humans (Vol. 8, pp. 189-198)

Appendix 6 (contd)

C.I. Name	C.I. No.	CAS Reg. No.	Use	Evaluation of carcinogenicity[a]
Food Red 6 (Ponceau 3R)	16155	3564-09-8	Wood staining	Sufficient evidence in animals; no data in humans (Vol. 8, pp. 199-204)
Food Red 9 (Amaranth)	16185	915-67-3	Leather and paper dyeing; wood staining	Inadequate data in animals; no data in humans (Vol. 8, pp. 41-51)
Food Red I (Ponceau SX)	14700	4548-53-2	Wood staining	Not carcinogenic in animals; no data in humans (Vol. 8, pp. 207-215)
Indigo	73000	482-89-3	Wood staining	
Induline	50400	8004-98-6	Wood staining	
Nitrosine			Wood staining	
Pigment Blue 27	77510		Carbon-paper dyeing	
Pigment Blue 29	77007		Wall-paper dyeing	
Rosaniline		632-99-5	Wood staining	
Solvent Brown I (Sudan Brown RR)	11285	6416-57-5	Wood staining	Inadequate data in animals; no data in humans (Vol. 8, pp. 249-252)
Solvent Orange 7 (Sudan II)	12140	3118-97-6	Wood staining	Inadequate data in animals; no data in humans (Vol. 8, pp. 233-240)
Solvent Orange 15 (Acridine Orange)	46005:1	494-38-2	Leather dyeing	Inadequate data in animals; no data in humans (Vol. 16, pp. 145-152)
Solvent Red 19 (Sudan Red 78)	26050	6368-72-5	Wood staining	Inadequate data in animals; no data in humans (Vol. 8, pp. 253-256)

Appendix 6 (contd)

C.I. Name	C.I. No.	CAS Reg. No.	Use	Evaluation of carcinogenicity[a]
Solvent Red 23 (Sudan III)	26100	85-86-9	Wood staining	Inadequate data in animals; no data in humans (Vol. 8, pp. 241-247)
Solvent Red 24 (Scarlet Red)	26105	85-83-6	Wood staining	Inadequate data in animals; no data in humans (Vol. 8, pp. 217-224)
Solvent Red 41	42510		Wood dyeing	
Solvent Yellow 14 (Sudan I)	12055	842-07-9	Wood staining	Sufficient evidence in animals; no data in humans (Vol. 8, pp. 225-231)
Solvent Yellow 34 (Auramine)	492808		Leather and paper dyeing	Sufficient evidence in animals; manufacture of auramine is carcinogenic to humans (Vol. 1, pp. 69-73; Supplement 1, p. 24)

GLOSSARY

alum — A double sulphate of aluminium and potassium

bagasse — dry refuse (crushed sugar-cane fibres) from sugar making; used as a fuel in sugar factories, and as a base in paper manufacture

bandsaw — a narrow, endless strip of saw-blading running over and driven by pulleys, as a belt

bate — a fermenting solution containing enzymes derived from the pancreas, or from synthetically prepared ferments; used for steeping light skins, prior to tanning, to render them smooth and flexible

beamhouse — place where skins are received, trimmed, sorted, washed, fleshed and unhaired, before tanning

board — timber cut to thickness of less than 50 mm and to any width from 100 mm upwards (see *plank*)

buff (to) — to grind down a surface (of wood, leather, etc.) in order to remove extrusions or to expose the underlying material
— to cover a surface (of wood) with a transparent varnish

butt-end — the squared-off end of a board or plank

calender — a machine, generally consisting of a number of vertical rollers (or bowls), heated or unheated, through which material is passed under pressure, to impart the desired finish (dull, glazed, etc.) or to ensure uniform thickness

cant — a log partially square-sawn, intended for re-sawing at right angles to its widest face

— edge of board cut at right angle

chipboard — a paperboard normally made from recycled paper stock, with a relatively low density, in various thicknesses

circular saw — a steel disc carrying teeth on its periphery, usually power-driven

cotton linters   -   short stiff fibres remaining on cotton seeds after removal of the longer fibres; removed before the seeds are crushed; used exclusively in the manufacture of rayon, gun cotton, absorbent cotton, etc.

couch roll   -   a cylinder covered with felt, used to press out water from the damp web of paper, and to cause the fibres to felt together more thoroughly

cross-cut saw   -   a saw designed for cutting timber across the grain

currier   -   one who dresses and colours tanned leather

curry (to)   -   to treat (dress) leather with grease mixtures to make it pliable

dandy roll   -   a wire-gauze cylinder which comes into contact with paper when in the wet stage; it impresses the ribs in 'laid' paper (writing and printing paper with a ribbed watermark), and any watermark required

edge (to)   -   to trim the edges off boards or leather

esparto   -   a paper made from a coarse grass of the same name obtained from southern Spain and northern Africa

fibreboard   -   a broad, generic term inclusive of sheet materials of widely varying densities manufactured from refined or partially refined wood (or other vegetable) fibres. Fibreboard as used in the construction and furniture industries is formulated from mechanically-produced wood fibres and formaldehyde-based urea, melamine or phenolic resins. In the shoe industry, fibreboard is produced from pulp fibres in combination with plastics such as polyethylene and polychloroprene. (See *chipboard, flakeboard, hardboard, particle-board.*)

filler   -   (1) a material used to fill in the pores of, or any holes in, wood, plaster, etc., which is to be painted, varnished or otherwise decorated

     -   (2) an extender, a substance added to synthetic resin adhesives to reduce the cost of gluing or to adjust viscosity, e.g., wood-flour, clay, mica, metal powders

     -   (3) mineral powder added to paper to improve quality and in some cases to lower costs, e.g., China clay, titanium dioxide

flakeboard - a panel manufactured from flakes of wood (see *particle-board*)

flesh (to) - to remove the subcutaneous coat of the derma from the inside of a hide before tanning

fluting medium - a coarse paper which has been passed through intermeshing, grooved, metal rolls and which forms the core for cardboard sheets or boxes

four cutter - a type of planing machine (q.v.)

frame saw - a thin-bladed saw, which is held taut in a special frame; also called a span saw

French polish - a solution of shellac dissolved in methanol

full (to) - to soften leather by imbuing it with water

gall - an abnormal growth formed on a plant following attack by a parasite, especially on oak, used in making ink and tannin

gang-saw - an arrangement of parallel saws secured in a frame to operate simultaneously in sawing a log into strips

groundwood - pulp produced by grinding wood; also called mechanical wood, to differentiate it from pulp produced chemically

hardboard - a generic term for a panel manufactured primarily from matted ligno-cellulosic fibres (usually wood), consolidated under heat and pressure in a hot press to a density of about 500 kg/m^3 or greater, and to which other materials may be added during manufacture

hardwoods - generally, one of the botanical groups of trees that have broad leaves, in contrast to the conifers or softwoods. The term has no reference to the actual hardness of the wood.

head-box - a constant-level tank situated before the machine wire on the Fourdrinier machine which controls the amount of paper stock flowing to the machine by means of its stuff tap

heartwood   - the wood extending from the pith to the sapwood, the cells of which no longer participate in the life processes of the tree. Heartwood may contain phenolic compounds, resins and other materials that usually make it darker and more decay-resistant than sapwood.

hollander   - a trough containing a beating roll with bars set parallel to the axis; used for reducing materials to the condition requisite for producing a particular class of paper

hydropulper - mixing tank equipped with large mechanical beaters to convert dry pulp to a water slurry of cellulose fibres

kiln   - a chamber with controlled air flow, temperature and relative humidity, for drying lumber, veneer and other wood products

kraft   - brown paper made from high-class sulphate wood pulp; used extensively as a dielectric, for gummed tape, wrappings, etc.

laminate   - a product made by bonding together two or more layers (laminations) of material(s)

last   - shoemaker's wooden model for shaping shoes, etc.

lasting   - strong twill cloth of hard-twisted cotton or worsted yarns, or cotton warp and worsted weft; used for boot and bag linings, etc.

lathe   - a machine tool for producing cylindrical work, facing, boring and screw-cutting

lathing   - softwood strips ~1 m long fixed to surfaces to provide a basis for plaster

lichens   - a large group of composite plants, consisting of an alga and fungus in intimate association, and divided into genera and species as if they were independent plants

lignin   - the second most abundant constituent of wood after cellulose, located principally in the secondary wall and the middle lamella, which is the thin cementing layer between wood cells. Chemically, it is an irregular polymer of substituted propylphenol groups, and thus no simple chemical formula can be written for it

liverworts   - a genus of ranunculaceous plants. The plant that bears the sexual organs
(Hepatica)   is a dichotomosing thallus. The capsule usually contains elaters (elon-
                      gated cells with spiral thickenings on walls) mixed with the spores.

mat   - of surfaces; dull, without lustre

mortiser   - a machine to cut slots into boards, planks or timber, usually edgewise, to
                      receive the tenon (q.v.) of another board, plank or timber to form a
                      joint

nip rolls   - a pair of steel rolls situated before the last section of drying cylinders of
                      the paper machine to give a high finish to the paper while still moist

pallet   - a low wood or metal platform on which material can be stacked to
                      facilitate mechanical handling, moving and storage

paperboard   - the distinction between paper and paperboard is not sharp, but, broadly
                      speaking, the thicker (>30 mm), heavier and more rigid grades of paper
                      are called paperboard.

particleboard   - a generic term for a panel manufactured from ligno-cellulosic materials
                      (commonly wood) essentially in the form of particles (as distinct from
                      fibres). These materials are bonded together with synthetic resin or
                      other suitable binder, under heat and pressure, by a process wherein the
                      interparticle bonds are created wholly by the added binder.

plane   - a wood-working tool used for smoothing surfaces and reducing the size
                      of wood

planing machine - a machine for producing large flat surfaces. It consists of a gear-driven
(planer)   reciprocating work-table sliding on a heavy bed, the stationary tool being
                      carried above it by a saddle, which can be traversed across a horizontal
                      rail carried by uprights.

plank   - a broad board, usually more than 2.5 cm thick, laid with its wide di-
                      mension horizontal and used as a bearing surface

plywood   - a composite panel or board made up of cross-banded layers of veneer
                      only or of veneer in combination with a core of lumber or of particle-
                      board bonded with an adhesive. Generally ,the grain of one or more
                      plies is roughly at right angles to the other plies, and almost always an
                      odd number of plies are used.

podophyllin   - extract from the mandrake *Podophyllum peltatum* (America) or *Emodi* (India), containing resins which act as strong purgatives

poromeric   - permeable to water-vapour; said of a polyurethane-base synthetic leather used in the manufacture of shoe uppers

ramie   - bast fibre; strong and very white, grown in Japan, India, China and other tropical countries. Once widely used for gas mantles, also for bank-note paper. Fibre length varies enormously and poor elasticity is a serious disadvantage

ret (to)   - to soak flax, straw or jute in water so that bacteria will soften the woody tissue thus enabling the fibres to be extracted

rip-saw   - a saw designed for cutting timber along the grain

router plane   - a plane adapted to work on circular sashes; operated in the manner of a spokeshave (a double-handled plane used to shape convex surfaces)

sander   - a machine fitted with abrasive paper, for polishing surfaces

saprophyte   - any bacterium which breaks up dead animal and vegetable matter and does not produce disease in the animal or plant which it inhabits; more generally, an organism which obtains its food from dead organic material

scour (to)   - to sand a surface

                   - to clean by flushing or flowing through or over water

scud (to)   - to remove the bulb of hair

shank   - a component used to reinforce the narrow middle (waist) of a boot or shoe sole; usually made of metal or wood

size (to)   - to add materials to paper to render it more resistant to penetration by liquids, particularly water

skive (to)   - to split or pare a skin, to reduce it in thickness

slat (sticker)   - strip or board used to separate the layers of lumber in a pile and thus improve air circulation *sleeper*   - a horizontal timber supporting a vertical post and distributing the load over the ground

slurry   - semi-fluid residue

sock   - material used to cover the insole of a shoe

spindle moulder - moulding cutter - a specially shaped cutting tool which, when revolving about its own axis, is capable of cutting a desired moulding profile

split   - a hide that has been split into two or more layers, parallel to the surface

square   - a piece of square-section timber of side up to 15 cm

staking machine - a machine in which leather undergoes a process of stretching and softening, to prevent cohesion of the fibres while drying

slushing   - the process of suspending sheets of pulp, paper or partially dried paper stock in water to give individual fibres (or fibre bundles)

sulphite process - the preparation of pulp by pressure digestion of wood with a liquor containing calcium bisulphite and free sulphur dioxide; also called the acid process

surfactant   - an abbreviated form of 'surface active agent', i.e., a substance which has the effect of altering the interfacial tension of liquids or solids, e.g., detergents or soap

tackifier   - an agent which renders varnishes, glues, etc. sticky

tall oil   - a mixture of fatty and resin acids that separate as insoluble salts during the concentration of kraft black liquor and are converted to the free acid forms with sulphuric acid to give crude tall oil. This is usually purified by vacuum distillation into fatty and resin acid fractions.

tenoner   - a machine to cut a tongue on the end of a member by cutting away from both sides one-third of the thickness of the member. The projecting part fits into a mortise (q.v.) to make a joint between them.

toe puff   - a stiffener for the toe area of some footwear
(boxtoe)

upper	- upper part of boot or shoe
vamp	- upper front part of boot or shoe
veldt	- method whereby the out-turned upper is sewn to an extended insole which is then stuck to the outsole
veneer	- a thin layer or sheet of wood
wane	- a defect in converted timber: either some of the original rounded surface of the tree remains along an edge or wood is lacking from an edge or corner
welt	- strip of leather sewn around edge of boot or shoe uppers to serve as attachment to sole

SUPPLEMENTARY CORRIGENDA TO VOLUMES 1-24

Corrigenda covering Volumes 1-6 appeared in Volume 7, others appeared in Volumes 8, 10-13, 15-23.

Volume 16

p. 333	last para, 10th line	*replace* Shimskaya *by* Shumskaya

Volume 17

p. 139	(*c*) *Rat*, 1st line	*replace* mg/rat *by* mg/kg bw
	Newborn and suckling rat, 2nd para, 4th line	*replace by* 0.125 mg/rat at 1 day of age and 0.125 mg/rat or 10 mg/kg bw at day 7 induced 63%

Volume 20

p. 53	1st para, last line	*replace* 35/20 *by* 32/50

Volume 21

p. 260	1st para, 3rd line	*replace* 100 thousand-1 million *by* 100-1000
p. 346	4th para	*delete last sentence* (In . . . . kg.)
p. 420	1st para, 5th line	*replace* 200 thousand to 2 million *by* 200-2000
p. 463	1st para, 3rd line	*replace* 100 thousand to 1 million *by* 100-1000
	1st para	*delete last sentence* (Imports . . . . each.)
p. 494	3rd para	*delete last sentence* (In . . . . kg.).

Supplementary Corrigenda (contd)

Volume 22

p. 47   Iceland   *replace* S + + + d_2 *by* S - + m_2 + d_2
replace C + + + d_2 *by* C - - -

p. 50   *add* m_2 only in certain dietetic foods;
maximum, 400 mg/kg

Volume 23

p. 5   List of members   *add* R. Althouse, University of
Oxford, Clinical Medical School,
Radcliffe Hospital, Oxford, UK

p. 7   Secretariat   *add* L. Simonato, Division of
Human Cancer and Field
Programmes

p. 186   1st para, 4th line   *replace* 1051 *by* 1951

Supplement 2

p. 18   2nd para, 9th line   *replace* exposure *by* effects
3rd para, 8th line   *replace* this *by* there

Numbers in bold indicate volume, and other numbers indicate page. References to corrigenda are given in parentheses. Compounds marked with an asterisk (*) were considered by the Working Groups, but monographs were not prepared because adequate data on their carcinogenicity were not available.

A

Acetamide	**7,** 197	
Acetylsalicyclic acid*		
Acridine orange	**16,** 145	
Acriflavinium chloride	**13,** 31	
Acrolein	**19,** 479	
Acrylic acid	**19,** 47	
Acrylic fibres	**19,** 86	
Acrylonitrile	**19,** 73	
Acrylonitrile-butadiene-styrene copolymers	**19,** 91	
Actinomycins	**10,** 29	
Adipic acid*		
Adriamycin	**10,** 43	
Aflatoxins	**1,** 145	(corr. **7,** 319)
		(corr. **8,** 349)
	10, 51	
Aldrin	**5,** 25	
Amaranth	**8,** 41	
5-Aminoacenaphthene	**16,** 243	
para-Aminoazobenzene	**8,** 53	
ortho-Aminoazotoluene	**8,** 61	(corr. **11,** 295)
para-Aminobenzoic acid	**16,** 249	
4-Aminobiphenyl	**1,** 74	(corr. **10,** 343)
2-Amino-5-(5-nitro-2-furyl)-1,3,4-thiadiazole	**7,** 143	
4-Amino-2-nitrophenol	**16,** 43	
2-Amino-4-nitrophenol*		
2-Amino-5-nitrophenol*		
6-Amino penicillanic acid*		
Amitrole	**7,** 31	

Amobarbital sodium*

Anaesthetics, volatile   **11,** 285

Aniline   **4,**   27   (corr. **7,** 320)

Anthranilic acid   **16,** 265

Apholate   **9,**   31

Aramite®   **5,**   39

Arsenic and arsenic compounds   **1,**   41

                                                    2,   48

                                                    23, 39

    Arsanilic acid
    Arsenic pentoxide
    Arsenic sulphide
    Arsenic trioxide
    Arsine
    Calcium arsenate
    Dimethylarsinic acid
    Lead arsenate
    Methanearsonic acid, disodium salt
    Methanearsonic acid, monosodium salt
    Potassium arsenate
    Potassium arsenite
    Sodium arsenate
    Sodium arsenite
    Sodium cacodylate

Asbestos   **2,**   17   (corr. **7,** 319)

                                                    14   (corr. **15,** 341)

                                                                    (corr. **17,** 351)

    Actinolite
    Amosite
    Anthophyllite
    Chrysotile
    Crocidolite
    Tremolite

Asiaticoside*

Auramine   **1,**   69   (corr. **7,** 319)

Aurothioglucose   **13,** 39

Azaserine   **10,** 73   (corr. **12,** 271)

Bis(1-aziridinyl)morpholinophosphine sulphide	**9,** 55	
Bis(2-chloroethyl)ether	**9,** 117	
N,N-Bis(2-chloroethyl)-2-naphthylamine	**4,** 119	
Bischloroethyl nitrosourea*		
Bis(2-chloroisopropyl)ether*		
1,2-Bis(chloromethoxy)ethane	**15,** 31	
1,4-Bis(chloromethoxymethyl)benzene	**15,** 37	
Bis(chloromethyl)ether	**4,** 231	(corr. **13,** 243)
Blue VRS	**16,** 163	
Boot and shoe manufacture and repair	**25,** 249	
Brilliant blue FCF diammonium and disodium salts	**16,** 171	
1,4-Butanediol dimethanesulphonate (Myleran)	**4,** 247	
Butyl-cis-9,10-epoxystearate*		
β-Butyrolactone	**11,** 225	
γ-Butyrolactone	**11,** 231	

C

Cadmium and cadmium compounds	**2,** 74	
	11, 39	
Cadmium acetate		
Cadmium chloride		
Cadmium oxide		
Cadmium sulphate		
Cadmium sulphide		
Calcium cyclamate	**22,** 58	(corr. **25,** 392)
Calcium saccharin	**22,** 120	(corr. **25,** 392)
Cantharidin	**10,** 79	
Caprolactam	**19,** 115	
Carbaryl	**12,** 37	
Carbon tetrachloride	**1,** 53	
	20, 371	
Carmoisine	**8,** 83	
Carpentry and joinery	**25,** 139	
Catechol	**15,** 155	
Chlorambucil	**9,** 125	
Chloramphenicol	**10,** 85	
Chlordane	**20,** 45	(corr. **25,** 391)